T0344419

Music Therapy

Research and Evidence-Based Practice

Music Therapy

Research and Evidence-Based Practice

OLIVIA SWEDBERG YINGER, PHD, MT-BC
University of Kentucky,
Lexington, KY
USA

ELSEVIER

Content Strategist: Kayla Wolfe
Content Development Manager: Taylor Ball
Content Development Specialist: Donald Mumford
Publishing Services Manager: Deepthi Unni
Project Manager: Janish Ashwin Paul
Designer: Renee Deunow

Printed in United States of America

Last digit is the print number: 9 8 7 6 5 4 3 2 1

Working together
to grow libraries in
developing countries

www.elsevier.com • www.bookaid.org

List of Contributors

Olivia Swedberg Yinger, PhD, MT-BC
Director of Music Therapy
Assistant Professor of Music Therapy
School of Music, College of Fine Arts
University of Kentucky
Lexington, KY, United States

Jayne M. Standley, PhD, MT-BC
Robert O. Lawton Distinguised Professor
Colleges of Music and Medicine
Florida State University
Tallahassee, FL, United States

Kimberly Sena Moore, PhD, MT-BC
Assistant Professor of Professional Practice
Department of Music Education and Music Therapy
Frost School of Music, University of Miami
Coral Gables, FL, United States

Michael R. Detmer, MME, MT-BC
Neonatal Intensive Care Unit Music Therapist
  (NICU-MT)
Adjunct Professor, Music Therapist
School of Music, University of Louisville
Norton Women's and Children's Hospital
Louisville, KY, United States

Lori F. Gooding, PhD, MT-BC
Assistant Professor of Music Therapy
College of Music, Florida State University
Tallahassee, FL, United States

Darcy DeLoach, PhD, MT-BC
Director of Music Therapy
Associate Professor of Music Therapy
School of Music, University of Louisville
Louisville, KY, United States

Meganne K. Masko, PhD, MT-BC/L
Assistant Professor of Music and Arts Technology
Department of Music and Arts Technology
Purdue School of Engineering and Technology
Indiana University-Purdue University Indianapolis
Indianapolis, IN, United States

Lorna E. Segall, PhD, MT-BC
Assistant Professor of Music Therapy
School of Music, College of Fine Arts
University of Kentucky
Lexington, KY, United States

Alejandra J. Ferrer, PhD, MT-BC
Coordinator of Music Therapy
Assistant Professor of Music Therapy
School of Music, Belmont University
Nashville, TN, United States

Foreword

Music therapy (MT) has been a research-based, degreed profession in the United States for almost 70 years. It began in residential settings for persons with mental illnesses and intellectual disabilities and spread rapidly to all rehabilitative settings. Today, a nationally qualified music therapist, MT-BC (Music Therapist-Board Certified), is an essential component of the interdisciplinary and multidisciplinary teams serving people in early childhood intervention, special education, mental health and counseling programs, hospice, hospitals, neurologic rehabilitation facilities, programs for the elderly, especially those with Alzheimer disease, and wellness programs. Despite its prevalent use, MT is widely misunderstood by some. It is not music performance or the teaching of music lessons for the purpose of eliciting pleasure, although many volunteer musicians provide this service. Nor is it music to improve aesthetic conditions in rehabilitative and medical settings, although volunteers in Arts in Medicine programs often do that. It is the use of music by highly trained professionals who are competent in research, neuroscience, psychology, counseling, therapy, teaching skills, and music for the purpose of alleviating distress, increasing learning, and/or improving the quality of people's lives.

Others using music in clinical settings are not doing MT. Although many non–music therapists use research in the field to sell products or justify beneficial claims for their music activities, no other professionals or volunteers have the training or multiple skills to understand, design, or practice clinical MT as do MT-BCs. Other professionals may select music for use in their work setting (physicians, nurses, social workers, teachers, etc.) with good intentions but often err by ignoring 50 years of research about how the brain processes music. One's discipline and training may also foster incorrect expectations. For example, the physician may believe that if music is therapeutic, one should be able to prescribe it like a pill with a particular composition used for a specific disease or symptom: recommend Bach for headaches or, if Mozart makes you smarter, prescribe it for neurologic applications. Counseling professionals may adopt principles of lyric analysis or songwriting without fully understanding the psychological

principles underlying the music involved. The MT-BC has the skill and training to design clinical applications of music that meet the needs of each individual client and facilitate the accomplishment of his/her therapeutic objective.

Unlike other professions, music therapists begin their training with studies in psychology of music and acoustics. Music is acoustically different from all other sounds, from the human voice speaking a language, from ambient sound in the environment, from white noise, from random tones. Unlike music, noise is inconsistent vibration, sound with no fixed pitch and inconsistencies of tension, stress, and configuration. Ambient noise is the composite of these inconsistent sounds in one's environment, to which the brain reacts with stress, anxiety, and fatigue. Research shows that the brain has a distinctive response to music and develops differently from exposure to it. The music-influenced neurologic pathways developed from a person's genetic structure and life experiences allow an MT-BC to assess and carefully select music stimuli to accomplish a wide array of therapeutic objectives.

Hearing is the first sense developed by the fetus, and auditory input is critical to neurologic development at its beginning (Cheour-Luhtanen et al., 1996). Music is multisensory and activates unique sensory processing skills. It is sound created by vibrations that exist across many parameters: high/low (pitch), loud/soft (volume), rough/smooth (timbre), and simple/complex (a single note vs. harmonics) (Wagner, 1994). Progressive changes of the tone and elements of music from moment to moment aid identification, affect perception, and elicit sustained attention across time. Acoustic properties change for recorded versus live production and this, too, affects perception. Research shows that MT is most effective when live music is utilized (Standley, 2000) and is effective in aiding the brain to sustain attention to therapeutic objectives.

Contemporary music is the result of centuries of composers and musicians selecting those sounds that invoke positive neurologic responses. Historical preference has led composers to the formulation of music theory and principles of music composition, consisting of the consonant sounds most preferred across time. Consonance in music is more pleasant, soothing, and interesting than noise or dissonance and increases preference (Bidelman & Krishnan, 2011). Even infants are capable of differentiating consonance and dissonance in music (Trainor & Heinmiller, 1997). Consonant music affects pleasure responses in the brain and releases soothing, beneficial hormones. Music-derived pleasure is integral to all hearing cultures, qualifying it as universal reinforcement.

Aural perception is the sensory translation of physical vibrations experienced and learned over time. The neurons of the central auditory system send multiple signals by different routes to the temporal lobes. Neurons in one path respond to high tones, whereas those along a different path respond to low tones. Music and rhythm are processed and stored separately from language and are processed simultaneously in multiple areas of the brain across both hemispheres via the corpus callosum (Peretz & Zatorre, 2005). Music exposure promotes neurologic wiring. In fact, music study increases the size of the corpus callosum to such an extent that recognition of a trained musician's brain is readily apparent (Sachs, 2007). Neurologic changes due to music facilitate its use for learning, enhancement of memory, reality orientation, and motor coordination. MT is an excellent cotreatment with speech therapy and physical therapy to facilitate neurologic rehabilitation (Thaut, 2005). Cotreating with MT combines multiple specialties and allows the patient to rehabilitate more quickly and with reduced costs.

Melodies are organized sound, successive intervals following a pattern of music composition. The brain perceives and stores that organization through repeated listening and then develops expectancies for future analyses of music content. It is theorized that the brain enjoys this process of analyzing and categorizing sound until fatigue sets in. This pleasure in processing and ordering music stimuli contributes to the ability to enjoy repetitions of music (accompanying repetitious physical therapy exercises) or to focus on music despite being in an unpleasant situation (such as music distraction during painful medical treatment).

Masking is the effect of one set of sounds impinging upon the perception of another set of sounds. Music, a pleasant set of sounds, is often deliberately used in therapy to mask aversive auditory stimuli. This is particularly effective in hospitals where ambient sound at a high level from medical machinery can exacerbate pain and stress and worsen medical outcomes for patients.

Music is multisensory and multilayered. It contains multiple cognitive stimuli or elements: melody, rhythm, harmony, timbre, form, style, and expressive characteristics. These are neurologically processed individually and/ or simultaneously while listening to music. For instance, two pitches are perceived very differently when heard sequentially, as in a melody, versus simultaneously, as in a chord. Also, people identify intervals in the low hearing range as "more dissonant" than the same interval in a higher octave. These facts are important in selection of music for MT clinical applications, especially for those with neurologic hypersensitivity: premature infants with an immature neurologic system, patients with traumatic brain injury, or those with dementia or attention-deficit disorder.

Music quickly and strongly affects humans' moods and activity levels. Research shows that mood responses are learned; therefore, no one piece of music functions consistently to stimulate happiness or high activity levels in everyone. However, each person responds to some type of music that elevates mood, alleviates depression, or motivates one to accomplish a therapeutic objective.

Although there are some common cultural responses to music (as has been shown through ethnomusicology research), preferences for concepts such as soothing music are individually determined by background and experience. An individual's preference is basic and the most important aspect of music selection for therapeutic purposes (Standley, 2000). Music therapists must have a vast music repertoire across genres, cultures, and patient age ranges to provide patient-preferred music in the therapeutic setting. Even during procedures with anesthesia-induced unconsciousness, the music should be the patient's preference, not the physician's, because the auditory system continues functioning even under anesthesia (Cheek, 1966; Newman, Boyd, Meyers, & Bonanno, 2010).

In summary, music is a multisensory, multilayered stimulus containing infinite variations of pitch, rhythm, harmony, style, and even language. The neurologic system responds to music differently from all other sound stimuli and there are established principles with the psychology of music that predict human responses. Each individual develops his or her personal experiences with music affected by history, gender, and age. Music is universally positive within all hearing cultures, eliciting cognitive, motor, social, and emotional responses learned over time; therefore, it is highly effective in facilitating therapeutic outcomes while promoting pleasure and aesthetic responses.

This book provides an overview of research and evidence-based clinical MT across a wide variety of therapeutic settings. It is written by outstanding clinicians, academics, and researchers and intended to inform other disciplines about MT. Its purpose, ultimately, is to reveal what the highly specialized field of evidence-based MT can add to treatment and how to incorporate MT to improve patient and client care. Olivia Yinger is an outstanding researcher and she has selected accomplished scholars to describe their specialties. This volume is a valuable resource for professionals in educational, clinical, and healthcare settings that will ultimately enhance a vast array of human services.

Jayne M. Standley, PhD, MT-BC
Neonatal Intensive Care Unit Music Therapist
(NICU-MT)

REFERENCES

Bidelman, G. M., & Krishnan, A. (2011). Brainstem correlates of behavioural and compositional preferences of musical harmony. *Neuroreport, 30*(5), 212–216. http://dx.doi.org/10.1097/WNR.0b013e328344a689.

Cheek, D. B. (1966). The meaning of continued hearing sense under general chemo-anesthesia: a progress report and report of a case. *American Journal of Clinical Hypnosis, 8,* 275–280. http://dx.doi.org/10.1080/00291757.1966.10402506.

Cheour-Luhtanen, M., Alho, K., Sainio, K., Rinne, T., Reinikainen, K., Pohjavuori, M., et al. (1996). The ontogenetically

earliest discriminative response of the human brain. *Psychophysiology, 33,* 478–481. http://dx.doi.org/10.1111/j.1469-8986.1996.tb01074.x.

Newman, A., Boyd, C., Meyers, D., & Bonanno, L. (2010). Implementation of music as an anesthetic adjunct during monitored anesthesia care. *Journal of Perianesthesia Nursing, 25,* 387–391. http://dx.doi.org/10.1016/j.jopan.2010.10.003.

Peretz, I., & Zatorre, R. J. (2005). Brain organization for music processing. *Annual Review of Psychology, 58,* 89–114. http://dx.doi.org/10.1146/annurev.psych.56.091103.070225.

Sachs, O. (2007). *Musicophilia: Tales of music and the brain.* New York, NY: Knopf.

Standley, J. (2000). Music research in medical treatment. In American Music Therapy Association (Ed.), *Effectiveness of music therapy procedures: Documentation of research and clinical practice* (3rd ed.) (pp. 1–64). Silver Spring, MD: American Music Therapy Association.

Thaut, M. (2005). *Rhythm, music, and the brain.* New York, NY: Routledge, Taylor & Francis Group.

Trainor, L. J., & Heinmiller, B. M. (1997). The development of evaluative responses to music: Infants prefer to listen to consonance over dissonance. *Infant Behavior and Development, 21,* 77–88. http://dx.doi.org/10.1016/S0163-6383(98)90055-8.

Wagner, M. (1994). *Introductory musical acoustics.* Raleigh, NC: Contemporary Publishing.

Preface

In the spring of 2016, Kellie Heap, acquisitions editor for Elsevier Clinical Solutions, contacted me to ask if I was interested in writing a short book on music therapy for professionals outside of the field of music therapy, and I jumped at the opportunity. During my training to become a music therapist, and at every music therapy conference I have attended over the past decade, the importance of educating others about our relatively young profession has been impressed upon me. I envisioned this book as an opportunity to raise awareness about music therapy among people with whom my fellow music therapists, my students, and I might someday get to work.

Overall awareness of music therapy seems to be growing in the United States. As a senior in high school, I had little exposure to music therapy. It was not until a friend shared a paper she wrote on music therapy that I even considered it to be a career option for me. At the time, I was trying to decide whether to major in music or psychology in college. A friend in my psychology class suggested that music therapy might be a profession in which I could combine my passion for the arts with my desire to help others. When I was an undergraduate student majoring in music therapy, several of my friends struggled to convince their parents that music therapy was a legitimate major that could lead to employment. (I was fortunate that my parents, both musicians, never questioned my decision to major in music therapy.) When I told someone what my major was, the most common response was this: "Music therapy?" followed by a pause, a furrowing of the brows, and a question such as "What is that, exactly? Is that like aromatherapy?" or "So you provide therapy for injured musicians?" I also heard statements like "I use music therapy every day on my way home from work when I listen to relaxing music in my car!" Rather than getting frustrated by the frequent questions or misunderstandings about my profession, I learned to see them as an opportunity to educate and advocate.

Now, more than 15 years later, many of the prospective students who come to my office at the University of Kentucky have had far more experiences with music therapy than I had had at their age. Recently, I met with a prospective student whose parents were clearly intent on having her major in music therapy because they had read about the growing number of job opportunities for music therapists, yet it was clear that the student was not interested in earning a music degree. I was surprised by what I perceived as a reversal of the usual parent/college student roles; however, I believe the increased support from parents regarding majoring in music therapy is indicative of greater awareness of music therapy as a legitimate profession. I am also pleased that over the years, these questions and statements indicative of a lack of understanding have become less frequent. Now, when people find out I am a music therapist, common responses include "My mother received music therapy when she was in hospice care, and it was such a wonderful service!" "My friend's daughter has autism and she gets music therapy at school" or "I've heard music therapy can be really helpful for people with Alzheimer's disease." I recently spoke to two surgical residents while at a conference in North Carolina, and they both not only knew what music therapy was but also were familiar with the advanced specialized training for music therapists who work in the neonatal intensive care unit (NICU-MT). It has been exciting to see awareness of music therapy grow over the past 15+ years.

Despite my perception of a growing awareness of music therapy among the general population, misconceptions still exist about the field today. One misconception about music therapy that still sometimes exists is that music listening is the same as music therapy, when in fact the practice of music therapy entails far more than just listening to music. A factor that perpetuates this misconception is the existence of a number of published peer-reviewed articles, particularly within the fields of nursing and medicine, that use the term *music therapy* when a music therapist was not involved in developing or administering the intervention. In most of these articles, the intervention entailed having the patient listen to recorded music selected either by the patient or a member of the healthcare team; this practice would be more accurately called *music medicine.*

Another challenge in conceptualizing music therapy stems from the fact that how one defines music therapy may vary depending on the country where one lives and one's specific approach to music therapy. As a music therapist trained in cognitive-behavioral music therapy practicing in the United States, I use the definition put forth by the American Music Therapy Association: "Music therapy is the clinical and evidence-based use of music interventions to accomplish individualized goals within a therapeutic relationship by a credentialed professional who has completed an approved music therapy program" (AMTA, 2017, para. 1).

When explaining to others what I do as a music therapist, I find it important to go beyond giving the basic definition of music therapy and to describe specific examples of what music therapists actually do. One way in which music therapy is often described is based on the settings or areas in which music therapists most commonly work, which include educational facilities, medical and psychiatric hospitals, hospice facilities, and elder care facilities. There are a number of other areas where music therapists often work (e.g., private practices, correctional facilities, community-based wellness programs), but the aforementioned facilities are where music therapists most frequently report working. Another way to describe the work that music therapists do is based on the domains addressed, which can be categorized broadly as cognitive, communicative, emotional, musical, physiologic, psychosocial, sensorimotor, or spiritual. Yet another way to describe music therapy practice is based on the populations with whom music therapists work. Populations can be defined by age (i.e., infants, toddlers, children, adolescents, adults, and older adults), and music therapists work with all age groups. Populations can also be organized based on diagnosis (although some individuals with whom music therapists work may not have a diagnosis) or a specific population, such as people receiving medical treatment, consumers of mental health services, individuals at the end of life and their families, children receiving special education services, at-risk youth, and older adults with dementia.

Because music therapists work with such a broad range of individuals, organizing the chapters in this book based on areas where music therapists most frequently work seemed to be the simplest way to describe music therapy practice. This way, professionals who work within educational, medical, psychiatric, hospice, or elder care settings can easily find the information they seek. There will necessarily be some overlap between chapters (for example, some patients receiving music therapy while undergoing medical treatment at a hospital may also have mental health needs). In addition, there will be some settings where music therapists

work that do not have entire chapters devoted to them, such as physical rehabilitation, corrections, or veteran's affair services.

In Chapter 1, Overview of the Music Therapy Profession, I expand upon the definition of music therapy, providing a brief history of music therapy in the United States and a description of the educational and clinical training requirements for music therapists. I describe the settings where music therapists most frequently work and provide a basic overview of common music therapy interventions. I outline the music therapy treatment process and cover the domains and goals that music therapists often address. A brief discussion of approaches to music therapy grounded in diverse philosophical orientations follows, leading to a discussion about advanced competencies in music therapy. Finally, I provide helpful information on differentiating music therapy from other music-based services.

Chapter 2, Neurologic Foundations of Music-Based Interventions, by Dr. Kimberly Sena Moore, provides a clear overview of the neurologic processes involved with music perception. Furthermore, Dr. Sena Moore describes ways in which music therapists use knowledge of how music affects the brain to tailor interventions that meet specific needs related to motor, cognitive, communicative, emotional, and social responses.

Chapters 3–8 each focus on a setting where music therapists commonly work. Each chapter includes an overview of populations served; a summary of the research; a description of evidence-based practices; case examples; information about provision of services, including information about funding, referral pathways, and collaboration with other disciplines; and areas for future research. In Chapter 3, Music Therapy in Educational Settings, Michael Detmer describes music therapy research and practice in educational settings, which often include K to 12 schools, early intervention programs, children's day care centers, and preschools. Chapter 4, Music Therapy in Mental Health Treatment by Dr. Lori Gooding, provides an overview of music therapy research and practice in mental health settings, which may include inpatient psychiatric units, child/adolescent treatment centers, community mental health centers, drug and alcohol programs, and forensic facilities. In Chapter 5, Music Therapy in Medical Treatment and Rehabilitation, Dr. Darcy DeLoach provides a rationale for the use of music therapy interventions featuring live, patient-preferred music in medical treatment and acute rehabilitation settings, which may include general hospitals, children's hospitals, home health agencies, oncology treatment facilities, outpatient clinics, and partial hospitalization programs.

Chapter 6, Music Therapy in Hospice and Palliative Care by Dr. Meganne Masko, highlights the similarities and differences between hospice and palliative care and describes ways in which music therapists address needs of patients nearing the end of life and their families. In Chapter 7, Music Therapy in Gerontology, I offer a description of music therapy services for older adults in various settings, including skilled nursing facilities, assisted living facilities, and adult day facilities. In Chapter 8, Music Therapy and Wellness, Dr. Lorna Segall describes music therapy practices across a variety of settings, including schools, universities, workplaces, and communities that are united by an approach to enhancing wellness.

In Chapter 9, Current Trends and Future Directions in Music Therapy, Dr. Alejandra Ferrer describes the music therapy profession in greater detail, delving into how the profession has grown over the past decade and providing suggestions and predictions for the future of the profession. I have provided at the end of the book a glossary of terms with which readers may be unfamiliar.

All of the contributors to this book are board-certified music therapists who have undergone advanced training and possess clinical and research experience in the areas covered within their chapters. I am deeply grateful to the contributors who devoted their time and effort to bring this book to fruition. Many thanks to the wonderful people at Elsevier, particularly senior development editor Donald Mumford, project manager Janish Paul, and content strategists Lauren Willis, Kayla Wolfe, and Kellie Heap. Finally, this book would not have been possible without the support and encouragement from numerous friends and family, particularly my dear friends and colleagues, Nicole, Martina, and Lorna; my exchange daughter, Helene; and my fantastic husband, Tim.

Olivia Swedberg Yinger, PhD, MT-BC

REFERENCE

American Music Therapy Association. (2017). *Definition and quotes about music therapy*. Retrieved from https://www.musictherapy.org/about/quotes/.

Contents

CHAPTER 1

Overview of the Music Therapy Profession

OLIVIA SWEDBERG YINGER, PHD, MT-BC

INTRODUCTION

An infant born prematurely is receiving intermediate care in the neonatal intensive care unit (NICU). To be discharged from the NICU, the infant must first be able to be bottle-fed, rather than receive feedings via an orogastric tube. Once the infant's gestational age is 34 weeks, a music therapist implements the use of the Pacifier Activated Lullaby device, which uses music contingently to improve nonnutritive sucking. This helps the infant bottle-feed faster and ultimately go home sooner.

A music therapist working with a group of 3-year-olds on school readiness might address skills for appropriate social interaction, such as listening, following directions, sharing, and appropriately greeting others by smiling, waving, and/or saying hello or goodbye.

A 10-year-old child with an intellectual disability has difficulty remembering his mother's phone number. A music therapist teaches it to him using a simple but engaging original song. The child and the music therapist practice the song together repeatedly until the child can sing in independently. After practicing the song for several weeks, the child is able to recite his mother's phone number fluently through speaking rather than singing.

A group of four teenagers in an acute behavioral healthcare facility are getting the care they need to better function in their lives outside the facility. To make the most of their brief time at the facility, the teens are expected to engage in group therapy, which can be awkward with people they do not know well who may be at the facility for vastly different reasons. A music therapist engages them in a conversation about the lyrics of a popular song and they realize that not only can they relate to the experience of the person who wrote the song, but also relate each other. This allows them to feel more comfortable sharing with each other when the music therapist guides the conversation to a discussion about stress reduction strategies and coping skills.

A 35-year-old patient is recovering from surgery and has been prescribed opioid medications for pain relief. He may self-administer pain medication as needed (within certain limitations) via a pain-medication pump. The patient's surgeon requests that a music therapist see the client once a day during recovery to see if teaching relaxation skills with music can reduce the amount of pain medication that the client self-administers in an effort to decrease the risk of opioid addiction.

A 72-year-old woman recently had a stroke and is working with a physical therapist at an inpatient rehabilitation facility on seated range of motion and endurance exercises. The physical therapist asks the music therapist to provide live instrumental music at a tempo appropriate for the pace at which the client can perform the physical exercises, and the rhythm of the music helps prime the client's motor system so that she is better able to perform the exercises.

An 89-year-old man is receiving hospice care because of terminal cancer. A music therapist meets with him and his wife in their home several times a week to help create a musical legacy project. This will allow his wife to have a meaningful gift to remember him by. Through the process of creating the legacy project, the couple is able to spend quality time together singing, listening to, and talking about their favorite music.

The aforementioned case examples illustrate some ways in which music therapists use carefully chosen music therapy interventions to address individualized goals of people at different stages of life with very diverse needs. Understanding evidence-based practice in music therapy requires some knowledge of where, with whom, why, and how music therapists practice. This chapter will provide readers with a basic understanding of music therapy professional practices in the United States. First, I will define music therapy and provide a brief history of how the music therapy profession came into existence in the United States. Next, I will describe education and clinical training requirements for board-certified

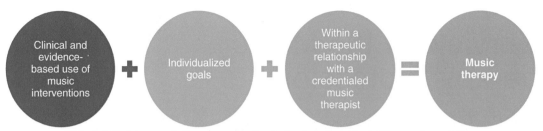

FIG. 1.1 Defining music therapy, according to the American Music Therapy Association.

music therapists and settings in which music therapists frequently work. Then, I will outline commonly used music therapy interventions, the music therapy treatment process, and domains addressed in music therapy practice. Finally, I will describe common approaches to music therapy, advanced music therapy practice, and how to differentiate music therapy from other types of music-based services.

DEFINING MUSIC THERAPY

The American Music Therapy Association (AMTA) defines music therapy as "...the clinical and evidence-based use of music interventions to accomplish individualized goals within a therapeutic relationship by a credentialed professional who has completed an approved music therapy program" (AMTA, 2016a, 1st para). There are key components of this definition that differentiate music therapy from other uses of music for wellness and healing. First, music therapy includes the evidence-based use of music interventions. Evidence-based practice is based on the best available research, clinical expertise, and the needs and choices of the individual client, patient, or student (McKibbon, 1998). Second, music interventions are used to accomplish individualized goals, meaning the music itself and the way the music is used are tailored to meet specific nonmusical objectives. Third, the music interventions are used within a therapeutic relationship with a credentialed professional who has completed an AMTA-approved music therapy program. Music is a tool used by music therapists, who are trained both as musicians and as therapists; however, in music therapy practice, both the music and the therapeutic relationship with the music therapist are key to helping accomplish individualized goals. Fig. 1.1 provides a summary of the AMTA's definition of music therapy.

BRIEF HISTORY OF THE PROFESSION

Although the concept of music as a healing agent has existed since antiquity, the profession of music therapy

in the United States was formed in the mid-20th century (AMTA, 2016b). Veterans hospitals serving veterans from World War I and World War II often brought in musicians to provide entertainment. Physicians and nurses observed that many veterans had positive emotional and physical responses upon hearing live music and asked that hospitals hire musicians. The need for musicians to be trained before working in a hospital setting resulted in the development of college music therapy programs, beginning with Michigan State College (now called Michigan State University) in 1944 and the formation of the National Association for Music Therapy (NAMT) in 1950 (AMTA, 2016b). The NAMT began publishing two peer-reviewed journals, both of which are still in publication today: *The Journal of Music Therapy* (1964 to present) and *Music Therapy Perspectives* (1982 to present). In 1971, a group of music therapists who used a different approach to music therapy practice established the American Association for Music Therapy (AAMT). The AAMT began publishing a peer-reviewed journal called *Music Therapy* in 1981 and continued to do so until 1996. The Certification Board for Music Therapists (CBMT) was formed in 1983 to ensure the proficiency of music therapists who hold the music therapist-board certified (MT-BC) credential. In 1998, the AMTA was formed when the NAMT merged with AAMT. Fig. 1.2 shows a timeline of key events in the development of the music therapy profession in the United States during the 20th century.

EDUCATION AND CLINICAL TRAINING OF MUSIC THERAPISTS

Music therapists undergo extensive training to provide high-quality, evidence-based services. An individual wishing to become a music therapist must first obtain an undergraduate degree in music therapy or the equivalent from an AMTA-approved university program or the equivalent. Some universities offer postbaccalaureate "equivalency" programs for students who have earned an undergraduate degree in an area of music other than

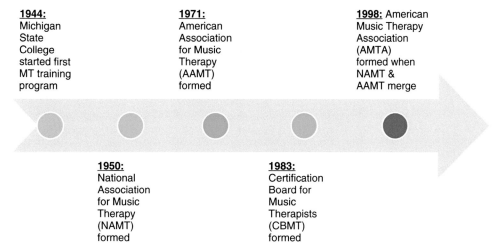

1944: Michigan State College started first MT training program

1971: American Association for Music Therapy (AAMT) formed

1998: American Music Therapy Association (AMTA) formed when NAMT & AAMT merge

1950: National Association for Music Therapy (NAMT) formed

1983: Certification Board for Music Therapists (CBMT) formed

FIG. 1.2 Timeline of key events in the development of music therapy in the United States during the 20th century.

music therapy (e.g., music education or music performance) who wish to become music therapists. For a university to offer an AMTA-approved undergraduate or equivalency program in music therapy, the university's music program must be accredited by the National Association of Schools of Music (NASM). The AMTA and NASM standards help ensure that music therapists are highly proficient musicians. Music therapy students take applied lessons on a principal instrument; perform in music ensembles; demonstrate proficiency on guitar, piano, and voice; and take coursework in music theory, music history, and conducting. In addition to taking music foundations coursework, music therapy students establish a solid clinical foundation by taking coursework in psychology, counseling, and anatomy/physiology. Finally, in music therapy core classes, students learn foundations and principles of music therapy practice and apply their knowledge in supervised clinical practice and internship experiences. To become board certified, music therapy students must complete 1200 clinical hours under the supervision of board-certified music therapists, gaining experience with multiple populations and across various settings in which music therapists work.

After completing an undergraduate training program in music therapy, which culminates in a 6-month clinical internship, students become eligible to take the board certification examination offered by CBMT. Only after passing the board certification examination may an individual begin using the credential MT-BC and the professional denotation "music therapist." To

maintain the MT-BC credential, one must complete 100 approved hours of continuing education every 5 years, including at least 3 h of ethics training. Fig. 1.3 provides an overview of the training and credentialing requirements for music therapists.

Board-certified music therapists must adhere to the CBMT Code of Professional Practice (CBMT, 2011) and work within the AMTA/CBMT Scope of Music Therapy Practice (AMTA & CBMT, 2015). Music therapists are also guided by the AMTA Code of Ethics (AMTA, 2015a) and Standards of Clinical Practice (AMTA, 2015b), which include general standards for music therapy clinical practice, as well as standards for music therapists working with specific populations (i.e., clients who have addictive disorders, intellectual and developmental disabilities, or physical disabilities and older adults), in specific settings (i.e., educational settings, medical settings, mental health settings, private practice, and wellness), or in a specific role (i.e., consultant).

SETTINGS WHERE MUSIC THERAPISTS WORK

Music therapists work with individuals of all ages, providing individual or group sessions in a variety of settings, most frequently in mental health, medical, hospice, geriatric, or educational facilities. Music therapists who are self-employed or who work in private practice may see individuals or groups at their own music therapy studio rather than at a facility, may have contracts with several facilities, or may have a

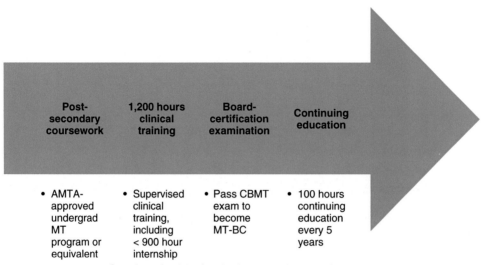

FIG. 1.3 Overview of training/credentialing requirements for music therapists.

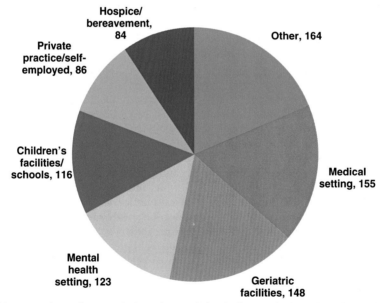

FIG. 1.4 Primary settings where music therapists work (excluding music therapists who work in colleges/universities), based on 2016 the American Music Therapy Association member survey and workforce analysis (AMTA, 2016c, p. 16).

combination of private clients and contracts with facilities. Some music therapists working in private practice specialize in one area of music therapy practice (e.g., children with disabilities), whereas others work with various populations. Each year, the AMTA publishes the results of a member survey and workforce analysis. After excluding music therapists who reported that they work in college/university settings (because their work in these settings is likely educational rather than clinical), the primary settings where music therapists reported working in 2016 are shown in Fig. 1.4 (AMTA, 2016c).

For the purpose of AMTA's survey, the category *children's facilities/schools* included children's day cares/preschools, early intervention programs, and schools (K to 12); *mental health settings* included child/adolescent treatment centers, community mental health centers, drug/alcohol programs, forensic facilities, and inpatient psychiatric units; *medical settings* included general hospitals, oncology, home health agencies, outpatient clinics, partial hospitalization, and children's hospitals or units; and *geriatric facilities* included adult day care, assisted living facilities, geriatric facilities-not nursing, geriatric psychiatric units, and nursing homes. The most frequently reported settings in the *other* category included community-based services, physical rehabilitation, state institutions, and group homes (AMTA, 2016c). This book contains chapters that discuss music therapy practices in the most common settings where music therapists practice (educational settings, medical settings, mental health settings, elder care facilities, and hospice/palliative care settings); Table 1.1 includes resources for those who wish to learn more about music therapy practices in settings where music therapists work less frequently (i.e., those grouped together in the

TABLE 1.1
Resources on Music Therapy Practices in Other Settings

Setting	Resources (Books, Online Fact Sheets, and Articles)
Community-based services	*Community Music Therapy* (Pavlicevic & Ansdell, 2004) Home-based music therapy - a systematic overview of settings and conditions for an innovative service in healthcare (Schmid & Ostermann, 2010)
Correctional facilities	*The Effect of a Music Therapy Intervention on Inmate Levels of Executive Function and Perceived Stress* (Segall, 2016)
Intermediate care facility/Developmental disabilities	Music therapy and developmental disabilities: A glance back and a look forward (Farnan, 2007)
Physical rehabilitation	Music Therapy and Rehabilitation: Selected References (AMTA, 2016d) *Music Therapy Methods in Neurorehabilitation: A Clinician's Manual* (Tamplin & Baker, 2006) *Clinical Guide to Music Therapy in Adult Physical Rehabilitation Settings* (Wong, 2004)
Veteran's affairs	Music Therapy and Military Populations (AMTA, 2014)

"other" category on AMTA's member survey and workforce analysis).

MUSIC THERAPY INTERVENTIONS

Interventions used in music therapy treatment may use live or recorded music. When deciding which music to use, music therapists consider the musical preferences of their client(s); the needs, goals, and abilities of the client(s); and the characteristics of the music (both musical elements and lyrical content). Numerous specific music therapy interventions exist, but they can be broadly categorized based on how the client engages with music: by listening to music, talking about music, making music, or moving to music. Some interventions involve clients with music in more than one way; for example, music-based patient education may involve listening to, talking about, and making music. Fig. 1.5 shows some commonly used music therapy interventions.

MUSIC THERAPY TREATMENT PROCESS

The music therapy treatment process may vary somewhat depending on the setting and population, but the general steps that are followed include (1) referral to music therapy services, (2) assessment and identification of goals and objectives, (3) treatment planning and implementation, (4) evaluation and documentation, and (5) termination of treatment (see Fig. 1.6). For an in-depth explanation of the music therapy treatment process, see Dr. Suzanne Hanser's book *The New Music Therapist's Handbook* (Hanser, 2000).

Referral

Music therapy referrals may come from a variety of sources, including the physicians, educators, nurses, other therapists, patients' family members, or even the patients themselves. In medical settings, physician approval for music therapy referrals is sometimes required, particularly if music therapy services are to be covered by third-party reimbursement. Documentation of the referral within the patient's medical chart is often required before initiation of music therapy services. Other terms sometimes used in medical settings in place of the term *referral* include *consult* and *order*.

In educational settings, parents of children with special needs, special educators, or classroom teachers often make referrals for music therapy. For a child with an Individualized Education Program (IEP) to receive music therapy, it must first be determined that the child can better achieve IEP goals with music therapy.

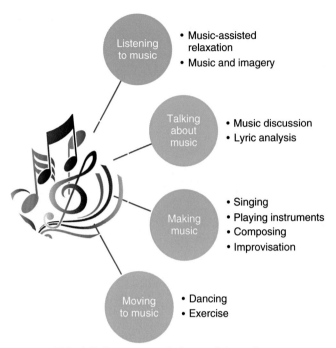

FIG. 1.5 Common music therapy interventions.

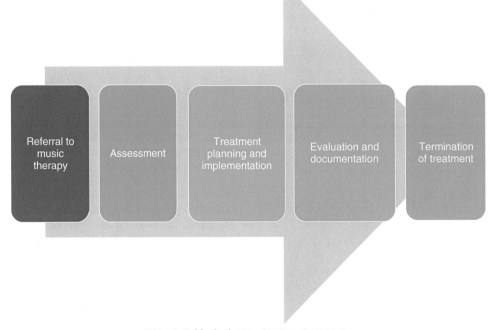

FIG. 1.6 Music therapy treatment process.

An independent music therapy evaluation, conducted by a music therapist who will not be the one providing music therapy treatment, is necessary to make this determination. This initial evaluation is an additional step in the referral process within educational settings.

In some community-based settings, patients self-refer and the referral process is less formal. This may also be the case in mental health settings, where patients who meet certain predetermined criteria are automatically eligible to receive group music therapy services, and they may choose from a variety of options for group treatment, including music therapy. Older adults in assisted living, skilled nursing, or memory care facilities may also choose whether or not to participate in group music therapy.

In private practice settings, music therapy referrals may come from the patients themselves, from family members, or from other healthcare professionals. The format for initiation and documentation of referrals varies greatly depending on the setting. Check-boxes, drop-down menus, fill-in-the-blank responses, and free response fields may all be used. Referrals may be received via email, hard copy, phone, pager, fax, electronic medical record, online forms, or face-to-face conversation.

Assessment

The assessment process also varies depending on the setting and the population. The areas being assessed sometimes depend on the reason for referral. In some settings, an assessment examines all areas of functioning for every referred client. In other situations, an assessment may focus only on areas of functioning related to the reason for referral. Assessment information may be collected through the use of standardized assessment tools or through the use of assessment forms created by the music therapist or the facility. Several music therapy–specific assessment tools exist, including the Special Education Music Therapy Assessment Profile and the Individual Music Therapy Assessment Profile. Whether or not a standardized assessment is used, music therapy assessments may include information about the following domains: cognitive, communicative, physical, psychological, social, and musical. There are several types of assessment, including initial assessment and ongoing assessment. Initial assessment is the process that most often occurs before the establishment of goals and initiation of treatment. Ongoing assessment occurs along with the implementation of treatment and is the process by which the music therapist evaluates the client's progress within the therapeutic setting.

In settings where patients may participate in only one music therapy session, such as acute-care medical or mental health settings, the assessment process is truncated and may be combined with the phase of treatment that includes setting goals and implementing treatment. A separate assessment session may not always be possible, because the music therapist has no way of knowing when a client will be discharged from the hospital, so short-term goals are established quickly and intervention may take place in the same session as assessment.

Treatment Planning and Implementation

Treatment planning may include the establishment of short-term and long-term goals and objectives. In music therapy practice, goals are directions for treatment progress, stated broadly, whereas objectives are specific, measurable, attainable, realistic, and time bound. In addition to establishing goals and objectives, a music therapy treatment plan will include strategies and interventions that will be used to work toward the goals and objectives. Strategies and interventions may include specific music therapy interventions, as well as techniques that are not music therapy specific, such as counseling techniques, alternative augmentative communication strategies, or behavior management approaches.

Music therapy objectives often follow a format that includes (1) specification of the circumstances under which a behavior should occur, (2) the behavior that is to be measured, (3) the number or times or percentage of time in which the behavior is set to occur, and (4) how the behavior will be measured. An operational definition for all behaviors being measured is crucial so that there is reliability regarding whether or not the target behavior or behaviors have occurred. Operational definitions must include clear descriptions of what constitutes a behavior and what does not, as well as examples of "borderline" behaviors (i.e., those about which there may be confusion). Ideally, reliability measures are taken by having multiple observers assess behaviors for a short period of time and calculating the rate of interobserver agreement.

Evaluation and Documentation

Several methods of documentation exist to record the results of ongoing assessment during implementation of music therapy treatment. Music therapists, particularly those working in medical, mental health, or hospice settings, may create structured progress notes using a format such as SOAP, PIE, DAR, DART, or DAP (Baird, 2014). Documentation may include check-boxes, drop-down menus, free-text notes, or any combination of these formats. In educational settings, documentation often follows the format of IEP goals and may include the number of times a behavior was observed or the percentage of times the behavior was observed out of a set number of trials. Behavioral observation, measurement of physiological variables, and recording of client-report measures are categories that may be documented to ascertain client progress. Often, a combination of measurements is used to provide additional validity. For example, a music therapist working with patients for whom relaxation is a goal might measure relaxation by observing the patients' behaviors (e.g., closing eyes and appearing to sleep); by monitoring their heart rate, respiration, and blood pressure; and by asking the patient to rate their level of relaxation on a scale of 0 to 10.

Results of ongoing assessment over time are periodically evaluated to determine whether progress is being made. Graphs are often useful to be able to see at a glance whether behaviors are increasing or decreasing. Results of ongoing assessments are often compiled into music therapy treatment reports and submitted to the client, to the client's treatment team, or the client's family member (particularly for children) and/or placed in the client's educational or medical record.

DOMAINS ADDRESSED BY MUSIC THERAPISTS

Music therapists create individualized treatment plans with goals based on the specific strengths and needs of the client. In Chapter 2, Kimberly Sena Moore describes the neurological foundations behind musical responses within the physiological, motor, cognitive, communicative, emotional, and social domains. In Chapter 5, Darcy DeLoach provides information about the use of music to decrease the perception of pain. Given the effects that music can have on each of these neurological systems, it follows that nonmusical goals addressed by music therapists would align with these domains (see Fig. 1.7). The case examples mentioned at the beginning of this chapter help illustrate some common goals that music therapists address with people in specific settings. When working with the infant in the NICU, contingent music is being used to strengthen the oral motor system. With 3-year-olds practicing attending, taking turns, and greeting each other, the cognitive, communicative, and social domains are being addressed. Cognitive and communicative goals are also the primary focus of the example with the child learning to recite his phone number. For adolescents in a behavioral health facility, the emotional domain would probably receive the most focus. These examples help illustrate the fact that multiple goals can be addressed simultaneously through music therapy treatment.

APPROACHES TO MUSIC THERAPY

Individual music therapists use a variety of approaches grounded in diverse philosophical orientations. Commonly used music therapy approaches include those informed by music education approaches, most frequently the Orff Schulwerk approach and less often the Dalcroze and Kodaly approaches. Other music

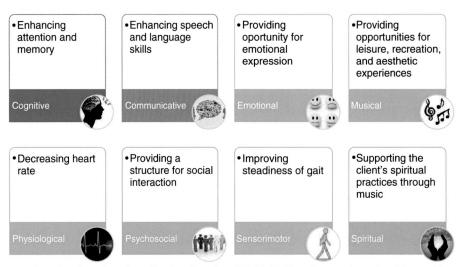

FIG. 1.7 Domains (from board certification domains; CBMT, 2015) and example goals addressed in music therapy practice.

therapists use approaches informed by psychology, including psychodynamic music therapy, behavioral music therapy, Nordoff-Robbins music therapy, and the Bonnie Method of Guided Imagery in Music (BMGIM). Still other common medical approaches to music therapy include the biomedical approach, the Neurologic Music Therapy (NMT) approach, and the wellness model. The decision regarding which music therapy approach to use may be based in part on the setting and the needs of the client population and in part on the music therapist's education, training, strengths, and therapeutic style. The book *Introduction to Approaches in Music Therapy*, edited by Alice-Ann Darrow (2008) provides an excellent overview of the most commonly used music therapy approaches. There are other approaches and philosophies of music therapy besides those outlined in Darrow's book. The CBMT board certification domains (CBMT, 2015), which are based on a practice analysis conducted in 2014, include several other theoretical orientations and music therapy treatment approaches that inform music therapy practice (see Box 1.1).

Those familiar with the various approaches to psychotherapy will likely have a basic understanding of the foundations of the music therapy approaches named after these approaches (e.g., behavioral, humanistic, psychodynamic). I will therefore briefly describe three of the approaches that readers are less likely to have heard of, namely, Orff Schulwerk music therapy, Nordoff-Robbins music therapy, and the BMGIM.

BOX 1.1
Theoretical Orientations and Music Therapy Treatment Approaches Listed in the CBMT Board Certification Domains (CBMT, 2015)

Theoretical Orientations That Inform Music Therapy Practice	Music Therapy Treatment Approaches
• Behavioral	• Behavioral
• Cognitive	• Culture centered
• Holistic	• Community music therapy
• Humanistic/existential	• Developmental
• Neuroscience	• Humanistic
• Psychodynamic	• Improvisational
	• Medical
	• Neurological
	• Psychodynamic

Orff Schulwerk

The Orff Schulwerk approach to music therapy is based on the music education approach of Carl Orff (1895-1982), a composer who created a philosophical framework and approach to teaching music to children in a developmentally appropriate way. The Orff Schulwerk approach to music education engages children in singing, chanting, moving, and playing instruments, providing them ample opportunities to experience music before labeling abstract theoretical musical concepts. When teaching using the Orff Schulwerk approach, the teacher (1) gives children opportunities to be creative and explore, incorporating the children's ideas into the lesson whenever possible; (2) invites them to imitate the teacher to teach basic skills; (3) asks children to improvise using the building blocks they have learned through imitation; and (4) guides the children through the process of creating a product in which they put together multiple elements to demonstrate what they have learned. Although the Orff Schulwerk approach was designed to teach children musical concepts, it has often been adapted for use in music therapy to help children accomplish nonmusical goals. In addition, the Orff Schulwerk approach has frequently been adapted for use in special music education settings, as the approach lends itself well to situations that require adaptation to meet the needs of diverse students. The Orff Schulwerk approach has also been used by music therapists outside of educational settings, including with bereaved children (Hilliard, 2007; Register & Hilliard, 2008), hospitalized children (Colwell, Edwards, Hernandez, & Brees, 2013), and college students (Detmer, 2015).

Nordoff-Robbins Music Therapy (Creative Music Therapy)

In 1959, American composer and pianist Paul Nordoff (1909–77) and British special educator Clive Robbins (1927–2011) developed a form of collaborative music making for children with disabilities that they called Creative Music Therapy. They believed that every child has inborn musicality and that by focusing on an individual's strengths using music as the primary clinical medium, they could provide opportunities for self-actualizing creativeness, courage, boldness, freedom, spontaneity, integration, and self-acceptance (Aigen et al., 2008). Goals commonly addressed through Creative Music Therapy include developing the client's inner potential, expressive freedom and creativity, peak experiences, growth motivation, and self-actualization. Clinical improvisation is the primary technique used in Creative Music Therapy. In the first issue of 2014 (volume 32), the journal *Music Therapy Perspectives* featured articles about Creative Music Therapy; this publication and the Nordoff-Robbins Website (https://www.nordoff-robbins.org.uk/) are excellent sources for more information on creative music therapy.

Bonny Method of Guided Imagery and Music

Helen Bonny (1921–2010) was a musician who had a peak experience while playing the violin. She was greatly influenced by the theories of Abraham Maslow, Carl Rogers, and Carl Jung, and those theories influenced her as she developed the BMGIM, a music-centered exploration of consciousness that uses specifically sequenced classical music programs (Burns & Woolrich, 2008). After listening to the specially selected classical music program, a music therapist would encourage the client to draw meaning and parallels with their own experiences from imagery evoked by the music. People who are looking for self-understanding and actualization who are able to distinguish reality from fantasy and generate imagery may benefit from BMGIM. The Association for Music and Imagery (AMI) Website (http://www.ami-bonnymethod.org/) is an excellent source for more information about BMGIM.

TABLE 1.2 Specialty Training Designations for Music Therapists	
Specialty Training Designation	**Party Responsible for Administering Training**
Fellows of the Association for Music and Imagery (FAMI)	Association for Music and Imagery http://www.ami-bonnymethod.org/
Hospice and Palliative Care Music Therapy (HPMT) certificate	Center for Music Therapy in End-of-Life Care http://www.hospicemusictherapy.org/
Neonatal Intensive Care Unit-Music Therapist (NICU-MT)	National Institute for Infant and Child Medical Music Therapy http://www.music.fsu.edu/NICU-MT
Neurologic Music Therapist (NMT)	The Academy of Neurologic Music Therapy https://nmtacademy.co/
Nordoff-Robbins Music Therapist (NRMT)	Nordoff-Robbins Center for Music Therapy http://steinhardt.nyu.edu/music/nordoff/training/

ADVANCED COMPETENCY IN MUSIC THERAPY

To become a board-certified music therapist, one must demonstrate professional competency according to AMTA's guidelines (AMTA, 2013); however, the AMTA has also outlined advanced competencies for those music therapists seeking to further their professional growth or seek specialized training (AMTA, 2015c). Music therapists may achieve an advanced level of practice by gaining extensive professional experience and/or further education or training, through engaging in clinical supervision, obtaining a graduate degree, or undertaking another type of advanced training. The AMTA has outlined guidelines for master's programs in music therapy to help music therapists achieve an advanced level of practice.

Several groups of music therapy professionals offer advanced training outside of graduate programs in music therapy that result in specialty training designations. Table 1.2 includes information about specialty training designations for advanced music therapists (Sena Moore, 2011). It is important to note that these specialty trainings are not offered by the AMTA or CBMT, although participants may receive continuing music therapy education credits

for earning specialty training designations. Although the AMTA and CBMT do not require that music therapists have specialized training to practice in specific settings (for example, the NMT designation is not required to practice in rehabilitation settings, nor is the HPMT designation required to practice in hospice and palliative care settings), some facilities or private practices may require or prefer specialty training designations when hiring music therapists. Similarly, although a master's degree is not currently required to become a board-certified music therapist, some employers may require or prefer that applicants possess a master's degree.

DIFFERENTIATING MUSIC THERAPY FROM OTHER MUSIC-BASED SERVICES

It is important to distinguish between music therapy and other uses of music in settings where music therapists work, particularly healthcare and older adult facilities. In the same way that physical therapists, massage therapists, and chiropractors all use manual therapy yet do so within different scopes of practice, music therapists are one group of professionals who use music within their specific scope of practice. This section will discuss the administration of recorded music in healthcare settings by other healthcare professionals, as well as the use of live music at bedside by musicians other than music therapists.

Music Medicine

As stated previously, music therapy involves the use of music and the therapeutic relationship with a credentialed music therapist to accomplish nonmusic goals. Music medicine, on the other hand, entails the use of recorded music listening in a healthcare setting, implemented by a healthcare professional who is not a music therapist (Dileo & Bradt, 2005). The definition of music therapy often varies from one country to another. Research conducted in countries in which music therapy has a different definition may classify an intervention as music therapy when in the United States the intervention would be classified as music medicine. For this reason, it is important for readers in the United States to understand the difference between music therapy and music medicine, and to make the distinction even when the terms are used interchangeably in the research literature. The terms passive music therapy and active music therapy are occasionally used in publications. Passive music therapy refers to interventions in which the client is listening to music, whereas active music therapy engages the client in music making. Passive music therapy is sometimes used incorrectly to refer to music medicine treatment. In music therapy practice, the term receptive music therapy is most often used instead of passive music therapy to describe music listening.

It should be noted that there are situations where recorded music is more appropriate than live music. It is not always possible to have a music therapist present, and when used appropriately, recorded music can bring about many benefits for clients. One advantage of having live music administered by a music therapist instead of music medicine is that the therapist may change the music in the moment in response to the client's needs. Live music also helps engage clients in treatment to a greater degree, and building the therapeutic relationship with the board-certified music therapist has numerous benefits in treatment.

Music & Memory

Music & Memory^{SM} is a program that was featured in the documentary Alive Inside. In the Music & Memory^{SM} program, older adults with dementia are given mp3 players with prerecorded music that was popular during their earlier years. There are numerous potential benefits of Music & Memory^{SM}; however, it is important to recognize how the Music & Memory^{SM} program differs from music therapy. Music therapy services involve interaction with a credentialed music therapist, whereas Music & Memory^{SM} programs may be implemented by other healthcare staff who work at a facility that has participated in Music & Memory^{SM} training. Music therapy services often involve the use of live music to address a specific goal. Music & Memory^{SM} services solely incorporate the use of recorded music. One benefit of the Music & Memory^{SM} program is that it may be used to allow clients to listen to music when it is not possible for a music therapist to be present. One drawback of the Music & Memory^{SM} program is that participants may experience strong emotions as a result of listening to music and may not have anyone with whom to process the deeply emotional experience. Individuals working with older adults with dementia are advised to be aware of the potential benefits and drawbacks of the Music & Memory^{SM} program and to use it with care (AMTA, 2015d).

Therapeutic Musicians

Other musicians who may work or volunteer in healthcare settings include certified music practitioners, harp therapists or harp practitioners, clinical musicians, therapeutic musicians, music healers or sound healers, and music thanatologists. Each of these groups has a different scope of practice and differences in training. Two characteristics that set music therapy apart from other types of therapeutic music are that (1) music therapy training is more extensive, requiring at least a bachelor's degree to practice, and (2) music therapists have a wider range of interventions within their scope of practice. The AMTA and the National Standards Board for Therapeutic Musicians (2015) created a chart that provides an overview of therapeutic music services. Descriptions of various music-based services are summarized in Table 1.3.

SUMMARY

Over the past 65 years, the music therapy profession has grown as generations of music therapists have contributed to the field through research, education, and clinical training. Music therapists use evidence-based music therapy practices to help people of all ages with diverse needs across a wide range of settings. Although music therapy approaches and interventions may vary, what all music therapists have in common is the use of music to address individualized goals within the therapeutic relationship.

TABLE 1.3
Summary of Music-Based Services

Music-Based Service	Use Live Music	Settings Include	Scope of Practice	Code of Ethics	Degree Program	Certification	State Licensure	Third-Party Reimbursement
Music therapy • Music Therapist-Board Certified (MT-BC)	✓	Medical and psychiatric hospitals, homes, hospice facilities, skilled nursing facilities, schools, early childhood centers, correctional facilities, veteran's care facilities, private practice	✓	✓	✓	✓	✓[a]	✓[b]
Therapeutic music • Certified Clinical Musician (CCM) • Certified Music Practitioner (CMP) • Certified Therapeutic Harp Practitioner (CTHP) • Certified Healing Musician (CHM)	✓	Hospitals, homes, hospice facilities, skilled nursing facilities	✓	✓	✗	✓	✗	✗
Music thanatology • Contemplative Musician (CM) • Music–Thanatologist (MTH) • Certified Music-Thanatologist (CM-TH)	✓	End-of-life care in hospitals, homes, and hospice facilities	✓	✓	✗	✓	✗	✗
Music medicine	✗	Medical hospitals and other healthcare facilities	✗	✗	✗	✗	✗	✗
Music & Memory^{SM}	✗	Skilled nursing, assisted living, and memory care facilities; homes	✗	✗	✗	✗[c]	✗	✗

[a]In some states.
[b]From some third-party payers.
[c]Facilities can be Music & Memory^{SM} certified; individuals cannot.

REFERENCES

Aigen, K., Miller, C. K., Kim, Y., Pasiali, V., Kwak, E. M., & Tague, D. B. (2008). Nordoff-Robbins music therapy. In A. A. Darrow (Ed.), *Introduction to approaches in music therapy* (2nd ed.) (pp. 61–77). Silver Spring, MD: American Music Therapy Association.

American Music Therapy Association. (2013). *Professional competencies.* Retrieved from https://www.musictherapy.org/about/competencies/.

American Music Therapy Association. (2014). *Music therapy and military populations: A status report and recommendations on music therapy treatment programs, research, and practice policy.* Retrieved from http://www.musictherapy.org/assets/1/7/MusicTherapyMilitaryPops_2014.pdf.

American Music Therapy Association. (2015a). *American music therapy association code of ethics.* Retrieved from https://www.musictherapy.org/about/ethics/.

American Music Therapy Association. (2015b). *AMTA standards of clinical practice.* Retrieved from https://www.musictherapy.org/about/standards/.

American Music Therapy Association. (2015c). *Advanced competencies.* Retrieved from https://www.musictherapy.org/members/advancedcomp/.

American Music Therapy Association. (2015d). *Clinical music therapy and the Music & Memory*^{SM} *program.* Retrieved from http://www.musictherapy.org/assets/1/7/ML-MM-MTFactSheet.pdf.

American Music Therapy Association. (2016a). *What is music therapy?* Retrieved from http://www.musictherapy.org/about/musictherapy/.

American Music Therapy Association. (2016b). *History of music therapy.* Retrieved from http://www.musictherapy.org/about/history/.

American Music Therapy Association. (2016c). *2016 AMTA member survey and workforce analysis.* Silver Spring, MD: AMTA.

American Music Therapy Association. (2016d). *Music therapy and rehabilitation: Selected references.* Retrieved from https://www.musictherapy.org/assets/1/7/NIHfactsheet_May2016.pdf.

American Music Therapy Association and Certification Board for Music Therapists. (2015). *Scope of music therapy practice.* Retrieved from https://www.musictherapy.org/about/scope_of_music_therapy_practice/.

American Music Therapy Association and National Standards Board for Therapeutic Musicians. (2015). *Therapeutic music services at-a-glance.* Retrieved from http://www.musictherapy.org/assets/1/7/TxMusicServicesAtAGlance_15.pdf.pdf.

Baird, B. N. (2014). *The internship, practicum, and field placement handbook: A guide for the helping professions* (7th ed.). Upper Saddle River, NJ: Pearson.

Burns, D., & Woolrich, J. (2008). The Bonny method of guided imagery and music. In A. A. Darrow (Ed.), *Introduction to approaches in music therapy* (2nd ed.) (pp. 49–59). Silver Spring, MD: American Music Therapy Association.

Certification Board for Music Therapists. (2011). *CBMT code of professional practice.* Retrieved from http://www.cbmt.org/about-certification/code-of-professional-practice/.

Certification Board for Music Therapists. (2015). *Board certification domains.* Retrieved from http://cbmt.org/.

Colwell, C., Edwards, R., Hernandez, E., & Brees, K. (2013). Impact of music therapy interventions (listening, composition, Orff-based) on the physiological and psychosocial behaviors of hospitalized children: A feasibility study. *Journal of Pediatric Nursing, 28,* 249–257. http://dx.doi.org/10.1016/j.pedn.2012.08.008.

Darrow, A. A. (2008). *Introduction to approaches in music therapy* (2nd ed.). Silver Spring, MD: AMTA.

Detmer, M. R. (2015). *Effect of Orff-based music interventions on state anxiety of music therapy students* (Master's thesis). Available from ProQuest Dissertations and Theses database (UMI No. 1583259).

Dileo, C., & Bradt, J. (2005). *Medical music therapy: A meta-analysis and agenda for future research.* Cherry Hill, NJ: Jeffrey Books.

Farnan, L. A. (2007). Music therapy and developmental disabilities: a glance back and a look forward. *Music Therapy Perspectives, 25,* 80–85. http://dx.doi.org/10.1093/mtp/25.2.80.

Hanser, S. B. (2000). *The new music therapist's handbook* (2nd ed.). Boston: Berklee Press.

Hilliard, R. E. (2007). The effects of Orff-based music therapy and social work groups on childhood grief symptoms and behaviors. *Journal of Music Therapy, 44,* 123–138. http://dx.doi.org/10.1093/jmt/44.2.123.

McKibbon, K. A. (1998). Evidence-based practice. *Bulletin of the Medical Library Association, 86,* 396–401.

Pavlicevic, M., & Ansdell, G. (2004). *Community music therapy.* London: Jessica Kingsley Publishers.

Register, D. M., & Hilliard, R. E. (2008). Using Orff-based techniques in children's bereavement groups: a cognitive-behavioral music therapy approach. *The Arts in Psychotherapy, 35,* 162–170. http://dx.doi.org/10.1016/j.aip.2007.10.001.

Schmid, W., & Ostermann, T. (2010). Home-based music therapy – A systematic overview of settings and conditions for an innovative service in healthcare. *BMC Health Services Research, 10,* 291–300. http://dx.doi.org/10.1186/1472-6963-10-291.

Segall, L. E. (2016). *The effect of a music therapy intervention on inmate levels of executive function and perceived stress.* (Unpublished doctoral dissertation). Tallahassee, FL: Florida State University.

Sena Moore, K. (2011, October 12). All you need to know about the designations behind a music therapist's name [Blog post]. Retrieved from http://www.musictherapymaven.com/acronyms-and-specialized-training-designations-for-the-professional-music-therapist/.

Tamplin, J., & Baker, F. (2006). *Music therapy methods in neurorehabilitation: A clinician's manual.* London: Jessica Kingsley Publishers.

Wong, E. (2004). *Clinical guide to music therapy in adult physical rehabilitation settings.* Silver Spring, MD: American Music Therapy Association.

FURTHER READING

Davis, W. B., Gfeller, K. E., & Thaut, M. H. (2008). *An introduction to music therapy theory and practice* (3rd ed.). Silver Spring, MD: American Music Therapy Association.

CHAPTER 2

Neurologic Foundations of Music-Based Interventions

KIMBERLY SENA MOORE, PHD, MT-BC

As an undergraduate student, I held a part-time job as a home health aide. One of my regular clients was "Johnny," a retired dentist and former 1930s big band leader who had Parkinson's disease. I assisted Johnny with food preparation and cleaning, kept him company, and helped in his mobility. Johnny lived in a long, 1950s-style ranch house. He began and ended his days in the bedroom located at one end of the house and spent the days in a TV room at the opposite end of the house. The route from one end of his home to the other involved Johnny walking from a carpeted surface to a smooth wood-floored foyer, then back to carpet. These flooring transitions were difficult for Johnny, who often "froze" and "got stuck" before moving from one surface to the next, a common challenge associated with Parkinson's disease. The visual change seemed to distract Johnny, and it was difficult for him to move smoothly from one floor type to the next. As the disease progressed and Johnny became weaker, he would freeze more often, whether or not the surface changed.

It was during this time that we discovered a trick. Once Johnny was positioned in the hallway at one end of the house, standing still with his hands on his walker, ready to begin the long trek down to the other end of the house, I would sing the introduction to the Sousa march *Stars and Stripes Forever*. A few beats into the introduction Johnny would start marching in place. The introduction is four measures long, followed by a pickup note to the first theme that begins on the downbeat of measure five. Once that first theme started, Johnny began his forward march. He continued marching in time as I sang him down the long hallway, and he would do so without stopping or freezing until he reached the other end of the house.

What I had unknowingly stumbled upon, with Johnny's help, was a strong link between music and the motor system. What I know now is that this connection is due to rhythmic entrainment, a phenomenon in which the human motor system synchronizes to a steady rhythmic pulse. However, this link is not the only one between music and human functioning—music also influences cognitive skills, emotional responses, social connections, serves as a communicative medium. These connections, are not learned; rather, they are biological phenomena that evolved and occur naturally. However, they can be leveraged in an intentional way, which is part of what music therapists do—we are trained to harness the influence of music on brain and behavior function in a purposeful way to effect therapeutic change. In this chapter, we explore some of these music, brain, and behavior connections. We will begin with an overview of music perception, review general principles that help explain how music influences brain functioning, and then explore neurologic foundations of music-based interventions that support and inform music therapy practice.

FROM ACOUSTIC TO ELECTRIC: MUSIC PERCEPTION

Hearing begins when acoustic sound waves enter the hearing apparatus and are transduced into an electric signal. The hearing apparatus has three parts: the outer ear, middle ear, and inner ear. The outer ear acts as a funnel; the pinna, or external part of our ear, captures the sound wave, which travels down the meatus (ear canal) to the tympanic membrane (ear drum). During this process, some of the sound wave is amplified and some attenuated, depending on the rate (frequency) and direction of the sound (Koelsch, 2013). The sound wave causes the tympanic membrane to vibrate. This membrane is connected to three small bones collectively referred to as the ossicles: the malleus (hammer, connected to the ear drum), incus (anvil), and stapes (stirrup, connected to the cochlea). When the tympanic membrane vibrates, it causes the ossicles to move, thus transmitting the vibrations from the air-filled outer ear to the fluid-filled inner ear, the cochlea.

The cochlea (Latin for "snail") is a fluid-filled structure in which the now mechanical vibrations

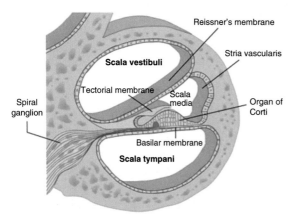

FIG. 2.1 Schematic of cross-section of the human cochlea

are transduced into electric signals. Much like its namesake, the cochlea is shaped like a coiled tube, with a bony outer shell filled with fluid and separated into three compartments (scala vestibuli, scala media, and scala tympani) by two membranes, the basilar membrane and Reissner membrane (see Fig. 2.1). Situated on the basilar membrane is the organ of Corti, which contains highly sensitive sensory receptors called "hair cells." Above the hair cells is the tectorial membrane. Outer hair cells help connect the organ of Corti to the tectorial membrane. As the ossicles vibrate, the stapes pushes against the oval window, a membrane into the cochlea. This mechanical energy changes the pressure of the fluid inside the cochlea, causing the basilar membrane to oscillate, an action that pushes the hair cells up against the tectorial membrane. The deflection of the hair cells causes them to depolarize (or hyperpolarize) and release glutamate, which stimulates the cochlear nerve, cranial nerve VIII.

The electric signal then travels via the cochlear nerve through various nuclei in the brainstem—the cochlear nucleus (CN), superior olivary complex (SOC), nuclei of the lateral lemniscus, and the inferior colliculus (IC)—before traveling through the medial geniculate body (MGB) in the thalamus to the primary auditory cortex for initial cortical processing. These subcortical nuclei conduct preliminary analyses of the auditory signal, and each seems responsible for examining a particular acoustic feature. For example, portions of the SOC are thought to be involved in discerning differences in intensity, or loudness levels (Hodges & Sebald, 2011). In addition, as the auditory signal travels through these subcortical pathways, it undergoes initial

processing responsible for certain subconscious behavioral responses:

- Motor-reticular response. Some auditory neurons project from the CN to the reticular formation, an area in the brainstem involved in generating reflexive motor responses. This connection partially explains how our motor system synchronizes to a steady rhythmic pulse (Koelsch, 2013). In other words, it enables us to dance and walk to the beat of a song and, because it occurs at the level of the brainstem, this synchronization occurs without learning or conscious awareness. This phenomenon of auditory-motor coupling is known as rhythmic entrainment.
- Visual-orienting response. Neurons in the IC project axons to the superior colliculus, an area in the brainstem involved in gaze control. When we hear a sudden sound, such as a loud crash coming from an intersection, we automatically turn our head and look in the direction from which the sound came. It is this connection between the inferior and superior colliculi that enables us to shift our eye gaze and the direction of our head toward an unexpected sound in a reflexive manner (Schnupp, Nelken, & King, 2011).
- Detection of danger. Neurons in the IC and MGB project to the amygdala, an area implicated in detecting emotional salience in the environment. This connection allows us to detect potential danger in our surroundings based on an auditory signal (Koelsch, 2013), such as when hearing a twig snap suddenly at night while camping alone in the woods.

For detailed descriptions of the hearing process and initial subcortical auditory processing, see Hodges and Sebald (2011), Koelsch (2013), and Schnupp et al. (2011).

CORTICAL PROCESSING OF MUSIC: GENERAL PRINCIPLES

The majority of the auditory signal travels via the MGB in the thalamus to the primary auditory cortex, an area located on the superior temporal gyrus in the temporal lobe. The primary auditory cortex is implicated in detecting and processing characteristics of the auditory signal. Specifically, the primary auditory cortex is involved with analyzing acoustic features of frequency, intensity, and timbre; storing auditory sensory memory; discriminating and organizing sounds and sound patterns (known as stream segregation); and transforming the acoustic features (e.g., frequency) into perceptual ones (e.g., pitch) (Koelsch, 2013). Surrounding the primary auditory cortex are belt areas that constitute auditory association areas, where the auditory signal undergoes further cortical processing. These primary and secondary auditory processing areas interact with multiple areas throughout the brain. However, before exploring these interactions and their corresponding behavioral responses, let us explore general principles associated with cortical processing.

Connectivity Between Neural Networks

Neural processing does not happen through the activation of isolated structures or areas in the brain. Rather, what underlies human behavior is the connectivity between neural networks. Neural networks are like "committees" of structures and areas in the brain responsible for a certain behavior or task. The concept of connectivity can be thought of as the communication between these committees. Connectivity is conceptualized and explored in different ways in the brain imaging field. For example, functional connectivity utilizes statistical measures such as correlations to investigate shared timing of neural activity in separate areas in the brain (Friston, 2011; Koelsch, 2013). Another branch explores effective connectivity, which describes the causal influence one neural structure or area has over another. Effective connectivity corresponds to the idea of coupling between networks (Friston, 2011; Stephan & Friston, 2010). In theory, the stronger the connectivity between two networks, the closer the relationship between the tasks for which those networks are responsible. For example, music is not processed solely in the primary auditory cortex; rather, the signal is distributed to a diverse set of neural networks, including, but not limited to, areas implicated in motor behaviors, emotional responses, and cognition (see "Overview of Musically Induced Neural Responses" section). In this way, the natural influence of music on nonmusical behaviors emerges in part from its connectivity— or close linkage—with a multitude of neural networks across both hemispheres.

Neurochemical Mechanisms

One emerging area of study focuses on the neurochemical mechanisms underlying music processing; that is, the shared chemical and hormonal changes that occur when engaged in music and influence nonmusical behaviors. The production and release of neurochemicals help mediate, at least in part, the connectivity between neural networks. In others words, they are partially responsible for how different neural areas and networks communicate and influence each other. Regarding the influence of music on human brain functioning, researchers have explored in particular the areas of reward, motivation, and pleasure; stress and arousal; and social affiliation (Chanda & Levitin, 2013; Huron, 2003), which correspond with, respectively, dopamine, cortisol, and oxytocin.

Dopamine is implicated in reward, motivation, and pleasure, as well as working memory and reinforcement learning (Stegemöller, 2014). There is evidence that listening to "happy" music or music deemed pleasurable activates neural areas associated with the release of dopamine (Blood & Zatorre, 2001; Menon & Levitin, 2005; Mitterschiffthaler, Fu, Dalton, Andrew, & Williams, 2007; Salimpoor, Benovoy, Larcher, Dagher, & Zatorre, 2011). Furthermore, a genetic marker has been identified that may help explain the variability in our responses to music on emotions (Quarto et al., 2017). These results indicate that music may not only lead to feelings of pleasure, but also assist in motivating human behavior and have a role in learning and memory through its connection with dopamine. Cortisol is associated with, among other things, activation of the hypothalamo-pituitary-adrenal axis, the neural network underlying the body's stress response. Sometimes referred to as the "stress hormone," cortisol serves to regulate and mediate our biological response to a real or perceived threat. There is evidence that music influences cortisol levels, although in different ways based on the type of music and the type of situation. For example, music listening and singing have been shown to reduce cortisol levels in individuals undergoing elective orthopedic surgery (Koelsch et al., 2011) or who are under psychological stress (Khalfa, Dalla Bella, Roy, Peretz, & Lupien, 2003), as well as in patients with cancer and their caregivers (Fancourt, Williamon, Carvalho, & Steptoe, 2016). In contrast, music paired with video game playing led to an increase in cortisol levels (Hébert, Béland, Dionne-Fournelle, Crête, & Lupien, 2005). Thus, although music may not always automatically decrease cortisol levels—and by extension reduce feelings of stress—it may serve an arousal- and stress-modulating function through its ability to influence cortisol levels. Finally, oxytocin is a neurohormone that, although typically associated with maternal behaviors, may hold a broader function in regulating social behavior. Although research is not extensive, there is preliminary evidence that singing may lead to oxytocin release (Grape, Sandgren, Hansson, Ericson, & Theorell, 2003), which suggests a connection between music and social behavior.

Neuroplasticity: Learning, Changing, and Training

A core concept underlying any learning, training, or rehabilitative effort is neuroplasticity. This term describes the brain's ability to change based on experience. In other words, the human brain continues to reorganize itself throughout the lifetime based on our environment, behaviors, thoughts, and emotions. Plasticity can occur at the neuronal level, where synaptic connections between two neurons are weakened, created, or strengthened, and it can occur at a more structural level, where connections between entire neural networks are weakened, created, or strengthened. Weakening occurs through synaptic pruning, a process by which the brain sheds connections that are old or weak because of lack of use. New synaptic connections can also be created between neurons and networks. Once created, these connections can be strengthened by continued use through the process of myelination. In this way, the brain is a dynamic organ as neural networks and their connectivity continue to be shaped, mapped, and remapped based on one's experiences.

Music engagement is an experience that helps promote neuroplasticity in the context of learning (e.g., education) and relearning (e.g., therapy). Although this assertion was originally supported through correlational studies, such as studies noting a relationship between music training and improved test scores, research exploring structural neural changes associated with regular music engagement is emerging. On the learning side, Kraus et al. (2014) reported that at-risk children involved in a community music education program demonstrated improved neural encoding of speech after a year of music training. In a more therapeutic context, Särkämo et al. (2014) reported structural neural changes in patients with stroke following 6 months of daily music listening. Given the ability for music engagement to shape the brain, Stegemöller (2014) presented a neuroplasticity model of music therapy. She proposed that music can boost neuroplasticity in one of three ways: by (1) increasing dopamine levels; (2) synchronizing neural firing patterns, which serves to create and strengthen connections between neurons; and (3) providing a clear signal that is easy for the human brain to process, because music is an acoustically organized and structured stimulus.

OVERVIEW OF MUSICALLY INDUCED NEURAL RESPONSES

Once the acoustic music signal is transduced into an electric impulse and begins its journey to the primary auditory cortex, it starts to engage a diffuse web of neural networks cortically and subcortically across both hemispheres. Through its connectivity with these networks, music not only is able to engage the brain, but also has the potential to change the brain. In this way—in its ability to promote neuroplasticity—music can serve as a way to produce functional therapeutic outcomes. Trained music therapists are expert at developing and facilitating music experiences designed to target therapeutic needs across the following treatment domains: motor, cognition, communication, emotion, and social. Thus, our exploration of the neurologic foundations of music-based interventions will be organized by treatment domain. As we identify neural mechanisms underlying the connection between music and these areas of functioning, a list of the structures and areas, their location, and their functions can be found in Table 2.1.

Motor Responses

Arguably one of the more systematically studied and well-understood connections is that between music and motor responses. As experienced with Johnny, the human motor system has the ability to synchronize to a rhythmic beat, even without conscious awareness or control. This coupling between the auditory and motor systems begins subcortically with the motor-reticular response (Koelsch, 2013), but it also involves other subcortical (cerebellum and basal ganglia) and cortical (supplementary motor area [SMA] and premotor cortex) motor regions of the brain. All four neural areas are implicated in some way in various rhythmic tasks (Grahn & Watson, 2013).

Subcortical areas

The cerebellum is a two-hemisphere, subcortical structure that sits at the base of the brain. Cerebellum is Latin for "little brain," and it is implicated in coordinating and regulating motor output. Regarding auditory-motor synchronization, the cerebellum appears to be important for absolute, or duration-based, timing tasks. These occur when one is explicitly measuring the time span of rhythmic intervals, as when comparing two interval lengths (Grahn & Watson, 2013). Furthermore, owing to the connections of the cerebellum with various cortical areas, its activation appears to also be associated with mediating conscious auditory-motor synchronization, modulating motor movements based on rhythmic changes (Thaut et al., 2009), and coordinating precisely timed movements (Chen, Penhune, & Zatorre, 2008).

The basal ganglia describes a subcortical cluster of nuclei with input and output connections to several

TABLE 2.1
Identification of Neural Areas and Their Location and Functions

Neural Area	Location	Functions
Amygdala	Subcortical (base of the temporal lobe)	Detects and assesses emotional salience
Anterior cingulate cortex	Frontal part of the cingulate cortex, which sits below the cortex and above the corpus callosum	Regulates attention, emotion, reward anticipation, decision making, and autonomic functions
Anterior frontomedian cortex	Cortical (frontal lobe)	Makes evaluative judgments, self-initiates cognitive processes[a]
Basal ganglia	Subcortical (large group of nuclei, include the striatum)	Mediate several aspects of voluntary motor movements, and involved in procedural learning and emotions
Broca's area	Cortical (frontal lobe, left hemisphere)	Responsible for expressive speech production
Cerebellum	Base of cortex	Coordinates and regulates motor movement and motor learning
Cochlear nerve (cranial nerve VIII)	Connects cochlea to the brainstem	Transmits auditory signal from the hearing mechanism to the central nervous system
Dorsolateral PFC	Cortical (upper side of the PFC)	Implicated in working memory, executive functions, motor planning, and social cognition
Heschl's gyrus	Cortical (temporal lobe)	Initial processing of incoming auditory information
Hippocampus	Subcortical	Involved in memory, particularly long-term memory
Hypothalamus	Subcortical	Produces hormones that govern homeostasis and coordinate the autonomic nervous system
Insula	Underneath temporal lobe	Integrates multiple systems involved in emotion, motor, and cognitive processing[b]
Nucleus accumbens	Subcortical (part of ventral striatum)	Involved in reward and motivation by mediating dopamine release
Orbitofrontal cortex	Cortical (on the medial underside of the PFC)	Implicated in emotion regulation, decision making, and sensory integration
Parietal lobe	Cortical	Involved in perception and integration of sensory stimuli
Parahippocampal gyrus	Surrounds the hippocampus	Involved in visuospatial processing, episodic memory, and processing contextual associations[c]
Prefrontal cortex (PFC)	Cortical (frontal lobe)	Linked to planning complex cognitive behaviors, personality expression, decision making, and mediating social behavior
Premotor cortex	Cortical (frontal lobe)	Motor planning of precise motor tasks and movement initiation
Primary motor cortex	Cortical (frontal lobe)	Generates voluntary motor movement instructions
Reticular formation	Brainstem (group of nuclei)	Implicated in awareness, consciousness, and reflexive motor responses
Rolandic operculum	Cortical (frontal lobe)	Represents motor movements of the lips, tongue, and pharynx muscles[d]
Substantia nigra	Brainstem/basal ganglia	Produces dopamine and plays a role in reward and motor movement
Supplementary motor area	Cortical (frontal lobe)	Motor planning and movement initiation

Continued

TABLE 2.1		
Identification of Neural Areas and Their Location and Functions—cont'd		
Neural Area	**Location**	**Functions**
Temporal poles	Cortical (front end of the temporal lobe)	Integrates complex perceptual information (auditory, olfactory, and visual) with emotions[e]
Ventral striatum	Basal ganglia	Mediates reward, reinforcement, and motivation
Ventral tegmental area	Brainstem (part of the reticular formation)	Involved in reward and motivation by producing dopamine
Ventromedial PFC	Cortical (on the medial underside of the PFC)	Implicated in emotion regulation, empathy, and social decision making

[a]Zysset, Huber, Ferstl, and von Cramon (2002).
[b]Chang, Yarkoni, Win Khaw, and Sanfey (2013).
[c]Aminoff, Kveraga, and Bar (2013).
[d]Brown, Ngan, and Liotti (2008).
[e]Olson, Plotzker, and Ezzyat (2007).

cortical and subcortical areas. These include the cortical motor response areas (SMA and premotor cortex), as well as the substantia nigra, an area in the brainstem that plays an important role in motor planning and, as it makes dopamine, in reward and motivation. Although the exact functions of the basal ganglia vary, it seems to play some role in regulating the intensity of motor movements, learning complex movement patterns, and initiating movements. The cerebellum is implicated in absolute timing, whereas the basal ganglia seems important for relative, or beat-based, timing, which occurs when we perceive the timing of rhythmic intervals based on an existing beat (Grahn & Watson, 2013).

Cortical areas

The SMA and premotor cortex are located in the frontal lobe and implicated in the planning and initiation of voluntary motor movements. In connection with the basal ganglia, the SMA and premotor cortex are activated during beat-based timing, as well as during beat perception (Grahn & Watson, 2013). Furthermore, research indicates that increased coupling between the auditory areas and premotor cortex exist during rhythm processing, particularly of complex rhythmic patterns (Chen et al., 2008; Grahn & Watson, 2013). These findings provide evidence as to the neurologic mechanisms underlying rhythmic entrainment and illustrate how we are able to synchronize our motor movements to a rhythmic pulse.

Cognitive Responses

I worked for several years in a medical facility, providing primarily bedside music therapy services to patients and their families (when present) in the oncology,

surgical, general medical, and transitional care units. Although most of the patients were adults, there was one unit on which pediatric patients would be placed. I once received a referral to work with a 4-year-old girl. I entered the room and found her sitting in bed being kept company by her grandmother. Also present were the young patient's 7-month-old twin sisters, who were playing with toys and interacting with each other on a second bed in the room. I directed my attention to the 4-year-old patient, and within a couple of minutes, I began singing. The most memorable moment of this particular session was what transpired next—the reactions of the 7-month-old twins. They immediately stopped their play and stared at me, enthralled and engaged throughout the 4 to 5 min I was singing to their sister. Then, once the song was over, their attention toward me ended, and they resumed their play. This interaction highlights the ability of music to grab and hold our attention, which is one type of cognitive response influenced by music.

Attention

Attention involves the ability to orient and focus on a stimulus or task, sustain that focus, and selectively control and switch the focus (Thaut & Gardiner, 2014). Music has the ability not only to reflexively grab our attention—visual-orienting response (Koelsch, 2013)—but, as a temporal stimulus, also to hold our attention over time. The initial orienting and focusing response involves areas in the parietal and frontal lobes, whereas the ability to control and switch our focus of attention involves various subcortical and cortical areas: the anterior cingulate cortex, the anterior insula, prefrontal areas in the frontal lobe, and the striatum, a part of the basal ganglia (Posner, Rothbart, Sheese, & Voelker, 2014). These same cortical and subcortical areas are also implicated in various music perception and production tasks. For example:

- Music listening activates the insula, striatum, cingulate cortex, and prefrontal cortex (PFC) (Blood & Zatorre, 2001; Fujisawa & Cook, 2011; Green, Bærentsen, Stødkilde-Jørgensen, Roepstorff, & Vuust, 2012; Koelsch, Fritz, Cramon, Müller, & Friederici, 2006; Limb, 2006);
- Music production (e.g., singing) activates the cingulate cortex, basal ganglia, and insula (Callan et al., 2006; Kleber, Bribaumer, Veit, Trevorrow, & Lotze, 2007); and
- Music improvisation influences activity in the cingulate cortex, PFC, and parietal and frontal lobes (Bengtsson, Csíkszentmihályi, & Ullén, 2007; Berkowitz & Ansari, 2008; Limb & Braun, 2008).

Thus, it seems that engaging in music, through listening, playing, or improvising, recruits similar neural areas and structures implicated in focusing, controlling, and shifting attention. There may also be a motivational mechanism involved. Not only is music a temporal stimulus, but it is also an emotionally salient one, which may serve to encourage us to maintain our attention on music and music tasks (Thaut & Gardiner, 2014).

Learning and memory

Learning involves the acquisition of knowledge or skills through experience, through study, or by being taught. Memory describes the capacity by which the mind stores and remembers knowledge or skills. Implicit, or procedural, memories generally involve the learning of an automatic or subconscious cognitive or motor skill, or of a conditioned response. These memories are mediated by the hippocampus, a subcortical neural structure, and the cerebellum. Both of these structures are also activated by music (Blood & Zatorre, 2001; Chen et al., 2008; Grahn & Watson, 2013; Thaut et al., 2009). Explicit, or declarative, memories involve the learning of conscious, verbal, and mental imagery information. These can include general knowledge of the world (semantic memory) and autobiographic information (episodic memory). Episodic memory is mediated by the hippocampus and PFC, areas also activated and modulated by music (Blood & Zatorre, 2001; Ford, Addis, & Giovanello, 2011; Janata, 2009; Nakamura et al., 1999; Särkämö, Altenmüller, Rodriguez-Fornells, & Peretz, 2016). Thus, as with attention, research indicates that music processing recruits neural areas implicated in learning and memory retrieval. Furthermore,

music is an organized stimulus that can be structured to chunk information, a quality that makes it easier to learn and remember information. For example, the melody in the familiar "Alphabet Song" takes the 26 letters of the American alphabet and groups them into four singable chunks (group 1: *A-B-C-D-E-F-G*, group 2: *H-I-J-K-L-M-N-O-P*, group 3: *Q-R-S-T-U-V*, group 4: *W-X-Y-Z*). This combination of the organizational structure of music and its ability to maintain our attention and motivate us may help facilitate the learning and memory process (Gardiner & Thaut, 2014a).

Executive functioning

Executive functioning (EF) is defined as the management of cognitive processes. It involves the ability to formulate goals, anticipate consequences, initiate behavior, plan and organize behavior, and monitor or adapt behavior to fit a particular task or context. Skills that underlie successful EF abilities include problem-solving, decision making, planning, goal setting, behavior regulation, attention regulation, organizing, and reasoning. These skills involve cognitive and emotional components, and there are distinct neural mechanisms underlying both types. Cognitive EF is associated with activation in the dorsolateral PFC and anterior cingulate, whereas emotional EF with activation in the ventromedial PFC (Robinson, Calamia, Gläscher, Bruss, & Tranel, 2014). Evidence exists that music training results in greater activation in the right ventromedial PFC (Zuk, Benjamin, Kenyon, & Gabb, 2014). In addition, mere exposure to music activates the dorsolateral PFC (Green et al., 2012), and, as mentioned when discussing music and attention, music listening and improvisation influence activity in the cingulate and prefrontal regions (Bengtsson et al., 2007; Berkowitz & Ansari, 2008; Blood & Zatorre, 2001; Fujisawa & Cook, 2011; Green et al., 2012; Limb, 2006; Limb & Braun, 2008). In these ways, it seems that music recruits similar cingulate and prefrontal areas implicated in both cognitive and emotional EF skills. In addition, the task of improvising and composing music requires similar skills used during EF, in particular decision making, planning, goal setting, organizing, and regulating behavior and attention (Gardiner & Thaut, 2014b). It follows, then, that improvisational and compositional experiences may help strengthen EF skills and abilities.

Communicative Responses

Early in my career, I worked as a backup music therapist on an inpatient rehabilitation unit. Patients on this unit typically had a stroke or traumatic brain injury, were placed here once medically stable, and after several days were discharged to a long-term rehabilitation center. The patient's daily schedule included several hours of therapy each morning and afternoon—physical therapy, occupational therapy, speech therapy, and music therapy. In addition to addressing motor-based rehabilitation goals, music therapy was also referred for clients with speech-related goals. Sessions with these clients incorporated lots of singing and followed a fairly typically structure. I begin with a highly familiar song such as *You Are My Sunshine* and, while singing, would drop the last word in each line (e.g., "You are my _____"). Even with no instructions, this omission would prompt clients to sing the missing word (e.g., "sunshine"), after which I would move on to the next line and repeat the process. This opening exercise functioned as a way to initiate speech production as cued by the musical pauses. Next, I would work with clients on speech-related exercises developed following a consultation with the speech-language pathologist. Depending on the client's specific goals, these exercises may have involved practicing articulation patterns, increasing respiratory strength and endurance, or rehearsing functional sentences (e.g., "I'm hungry") by singing them. Sessions ended by singing a song familiar to the client and encouraging him or her to sing throughout, an exercise designed to build the client's endurance. These examples illustrate the close connection between music, particularly singing, and speech production, a communication skill.

Communication is a broad construct that involves the meaningful conveyance of information, ideas, or feelings through verbal or nonverbal means. Although joint music making, in particular music improvisation, can be used as a way to stimulate and train nonverbal communicative behaviors (Thaut, 2014), most of the neuroscience research has focused on the similarities and differences between music processing and speech and language processing.

Music production (singing) and speech production (speaking) involve shared neural mechanisms, with distinct variations in activation patterns. Research indicates that singing and speaking activate nearly identical cortical and subcortical areas in the brain—the primary motor cortex, SMA, Broca area, anterior insula, primary and secondary auditory cortices, temporal pole, basal ganglia, ventral thalamus, and posterior cerebellum (Brown, Martinez, & Parsons, 2006; Callan et al., 2006; Jeffries, Fritz, & Braun, 2003). Interestingly, however, there seem to be lateralization differences between the two; namely, that speaking favors the left hemisphere, whereas singing favors the right (Brown et al., 2006;

Callan et al., 2006). However, from a rehabilitative perspective this difference in activation patterns gives music a unique advantage. Should a person's speech processing areas be damaged (e.g., because of a stroke), there is the potential that a singing-based intervention can help rewire the brain for functional speech (Thaut, Thaut, & McIntosh, 2014), which helps explain why those on the inpatient rehabilitation unit benefited from music therapy services.

Emotional Responses

One common response I receive from people who learn I am a music therapist is, "So, you use music to help people feel better?" In my experience, most people have felt the pull of music on their emotions. We use it to self-regulate our emotions by, for instance, listening to music that makes us feel sad to experience that feeling of sadness. We also find our emotional states changed during music experiences. For example, we may find ourselves experiencing chills while listening to a particularly moving song. Given these experiences, people who first hear the term "music therapy" commonly assume that my job involves improving people's quality of life by changing their emotional states. Although this characterization does not encompass the extent of what a music therapist can provide, it is accurate to state that music influences our emotions. Furthermore, this particular phenomenon is of long-lasting and growing interest among researchers (Juslin & Sloboda, 2010).

Emotion processing is a complex phenomenon, involving multiple components that are mediated by a diverse network of cortical and subcortical areas. Some are implicated in reward and motivation, in particular the nucleus accumbens in the ventral striatum and ventral tegmental area in the midbrain (Blood & Zatorre, 2001; Menon & Levitin, 2005), both associated with the production and release of dopamine (Blood & Zatorre, 2001; Menon & Levitin, 2005; Mitterschiffthaler et al., 2007; Salimpoor et al., 2011). Other neural areas help mediate emotion regulation processes. These include the amygdala, implicated in assessing emotional salience, and cognitive control and monitoring areas such as the anterior cingulate cortex, orbitofrontal cortex, and lateral PFC (Gyurak, Gross, & Etkin, 2011; McRae et al., 2010; Ochsner & Gross, 2005; Rempel-Clower, 2007). Finally, the amygdala, hypothalamus, insula, orbitofrontal cortex, and ventromedial PFC are activated during emotion-based physiologic arousal (Blood & Zatorre, 2001; Menon & Levitin, 2005). Although evidence exists that listening to music influences activity in all these neural areas associated with emotions, arousal, reward and motivation, and emotion regulation (Blood & Zatorre, 2001; Menon & Levitin, 2005; Mitterschiffthaler et al., 2007; Salimpoor et al., 2011; Sena Moore, 2013), researchers are also exploring differences in activation patterns based on the type of music and on the emotional states it induces.

Listening to music deemed unpleasant is associated with increased activation in the amygdala, hippocampus, parahippocampal gyrus, and temporal poles, all areas that are implicated in processing negative emotions. In contrast, music deemed pleasant shows increased activation in the insula, ventral striatum, Heschl gyrus, and Rolandic operculum, areas implicated in reward and motor-related responses to music (Koelsch et al., 2006). There also seem to be hemispheric differences in processing pleasant and unpleasant music. For example, neural activity increases in the left hemisphere when listening to music deemed pleasant and in the right hemisphere when the music is deemed unpleasant. Researchers have attributed this difference to the role of the right hemisphere in processing novel situations and the left hemisphere in processing predictable ones (Flores-Gutiérrez et al., 2007). Such results lend neural-based support for using music as a way to increase motivation, modulate emotions, and influence arousal levels.

As a final consideration, it is common practice in the music therapy profession to incorporate client-preferred music in clinical work. The thought process underlying this practice is that using client-preferred music may increase a client's motivation to be involved in the therapeutic experience. However, according to neuroscience this convention may not be necessary, as research indicates that unfamiliar music deemed pleasant also activates similar neural networks implicated in emotion and reward processing (Brown, Martinez, & Parsons, 2004). This finding suggests that familiar, client-preferred music is not always necessary, as long as the client deems the music enjoyable.

Social Responses

One simple yet surprisingly effective music experience I have used to begin a group session is the musical check-in. A "check-in" is a brief process during which clients identify and share their current emotional and/or cognitive state, and music therapists commonly incorporate instrument playing as the way in which clients express this state. Musical check-ins work with both children and adults and they function in part as a way to transition clients emotionally and mentally to the group session. There are several variations to the

musical check-in, and one of my favorites incorporates the shekere, a West African instrument made by taking a dried hollow gourd and covering it with a netting of beads. The shekere can be shaken like a rattle, the bottom can be pounded like a drum, and the netting can be smoothed over the gourd like a cabasa. Through this variety in playing styles the shekere can create sounds ranging from a quiet "shh"-ing to a deep, pounding rattle. I begin the musical check-in by introducing the group to the shekere and demonstrating the different sounds it can create. We then pass the shekere around to each group member, who are directed to play how they feel in that moment, no right or wrong. The group then guesses that client's emotion based on how he or she played the shekere. Once the correct emotion has been identified, the client passes the instrument to the next group member and the process begins again. Although this musical check-in serves as a way for clients to identify and express their current emotional state, it also promotes identification of emotions in others (a precursor to feeling empathy) and provides a way for clients to interact with each other, both of which constitute social behaviors.

Humans are inherently social creatures—we crave connections and interactions. This need is evident in infancy through the interactions between parents and children, and it continues through end-of-life situations, when individuals often wish to have family and loved ones nearby. We engage in group-oriented experiences, such as participating in spiritual services, watching sports games, and eating family meals. Furthermore, in addition to our ability to be adaptable thinkers and problem-solvers, being part of a cohesive social unit was necessary for human survival (Hodges & Sebald, 2011). Music, in particular music making, evolved as a social activity (Koelsch, 2013), and some suggest its survival benefits are based in part on promoting parent-infant bonding and facilitating social organization (Hodges & Sebald, 2011). To date, much of the research exploring the intersection between music and social behaviors has emerged from behavioral and anthropologic perspectives. However, through a neurologic lens, this intersection can be examined first through understanding the neural correlates of certain social behaviors (e.g., empathy), followed by exploring any shared neural activity between music and social behaviors.

Empathy describes the capacity to be aware of and understand another person's feelings and emotions. Although the ability to empathize is commonly thought of as a skill under the emotion domain, it has social implications in that it augments helping behaviors and can be considered a precursor to social behaviors. One structure implicated in empathy is the medial PFC (Rameson, Morelli, & Lieberman, 2012), an area also activated when listening to music deemed pleasant (Blood & Zatorre, 2001; Menon & Levitin, 2005). Another skill in this domain is social cognition, which describes the mental processes underlying social interactions. More specifically, it refers to our capacity to predict other people's intentions, motivations, and actions and how this ability influences social practices. Neural areas implicated in social cognition include the anterior frontomedian cortex, temporal poles, and superior temporal sulcus (Koelsch, 2015), some of which are also activated during music listening (temporal poles; Koelsch et al., 2006) and music improvisation (superior temporal sulcus; Limb & Braun, 2008). Finally, from a neurochemical perspective, one neurohormone implicated in social behavior and trust is oxytocin (Roth & Keeler, 2016). Evidence exists that singing and group vocal improvisation may lead to oxytocin release (Grape et al., 2003; Roth & Keeler, 2016). Together, these types of results provide preliminary evidence to support the overlap between music and social behavior processing in the brain.

IMPLICATIONS FOR MUSIC THERAPY CLINICAL PRACTICE

As this brief review demonstrates, current neuroscience research provides evidence that engaging in music experiences activates neural networks and mechanisms implicated in various nonmusical skills and behaviors, including motor movement, attention, learning and memory, EF, verbal communication, emotion regulation, emotion processing, empathy, and prosocial behaviors. These results provide a preliminary rationale to support the use of music as a therapeutic option. Furthermore, through the phenomenon of neuroplasticity, regular engagement in music experiences has the potential to promote structural changes in the neural networks underlying these skills, which would be evidenced behaviorally as changes in functional nonmusical abilities. Arguably, this type of behavioral change would be more potent if the music experiences were intentionally designed and facilitated to target specific functional therapeutic outcomes, all skills that fall under the education, clinical training, and scope of professional music therapists.

Research on music and the brain also provides emerging recommendations for how to structure a music experience to meet a certain need, providing an additional neurologically based rationale to support the use of music in therapy. For example, given the coupling that occurs between the auditory and motor systems (Chen et al., 2008; Grahn & Watson, 2013; Koelsch, 2013; Thaut et al., 2009), music designed to target a motor-based therapeutic goal should have a clear steady beat, one that can be used to cue and pace the motor movement. There is also support for music's ability to activate neural mechanisms implicated in reward and motivation (Blood & Zatorre, 2001; Menon & Levitin, 2005; Mitterschiffthaler et al., 2007; Salimpoor et al., 2011). Although at first glance this connection may seem to promote the notion that music deemed enjoyable helps us "feel better," for the clinician it also provides support for the idea that the music experiences we facilitate must be aesthetically pleasing. This practice will serve to help motivate clients to engage in the therapy, and it also speaks to the need for professional music therapists to be skilled musicians.

Interest in understanding the neurologic mechanisms of music processing is strong in the music therapy and neuroscience fields, and the body of research keeps growing. However, it should be noted that there are limitations to using neuroscience as the only way to explain music therapy. For example, there are certain methodological characteristics of neuroscience research that do not accurately reflect clinical music therapy practice (O'Kelly, 2016). These include the lack of diversity in music experiences (most research paradigms are limited to using music listening, and some incorporate music improvisation) and the physical constraints involved during the brain imaging process (i.e., laying down and staying still). Neither characteristic mirrors what occurs in music therapy treatment, which often involves multiple types of music experiences (e.g., listening, singing, instrument playing, composition, moving to music, improvisation) and which emphasizes interacting and relating through shared music experiences—interactions that would not be possible without physical movement (e.g., through singing or playing instruments together). Nevertheless, there are benefits to both the music therapy and neuroscience fields in understanding the neurologic foundations of music processing.

Given that music activates a diverse network of subcortical and cortical structures, it is a prime stimulus to use when exploring brain functions across motor, cognitive, communicative, emotional, and social behaviors. This realization is one reason why music was included even in early neuroscience research (Thaut & McIntosh, 2010). In addition, clinical music therapists can apply findings from the neuroscience field not only to support the use of music as a medium in therapy treatment, but also to inform the development of functional therapeutic music experiences. Ultimately, this type of relationship between the music therapy and neuroscience professions is advantageous to clients who receive music therapy services, as well as to those who, like Johnny, look to incorporate music-based ways to help them function during the day.

REFERENCES

Aminoff, E. M., Kveraga, K., & Bar, M. (2013). The role of the parahippocampal cortex in cognition. *Trends in Cognitive Science*, 17(8), 379–390. http://dx.doi.org/10.1016/j.tics.2013.06.009.

Bengtsson, S. L., Csíkszentmihályi, M., & Ullén, F. (2007). Cortical regions involved in the generation of musical structures during improvisation in pianists. *Journal of Cognitive Neuroscience*, 19(5), 830–842.

Berkowitz, A. L., & Ansari, D. (2008). Generation of novel motor sequences: the neural correlates of musical improvisation. *NeuroImage*, 41, 535–543. http://dx.doi.org/10.1016/j.neuroimage.2008.02.028.

Blood, A. J., & Zatorre, R. J. (2001). Intensely pleasurable responses to music correlate with activity in brain regions implicated in reward and emotion. *Proceedings of the National Academy of Sciences*, 98, 11818–11823.

Brown, S., Martinez, M. J., & Parsons, L. M. (2004). Passive music listening spontaneously engages limbic and paralimbic systems. *NeuroReport*, 15(13), 2033–2037.

Brown, S., Martinez, M. J., & Parsons, L. M. (2006). Music and language side by side in the brain: a PET study of the generation of melodies and sentences. *European Journal of Neuroscience*, 23, 2791–2803.

Brown, S., Ngan, E., & Liotti, M. (2008). A larynx area in the human motor cortex. *Cerebral Cortex*, 18, 837–845. http://dx.doi.org/10.1093/cercor/bhm131.

Callan, D. E., Tsytsarev, V., Hanakawa, T., Callan, A. M., Katsuhara, M., Fukuyama, H., et al. (2006). Song and speech: brain regions involved with perception and covert production. *NeuroImage*, 31, 1327–1342. http://dx.doi.org/10.1016/j.neuroimage.2006.01.036.

Chanda, M. L., & Levitin, D. J. (2013). The neurochemistry of music. *Trends in Cognitive Sciences*, 17(4), 179–193. http://dx.doi.org/10.1016/j.tics.2013.02.007.

Chang, L. J., Yarkoni, T., Win Khaw, M., & Sanfey, A. G. (2013). Decoding the role of the insula in human cognition: functional percolation and large-scale reverse inference. *Cerebral Cortex*, 23, 739–749. http://dx.doi.org/10.1093/cercor/bhs065.

Chen, J. L., Penhune, V. B., & Zatorre, R. J. (2008). Moving on time: brain network for auditory-motor synchronization is modulated by rhythm complexity and musical training. *Journal of Cognitive Neuroscience*, 20(2), 226–239.

Fancourt, D., Williamon, A., Carvalho, L. A., & Steptoe, A. (2016). Singing is associated with modulations in cortisol, cytokine, beta-endorphin and oxytocin activity in cancer patients and carers. *Abstracts/Brain, Behavior, and Immunity*, 57, e1–e43. http://dx.doi.org/10.1016/j.bbi.2016.07.014.

Flores-Gutiérrez, E. O., Díaz, J., Barrios, F. A., Favila-Humara, R., Guevara, M. Á., del Río-Portilla, Y., et al. (2007). Metabolic and electric brain patterns during pleasant and unpleasant emotions induced by music masterpieces. *International Journal of Psychophysiology*, 65, 69–84. http://dx.doi.org/10.1016/j.ijpsycho.2007.03.004.

Ford, J. H., Addis, D. A., & Giovanello, K. S. (2011). Differential neural activity during search of specific and general autobiographical memories elicited by musical cues. *Neuropsychologia*, 49, 2514–2526. http://dx.doi.org/10.1016/j.neuropsychologia.2011.04.032.

Friston, K. J. (2011). Functional and effective connectivity: A review. *Brain Connectivity*, 1(1), 13–36. http://dx.doi.org/10.1089/brain.2011.0008.

Fujisawa, T. X., & Cook, N. D. (2011). The perception of harmonic triads: an fMRI study. *Brain Imaging and Behavior*, 5, 109–125. http://dx.doi.org/10.1007/s11682-011-9116-5.

Gardiner, J. C., & Thaut, M. H. (2014a). Musical mnemonics training (MMT). In M. H. Thaut, & V. Hoemberg (Eds.), *Handbook of neurologic music therapy* (pp. 294–310). Oxford: Oxford University Press.

Gardiner, J. C., & Thaut, M. H. (2014b). Musical executive function training (MEFT). In M. H. Thaut, & V. Hoemberg (Eds.), *Handbook of neurologic music therapy* (pp. 279–293). Oxford: Oxford University Press.

Grahn, J. A., & Watson, S. L. (2013). Perspectives on rhythm processing in motor regions of the brain. *Music Therapy Perspectives*, 31, 25–30. http://dx.doi.org/10.1093/mtp/31.1.25.

Grape, C., Sandgren, M., Hansson, L., Ericson, M., & Theorell, T. (2003). Does singing promote well-being? An empirical study of professional and amateur singer during a singing lesson. *Integrative Physiological & Behavioral Science*, 38(1), 65–74. http://dx.doi.org/10.1007/BF02734261.

Green, A. C., Bærentsen, K. B., Stødkilde-Jørgensen, H., Roepstorff, A., & Vuust, P. (2012). Listen, learn, like! Dorsolateral prefrontal cortex involved in the mere exposure effective in music. *Neurology Research International*, 2012, 846270. http://dx.doi.org/10.1155/2012/846270.

Gyurak, A., Gross, J. J., & Etkin, A. (2011). Explicit and implicit emotion regulation: a dual-process framework. *Cognition & Emotion*, 25, 400–412. http://dx.doi.org/10.1080/02699931.2010.544160.

Hébert, S., Béland, R., Dionne-Fournelle, O., Crête, M., & Lupien, S. J. (2005). Physiological stress response to video-game playing: the contribution of built-in music. *Life Sciences*, 76, 2371–2380. http://dx.doi.org/10.1016/j.lfs.2004.11.011.

Hodges, D. A., & Sebald, D. C. (2011). *Music in the human experience: An introduction to music psychology*. New York, NY: Routledge.

Huron, D. (2003). Is music an evolutionary adaptation? In I. Peretz, & R. Zatorre (Eds.), *The cognitive neuroscience of music* (pp. 57–75). Oxford: Oxford University Press.

Janata, P. (2009). The neural architecture of music-evoked autobiographical memories. *Cerebral Cortex, 19,* 2579–2594. http://dx.doi.org/10.1093/cercor/bhp008.

Jeffries, K. J., Fritz, J. B., & Braun, A. R. (2003). Words in melody: An H2^15O PET study of brain activation during singing and speaking. *NeuroReport, 14,* 749–754. http://dx.doi.org/10.1097/00001756-200304150-00018.

Juslin, P. N., & Sloboda, J. A. (2010). Introduction: aims, organization, and terminology. In P. N. Juslin, & J. A. Sloboda (Eds.), *Handbook of music and emotion: Theory, research, applications* (pp. 3–12). Oxford: Oxford University Press.

Khalfa, S., Dalla Bella, S., Roy, M., Peretz, I., & Lupien, S. J. (2003). Effects of relaxing music on salivary cortisol level after psychological stress. *Annals of the New York Academic of Sciences, 999,* 374–376. http://dx.doi.org/10.1196/annals.1284.045.

Kleber, B., Bribaumer, N., Veit, R., Trevorrow, T., & Lotze, M. (2007). Overt and imagined singing of an Italian aria. *NeuroImage, 36,* 889–900. http://dx.doi.org/10.1016/j.neuroimage.2007.02.053.

Koelsch, S. (2013). *Brain & music.* West Sussex, UK: Wiley-Blackwell.

Koelsch, S. (2015). Music-evoked emotions: principles, brain correlates, and implications for therapy. *Annals of the New York Academy of Sciences, 1337,* 193–201. http://dx.doi.org/10.1111/nyas.12684.

Koelsch, S., Fritz, T., Cramon, Y. V., Müller, K., & Friederici, A. D. (2006). Investigating emotion with music: an fMRI study. *Human Brain Mapping, 27,* 239–250. http://dx.doi.org/10.1002/hbm.20180.

Koelsch, S., Fuermetz, J., Sack, U., Bauer, K., Hohenadel, M., Wiegal, M., et al. (2011). Effects of music listening on cortisol levels and propofol consumption during spinal anesthesia. *Frontiers in Psychology, 2,* 1–9. http://dx.doi.org/10.3389/fpsyg.2011.00058.

Kraus, N., Slater, J., Thompson, E. C., Hornickel, J., Strait, D. L., Nicol, T., et al. (2014). Music enrichment programs improve the neural encoding of speech in at-risk children. *The Journal of Neuroscience, 34*(36), 11913–11918. http://dx.doi.org/10.1523/jneurosci.1881-14.2014.

Limb, C. J. (2006). Structural and functional neural correlates of music perception. *The Anatomical Record Part A Discoveries in Molecular Cellular and Evolutionary Biology, 288*(4), 435–446. http://dx.doi.org/10.1002/ar.a.20316.

Limb, C. J., & Braun, A. R. (2008). Neural substrates of spontaneous musical performance: an fMRI study of jazz improvisation. *PLoS One, 3*(2), e1679. http://dx.doi.org/10.1371/journal.pone.0001679.

McRae, K., Hughes, B., Chopra, S., Gabrieli, J. D. E., Gross, J. J., & Ochsner, K. N. (2010). The neural bases of distraction and reappraisal. *Journal of Cognitive Neuroscience, 22,* 248–262. http://dx.doi.org/10.1162/jocn.2009.21243.

Menon, V., & Levitin, D. (2005). The rewards of music listening: response and physiological connectivity of the mesolimbic system. *NeuroImage, 28,* 175–184. http://dx.doi.org/10.1016/j.neuroimage.2005.05.053.

Mitterschiffthaler, M. T., Fu, C. H. Y., Dalton, J. A., Andrew, C. M., & Williams, S. C. R. (2007). A functional MRI study of happy and sad affective states induced by classical music. *Human Brain Mapping, 28,* 1150–1162. http://dx.doi.org/10.1002/hbm.20337.

Nakamura, S., Sadato, N., Oohashi, T., Nishina, E., Fuwamoto, Y., & Yonekura, Y. (1999). Analysis of music-brain interaction with simultaneous measurement of regional cerebral blood flow and electroencephalogram beta rhythm in human subjects. *Neuroscience Letters, 275,* 222–226. http://dx.doi.org/10.1016/S0304-3940(99)000766-1.

Ochsner, K. N., & Gross, J. J. (2005). The cognitive control of emotion. *Trends in Cognitive Sciences, 9,* 242–249. http://dx.doi.org/10.1016/j.tics.2005.03.010.

Olson, I. R., Plotzker, A., & Ezzyat, Y. (2007). The enigmatic temporal pole: a review of findings on social and emotional processing. *Brain, 130,* 1718–1731. http://dx.doi.org/10.1093.brain/awm052.

O'Kelly, J. (2016). Music therapy and neuroscience: opportunities and challenges. *Voices: A World Forum for Music Therapy, 16*(2). http://dx.doi.org/10.15845/voices.v16i2.872.

Posner, M. I., Rothbart, M. K., Sheese, B. E., & Voelker, P. (2014). Developing attention: behavioral and brain mechanisms. *Advances in Neuroscience, 2014,* 405094. http://dx.doi.org/10.1155/2014/405094.

Quarto, T., Fasano, M. C., Taurisano, P., Fazio, L., Antonucci, L. A., Gelao, B., et al. (2017). Interaction between DRD2 variation and sound environment on mood and emotion-related brain activity. *Neuroscience, 341,* 9–17. http://dx.doi.org/10.1016/j.neuroscience.2016.11.010.

Rameson, L. T., Morelli, S. A., & Lieberman, M. D. (2012). The neural correlates of empathy: experience, automaticity, and prosocial behavior. *Journal of Cognitive Neuroscience, 24,* 235–245. http://dx.doi.org/10.1162/jocn_a_00130.

Rempel-Clower, N. L. (2007). Role of orbitofrontal cortex connections in emotion. *Annals of the New York Academy of Sciences, 1121,* 72–86. http://dx.doi.org/10.1196/annals.1401.026.

Robinson, H., Calamia, M., Gläscher, J., Bruss, J., & Tranel, D. (2014). Neuroanatomical correlates of executive functions: a neuropsychological approach using the EXAMINER battery. *Journal of the International Neuropsychological Society, 20,* 52–63. http://dx.doi.org/10.1017/S135561771300060X.

Roth, E. A., & Keeler, J. R. (2016, July). *Neurobiological changes associated with social bonding, stress, and flow-state in vocal improvisation.* Paper presented at the International Conference on Music Perception and Cognition, San Francisco, CA.

Salimpoor, V. N., Benovoy, M., Larcher, K., Dagher, A., & Zatorre, R. J. (2011). Anatomically distinct dopamine release during anticipation and experience of peak emotion to music. *Nature Neuroscience, 14,* 257–264. http://dx.doi.org/10.1038/nn.2726.

Särkämö, T., Altenmüller, E., Rodriguez-Fornells, A., & Peretz, I. (2016). Editorial: Music, brain, and rehabilitation: emerging therapeutic applications and potential neural mechanisms. *Frontiers in Human Neuroscience, 10,* 103. http://dx.doi.org/10.3389/fnhum.2016.00103.

Schnupp, J., Nelken, I., & King, A. (2011). *Auditory neuroscience: Making sense of sound.* Cambridge, MA: The MIT Press.

Sena Moore, K. (2013). A systematic review of the neural effect of music on emotion regulation: implications for music therapy practice. *Journal of Music Therapy, 50,* 198–242. http://dx.doi.org/10.1093/jmt/50.3.198.

Stegemöller, E. (2014). Exploring a neuroplasticity model of music therapy. *Journal of Music Therapy, 51,* 211–227. http://dx.doi.org/10.1093/jmt/thu023.

Stephan, K. E., & Friston, K. J. (2010). Analyzing effective connectivity with fMRI. *Wiley Interdisciplinary Reviews. Cognitive Science, 1,* 446–459. http://dx.doi.org/10.1002/wcs.58.

Thaut, C. P. (2014). Symbolic communication training through music (SYCOM). In M. H. Thaut, & V. Hoemberg (Eds.), *Handbook of neurologic music therapy* (pp. 217–220). Oxford: Oxford University Press.

Thaut, M. H., & Gardiner, J. C. (2014). Musical attention control training. In M. H. Thaut, & V. Hoemberg (Eds.), *Handbook of neurologic music therapy* (pp. 257–269). Oxford: Oxford University Press.

Thaut, M., & McIntosh, G. (2010, March 24). *How music helps to heal the injured brain: Therapeutic use crescendos thanks to advances in brain science.* Retrieved from http://dana.org/Cerebrum/2010/How_Music_Helps_to_Heal_the_Injured_Brain__Therapeutic_Use_Crescendos_Thanks_to_Advances_in_Brain_Science/.

Thaut, M. H., Stephan, K. M., Wunderlich, G., Schicks, W., Tellmann, L., Herzog, H., et al. (2009). Distinct cortico-cerebellar activations in rhythmic auditory motor synchronization. *Cortex, 45,* 44–53. http://dx.doi.org/10.1016/j.cortex.2007.09.009.

Thaut, M. H., Thaut, C. P., & McIntosh, K. (2014). Melodic intonation therapy (MIT). In M. H. Thaut, & V. Hoemberg (Eds.), *Handbook of neurologic music therapy* (pp. 140–145). Oxford: Oxford University Press.

Zuk, J., Benjamin, C., Kenyon, A., & Gabb, N. (2014). Behavioral and neural correlates of executive functioning in musicians and non-musicians. *PLoS One, 9*(6), e99868. http://dx.doi.org/10.1371/journal.pone.0099868.

Zysset, S., Huber, O., Ferstl, E., & von Cramon, D. Y. (2002). The anterior frontomedian cortex and evaluative judgement: an fMRI study. *NeuroImage, 15,* 983–991. http://dx.doi.org/10.1006/nimg.2001.1008.

CHAPTER 3

Music Therapy in Educational Settings

MICHAEL R. DETMER, MME, MT-BC*

INDIVIDUALS SERVED IN EDUCATIONAL SETTINGS

Music therapists are integral members of the interdisciplinary team in many educational settings across the United States. According to the 2016 workforce analysis of music therapists (American Music Therapy Association, 2016a), 12% of music therapy respondents provide services within children's facilities and schools, with an even higher percentage, 56%, working with school-aged individuals in various settings. Music therapy is recognized as a related service in the Individualized Education Program (IEP) (U.S. Department of Education, 2010a)—a legally required individualized student document that guides the delivery of special education supports and services—and research and clinical evidence suggest that music therapy can help students reach their IEP goals. This chapter will (1) provide an overview of those served by music therapists in the educational setting; discuss foundational evidence and current research supporting the integration of music therapy in educational settings; (2) describe evidence-based music therapy practices; (3) share case examples; explore the provision of services, including funding, referral pathways, and interdisciplinary collaboration; and finally, (4) identify areas for future research.

Major tenets of music therapy practice include a strong therapeutic relationship between the client and therapist, treatment planning for individualized goal areas, and the therapeutic design and implementation of musical elements. It is because of these unique properties that music therapy intervention can foster the simultaneous development of multiple domain areas, including cognitive, communicative, emotional, psychosocial, and sensorimotor functioning. Moreover, all of this can be done in compliance with the Individuals

with Disabilities Education Act (IDEA) of 2004, which requires education be provided in the "least restrictive environment" (U.S. Department of Education, 2006, §300.114). In essence, a least restrictive environment provides students with disabilities—with the use of supplementary aids and services—access to education in the most typical educational environment with students without disabilities, unless the severity of the disability prevents satisfactory education.

To better understand the context in which students with disabilities have access to special education services and why and how supportive services are implemented, it is important to have a basic knowledge of IDEA. On November 29, 1975, President Gerald Ford signed into law the Education for All Handicapped Children Act, which, now with subsequent amendments, is known as the Individuals with Disabilities Education Act (IDEA). IDEA provides "access to a free, appropriate, public education in the least restrictive environment to every child with a disability" (U.S. Department of Education, 2015). According to the most recently available data, IDEA has allowed 62% of students with disabilities to receive education in general education classrooms during 80% or more of their school day (U.S. Department of Education, 2015). As a nation, the United States has gone from excluding nearly 1.8 million students with disabilities from public schools (before 1975) to providing over 6.9 million students with disabilities special education and related services targeting their individual needs and preparing them for further education, employment, and independent living (U.S. Department of Education, 2015). Since the enactment in 1975, students with disabilities are achieving at levels that would have not been possible in decades prior. Indeed, more individuals with disabilities are now

- attending their neighborhood schools and learning from the general education curriculum,
- graduating high school,
- enrolled in postsecondary programs, and
- employed (U.S. Department of Education, 2010b).

*This author does not hold any commercial or financial conflicts of interest, and no funding sources were utilized for the development of this chapter.

Music therapists working in educational settings (or addressing educational goals in other settings) work with three main groups of individuals: (1) infants and toddlers under the age of 3 years with disabilities as defined in part C of IDEA; (2) children and young adults, ages 3 to 21 years, with a disability as defined in part B of IDEA; and (3) those with developmental needs who may not have an IEP, have limited access to supportive services, or are utilizing private therapeutic services.

According to the 2016 report to the US Congress on the implementation of IDEA, 350,581 infants and toddlers were served under part C in 2014 (U.S. Department of Education, 2016). Part C of IDEA states infants and toddlers under the age of 3 years may need early intervention services because they

1. are experiencing developmental delays, as measured by appropriate diagnostics and procedures, in one or more of the following areas:
   a. physical development,
   b. cognitive development,
   c. communication development,
   d. social or emotional development, and
   e. adaptive development; or
2. have a diagnosed physical or mental condition that has a high probability of resulting in developmental delay; or
3. are, at the state's discretion, infants or toddlers who are at risk of experiencing a substantial developmental delay if they did not receive early intervention services, or are children with disabilities who previously received services under part C of IDEA (U.S. Department of Education, 2006, §300.25).

Once a child reaches age 3 years, he or she may be eligible for services under part B of IDEA. In 2014, 6,697,938 students aged 3 to 21 years were served under part B. According to IDEA, a child with a disability means a child with

1. mental retardation,[a] hearing impairments including deafness, speech or language impairments, visual impairments including blindness, serious emotional disturbance, orthopedic impairments, autism, traumatic brain injury, other health impairments, or specific learning disabilities; and
2. who, by reason thereof, needs special education and related services (U.S. Department of Education, 2006, §300.8 (a)).

At the discretion of the state and local educational agency, a child aged 3 to 9 years, however, may qualify for services under part B of IDEA if they meet the following two criteria:

1. experiencing developmental delays, as defined by the state and as measured by appropriate diagnostic instruments and procedures in one or more of the following areas: physical development, cognitive development, communication development, social or emotional development, or adaptive development; and
2. who, by reason thereof, needs special education and related services (U.S. Department of Education, 2006, §300.8 (b)(1-2)).

The third group of individuals served by music therapists may not be explicitly defined within IDEA, or may not be receiving music therapy under an IEP because of the absence of a music therapist within their school setting, but may still receive music therapy services to promote developmental and educational achievement in alignment with typical IEP goal areas. This group includes, but is not limited to, children and young adults who

- see a private music therapist outside of the school setting, either individually or in a cotreatment situation with another therapist (e.g., physical therapy, speech therapy, occupational therapy), to address a range of goals, including improved self-esteem, coping strategies, compliance with treatment, or socialization;
- are juvenile offenders who attend individual or group-based music therapy in a residential treatment setting;
- take adaptive music lessons from a music therapist who tailors the educational approach and environment to the student's developmental and behavioral needs;
- have limited access to supportive education services because of parental placement in a private school; or
- are chronically hospitalized patients who see a music therapist as part of their inpatient hospital stay to offset developmental delay (see Chapter 5 for more information on medical music therapy).

As described in the previous paragraphs, there are many types of disabilities that can affect a student's success in the classroom. Boxes 3.1–3.9 have been compiled and adapted from Snell's (2006) disability charts, Adamek and Darrow's (2005) disability chapters, IDEA (U.S. Department of Education, 2006), and the Diagnostic and Statistical Manual of Mental Disorders, Fifth Edition (DSM-5) (American Psychological Association,

---

[a] "Mental retardation" is now termed "intellectual disability" in the DSM-5 (2013, p. 33).

BOX 3.1
Disability Overview: Autism Spectrum Disorder

AUTISM SPECTRUM DISORDER

IDEA Definition

A developmental disability significantly affecting verbal and nonverbal communication and social interaction, generally evident before age 3 years, that adversely affects a child's educational performance. Other characteristics often associated with autism are engagement in repetitive activities and stereotyped movements, resistance to environmental change or change in daily routines, and unusual responses to sensory experiences.

Autism does not apply if a child's educational performance is adversely affected primarily because the child has an emotional disturbance.

A child who manifests the characteristics of autism after age 3 years could be identified as having autism if the aforementioned criteria are met.

(U.S. Department of Education, 2006, §300.8 (c) (1))

Characteristics	Possible Music Therapy Supports
• Nonverbal, echolalic, and/or verbal with impaired expressive and receptive language • Compulsive, ritualistic, or repetitive patterns of behavior • Preoccupied with unusual objects or perseverative interests • Resistant to change • Hyper- or hyporeactivity to sensory input with potential for self-injurious behavior and/or unusual interest in sensory aspects of the environment • Minimal direct eye contact • Difficulty regulating behavior and emotional responses	• Use social story songs to teach meaningful interaction skills (e.g., taking turns, greetings) • Use musical elements (e.g., form, rhythmic pattern) to support predictability and motor planning in multistep tasks • Pair original songs with greetings and transition periods to support predictability in routines • Use musical prompts within familiar songs to bid for interaction or cue vocalization • Use contingent music to increase sustained attention to tasks or as positive reinforcement • Reinforce the use of music as a self-soothing activity during periods of dysregulation • Redirect to active music making as a replacement behavior for unproductive or potentially harmful physical movement

Note. "Autism spectrum disorder" as termed in the DSM-5 (American Psychological Association, 2013) is termed "autism" in IDEA (U.S. Department of Education, 2006).

2013) to provide a brief overview of common disabilities and how they are served by music therapists in the educational setting. They are not comprehensive, are not diagnostic tools, and do not apply to the entirety of every individual. It is recommended that the reader refer to further information in this chapter, as well as other applicable resources, for more information. Of note, some differences in terminology exist between IDEA (2006) and the DSM-5 (American Psychological Association, 2013), including the updated terms "autism spectrum disorder" (ASD) and "intellectual disability," which were termed "autism" and "mental retardation", respectively, in IDEA (2006).

SUMMARY OF RESEARCH

Music is a powerful, nonthreatening, inclusive, and accessible tool, and when applied in a therapeutic manner by a certified music therapist, it can produce unparalleled outcomes in students with disabilities. As indicated in the figures of the previous section, music therapists can facilitate improvements in multiple domain areas by targeting cognitive, communicative, emotional, psychosocial, and sensorimotor objectives. Because music is processed by a different area of the brain than speech and language, children can more easily learn new information and skills through the use of music. As a contingency, a prompt for a targeted response, or the structure for a multistep task, music helps students with disabilities demonstrate increased on-task behavior, sustained attention, and motivation to respond, learn, and practice new skills (Humpal & Colwell, 2006). A music therapist might initially use elements of music such as melody and rhythm to cue a student to engage in a behavior, but as the student learns to perform the behavior consistently and independently, the music therapist would fade the musical cues to aid in skill generalization and the transfer to other learning environments.

DEAF-BLINDNESS AND MULTIPLE DISABILITIES

IDEA Definition

Deaf-blindness

Concomitant hearing and visual impairments, the combination of which causes such severe communication and other developmental and educational needs that they cannot be accommodated in special education programs solely for children with deafness or children with blindness.

(U.S. Department of Education, 2006, §300.8 (c) (2))

Multiple disabilities

Concomitant impairments (such as mental retardation-blindness or mental retardation-orthopedic impairment), the combination of which causes such severe educational needs that they cannot be accommodated in special education programs solely for one of the impairments. Multiple disabilities does not include deaf-blindness.

(U.S. Department of Education, 2006, §300.8 (c) (7))

Characteristics	Possible Music Therapy Supports
Deaf-blindness: • impairments in hearing and vision • poor expressive language • limited ability to grasp abstract concepts requiring comprehension of visual and auditory stimuli • limited opportunities for interaction with others and the environmentMultiple-disabilities: • various combinations of disabilities • any number of behavioral manifestations present in the other disability overview figures in this section • cognitive abilities range from normal to profound	• Use music paired with multimodal sensory stimulation to elicit optimal participation and learning behavior • Apply and tailor complexity of music to motivate or calm during periods of agitation • Use structured music activities to provide age-appropriate, meaningful interactions • Use active music making to promote expression • Redirect to active music making as a replacement behavior for unproductive or potentially harmful physical movement • Use vibroacoustic elements of music to provide sensory input during times of dysregulation, sensory seeking behavior, or as a distraction technique

BOX 3.3
Disability Overview: Emotional Disturbance

EMOTIONAL DISTURBANCE

IDEA Definition

A condition exhibiting one or more of the following characteristics over a long period of time and to a marked degree that adversely affects a child's educational performance:

• an inability to learn that cannot be explained by intellectual, sensory, or health factors;

• an inability to build or maintain satisfactory interpersonal relationships with peers and teachers;

• inappropriate types of behavior or feelings under normal circumstances;

• a general pervasive mood of unhappiness or depression; or

• a tendency to develop physical symptoms or fears associated with personal or school problems.

Emotional disturbance includes schizophrenia. The term does not apply to children who are socially maladjusted, unless it is determined that they have an emotional disturbance according to the criteria listed earlier.

(U.S. Department of Education, 2006, §300.8 (c) (4))

Characteristics	Possible Music Therapy Supports
• Hyperactivity or impulsiveness • Limited attention span • Easily frustrated • Poor behavior regulation • Poor coping skills • Aggressive or attention-seeking behavior • Incongruent affect • High anxiety • Verbal manipulation of peers and elders • Low self-esteem or presentation of a (false) high-self esteem	• Use preferred music or music activities as positive reinforcement for appropriate behaviors • Use active music engagement as a distraction technique from problem behaviors • Use music (e.g., lyric analysis) to discuss and reinforce coping strategies • Use structured group music making to promote opportunities for positive social interaction • Use active music making (e.g., drumming) as an outlet for physical aggression

BOX 3.4
Disability Overview: Intellectual Disability

INTELLECTUAL DISABILITY

IDEA Definition

Significantly subaverage general intellectual functioning, existing concurrently with deficits in adaptive behavior and manifested during the developmental period, that adversely affects a child's educational performance.

(U.S. Department of Education, 2006, §300.8 (c) (6))

Characteristics	Possible Music Therapy Supports
• Deficits in reasoning, problem-solving, planning, abstract thinking, and judgment • Poor adaptation skills • Limited independence • Poor communication • Limited social engagementSeverity levels (determined by adaptive functioning skills, not IQ scores): • mild • moderate • severe • profound	• Use music paired with multimodal sensory stimulation to elicit optimal participation and learning behavior • Use music contingencies to provide immediate or simultaneous nonverbal, positive reinforcement for appropriate behaviors • Use music to support developmental learning experiences • Use structured music activities to provide age-appropriate, meaningful interactions • Use music to improve learning behavior, response time, memory, feelings of success, and attention span

Note. "Intellectual disability" as termed in the DSM-5 (American Psychological Association, 2013) is termed "mental retardation" in IDEA (U.S. Department of Education, 2006).

ORTHOPEDIC IMPAIRMENT AND OTHER HEALTH IMPAIRMENTS

IDEA Definition

Orthopedic impairment

A severe orthopedic impairment that adversely affects a child's educational performance. The term includes impairments caused by a congenital anomaly, impairments caused by disease (e.g., poliomyelitis, bone tuberculosis), and impairments from other causes (e.g., cerebral palsy, amputations, and fractures or burns that cause contractures).

(U.S. Department of Education, 2006, §300.8 (c) (8))

Other health impairments

Having limited strength, vitality, or alertness, including a heightened alertness to environmental stimuli, which results in limited alertness with respect to the educational environment, that

• is due to chronic or acute health problems, such as asthma, attention-deficit disorder or attention-deficit hyperactivity disorder, diabetes, epilepsy, a heart condition, hemophilia, lead poisoning, leukemia, nephritis, rheumatic fever, sickle cell anemia, and Tourette syndrome; and

• adversely affects a child's educational performance.

(U.S. Department of Education, 2006, §300.8 (c) (9))

Characteristics	Possible Music Therapy Supports
• Disturbances in gait, balance, or use of one or more extremities • Hypo- or hypertonic muscles • Deficits in vision, hearing, or speech • Spasms, seizures, or involuntary physical movement • Short attention span • Limited fine and/or gross motor skills • Impaired social skills • Poor self-esteem • Hyper- or hyporesponsiveness to stimuli • Limited physical endurance	• Use music elements (e.g., rhythm, tempo) to improve physical strength/endurance, motor planning, or sensorimotor responses • Use music activities to facilitate dynamic movement opportunities • Use music to facilitate meaningful social interaction and adaptive social skills • Use active music making and music-based discussion to highlight individual strengths • Use music to improve learning behavior, response time, memory, feelings of success, and attention span • Use of music as an outlet for self-expression • Utilize adaptive music equipment to facilitate optimal participation and create feelings of success

---

BOX 3.6
Disability Overview: Specific Learning Disability

SPECIFIC LEARNING DISABILITY

IDEA Definition

A disorder in one or more of the basic psychological processes involved in understanding or in using language, spoken or written, that may manifest itself in the imperfect ability to listen, think, speak, read, write, spell, or do mathematical calculations, including conditions such as perceptual disabilities, brain injury, minimal brain dysfunction, dyslexia, and developmental aphasia.

Specific learning disability does not include learning problems that are primarily the result of visual, hearing, or motor disabilities, of mental retardation, of emotional disturbance, or of environmental, cultural, or economic disadvantage.

(U.S. Department of Education, 2006, §300.8 (c) (10))

Characteristics	Possible Music Therapy Supports
• Difficulty with sequencing tasks and problem-solving • Poor retrieval of information • Limited attention span • Impulsive • Poor expressive language (verbal and written) • Difficulty with time and math concepts • Poor self-image and self-esteem • Social withdrawal • Auditory processing problems • Hyperactive • Easily frustrated	• Facilitate individual and group music therapy interactions to highlight individual strengths • Use active music engagement to pair motor movement with thinking skills • Use music to improve learning behavior, response time, memory, feelings of success, and attention span • Use structured music activities to provide age-appropriate, meaningful interactions • Use music to develop coping strategies for improved behavior regulation

---

BOX 3.7
Disability Overview: Speech or Language Impairment

SPEECH OR LANGUAGE IMPAIRMENT

IDEA Definition

A communication disorder, such as stuttering, impaired articulation, a language impairment, or a voice impairment, that adversely affects a child's educational performance.

(U.S. Department of Education, 2006, §300.8 (c) (11))

Characteristics	Possible Music Therapy Supports
• Poor vocal function • Impaired articulation or fluency • Impaired auditory processing skills, difficulty learning via verbal presentation • Limited expressive language • Difficulty with sequences and memory recall • Poor social interactions and ability to follow rules of conversation • Low frustration threshold • Low self-esteem	• Use music elements (rhythm, cadence, melody, form) to facilitate improved access to speech/language learning • Use singing to address and reinforce speech function (volume, articulation, contour, etc.) • Use music (e.g., songwriting, singing) as a mode of expression • Facilitate individual and group music therapy interactions to highlight individual strengths • Use verbal directives embedded in singing to improve receptive language skills

---

Music has been used in the classroom as early as the 1700s, and positive benefits of music with students with disabilities have been noted as early as 1878 (Doren, 1879). By the 1920s, it was evident that music made a therapeutic impact in the special education classroom, and the 1975 passage of Public Law 94-142, the Education for All Children Act, marked the beginning of an era in which music therapy research and practice in educational settings has flourished (Brown & Jellison, 2012). In fact, since 1975, significant positive effects in over 50 experimental studies (including those in which participants

---

BOX 3.8
Disability Overview: Traumatic Brain Injury

TRAUMATIC BRAIN INJURY

IDEA Definition

An acquired injury to the brain caused by an external physical force, resulting in total or partial functional disability or psychosocial impairment, or both, that adversely affects a child's educational performance. Traumatic brain injury applies to open or closed head injuries resulting in impairments in one or more areas such as cognition; language; memory; attention; reasoning; abstract thinking; judgment; problem-solving; sensory, perceptual, and motor abilities; psychosocial behavior; physical functions; information processing; and speech. Traumatic brain injury does not apply to brain injuries that are congenital or degenerative or to brain injuries induced by birth trauma.

   (U.S. Department of Education, 2006, §300.8 (c) (12))

Characteristics	Possible Music Therapy Supports
• Speech, vision, or other sensory impairments • Decreased fine/gross motor skills • Uncoordinated motor planning • Muscle spasticity • Paralysis on one or both sides of the body • Easily frustrated, aggressive • Low self-esteem, mood swings, and depression • Poor judgment, problem-solving skills, and sequencing ability • Short attention span • Impaired memory • Difficulty understanding abstract concepts • Limited social skills • Low motivation	• Use music to improve learning behavior, response time, memory, feelings of success, and attention span • Facilitate individual and group music therapy interactions to highlight individual strengths • Use music (e.g., songwriting, singing) as a mode of self-expression • Use structured music activities to provide age-appropriate, meaningful interactions • Use music to develop coping strategies for improved behavior regulation and adaptive responses

---

BOX 3.9
Disability Overview: Visual Impairment Including Blindness

VISUAL IMPAIRMENT INCLUDING BLINDNESS

IDEA Definition

Impairment in vision that, even with correction, adversely affects a child's educational performance. The term includes both partial sight and blindness.

   (U.S. Department of Education, 2006, §300.8 (c) (13))

Characteristics	Possible Music Therapy Supports
• Intelligence is not related to individual's visual ability • Frequent headaches • Difficulty comprehending abstract concepts that require visual stimuli • Physical appearance of eyes may be disfigured, discolored, or blank/incongruent with emotion • Mobility and orientation difficulties • Limited opportunities for social engagement	• Use music paired with multimodal sensory stimulation to elicit optimal participation and learning behavior • Use structured group music making to promote opportunities for positive social interaction • Use active music engagement to facilitate the combined use of motor, thinking, and social skills • Use music as a stimulus cue or prompt for sound localization

---

acted as their own control) that investigated the use of music to reach a therapeutic, nonmusic objective with students with disabilities have been published in peer-reviewed journals (Brown & Jellison, 2012; Klein, 2010).

Benefits from music therapy across the disability spectrum have been documented in areas including (1) attentive behaviors (Robb, 2003; Sussman, 2009); (2) communication (Register, 2001; Whipple, 2012); (3) learning and retention of verbal information

(Wolfe & Hom, 1993); (4) motivation, attention, and hostility (Montello & Coons, 1998); (5) restlessness and impulsivity (Rickson, 2006); and (6) social functioning (Gooding, 2011; Whipple, 2012). These are only a select few of the many studies that support the use of music therapy in education settings; Humpal and Colwell (2006) identified over 170 studies within music therapy journals and categorized them by disability.

Increasing adaptive behaviors and decreasing detrimental behaviors in those with disabilities can be done through the use of contingent music. This was demonstrated by Standley's (1996) landmark meta-analysis on the effects of music as a reinforcement for education/therapy objectives. Contingent music for this study was defined as (1) the use of music listening initiation (e.g., beginning to play music immediately following a desired behavior), (2) music interruption (e.g., stopping music with the onset of an undesirable behavior), and (3) music performance (e.g., an opportunity to actively engage in music making following a desirable behavior). Between 1962 and 1993, 98 studies on 208 dependent variables were included in the meta-analysis, and the dependent variables ranged from academics to transportation to physical rehabilitation. Special education studies included in this analysis used music contingencies to teach self-feeding skills; decrease stereotypical or disruptive behavior; decrease out-of-seat behavior; and increase direction following, imitating, and eye contact.

To synthesize the results of each individual study and the corresponding variable effects, it is standard practice in meta-analyses to convert all variables to "effect sizes" (ES) via a statistical formula, which then allows the researcher(s) to compare and generalize the data. Without conversion to effect sizes, one may say, "you would be comparing apples to oranges." Overall, Standley found the benefits of contingent music were almost three standard deviations greater than control/baseline conditions ($ES = 2.90$). The further away from 0 an effect size is, the larger the effect. In behavioral sciences, 0.20 is considered a small effect, 0.50 is considered a medium effect, and 0.80 or higher is considered a large effect (Cohen, 1988). In addition to Standley's finding of an extremely large effect for contingent music, many other interesting outcomes emerged.

The immediate reward of music showed greater effects than delayed rewards, such as the collection of tokens for later "purchase" of music or those that required sustained correct responses for an extended period before participation in music activities. Of all 208 variables, the effects were greatest for those related to physical rehabilitation and developmental behaviors. Also, studies using subjects with mental disabilities (now termed "intellectual disabilities") showed the greatest effects, which is interesting because the majority of these studies used participants who had a profound mental disability or multiple disabilities. In summary, Standley found contingent music reinforcement was (1) more effective than other contingent nonmusic stimuli, (2) more effective than music played continuously (i.e., not in direct response to a targeted behavior), and (3) less effective if paired with other stimuli (e.g., food, toys) (Standley, 1996).

A more recent meta-analysis highlighted the effects of music therapy for children with ASD (Whipple, 2012). Eight peer-reviewed published studies met inclusion criteria for the analysis, which included studies that (1) used group or individual experimental treatment designs, (2) used subjects 5 years or younger and diagnosed with ASD, (3) compared music therapy versus a no-music control condition, and (4) used a certified music therapist to facilitate the intervention. All but one study utilized live music and active involvement of the children. Most of the interventions used music play and/or original songs composed specifically for the children of the studies. Whipple revealed that, when compared with nonmusic conditions, music therapy for children with ASD had an effect size of $d = 0.76$, which was also considered to be statistically significant. These results indicate music therapy is an extremely effective treatment for young children with ASD for developing communication, interpersonal skills, personal responsibility, and play skills. Considering the similarities in intervention delivery to address communication and social skills deficits in students with ASD and speech and language impairments, this meta-analysis has many implications for educators, researchers, and administrators, particularly because ASD and speech and language impairments are among the top four most prevalent disabilities served under IDEA, according to the most recent annual report to congress (U.S. Department of Education, 2016, pp. xxiii–xxv).

EVIDENCE-BASED PRACTICES

The American Music Therapy Association and the Certification Board for Music Therapists both describe music therapy as an evidence-based healthcare profession. "Evidence-based practice" (EBP) is a widely used term in healthcare, education, and other fields, but no one definition has satisfied all professions (Kern, 2010). The ultimate aim of EBP is to bridge the gap between research and practice to provide the best possible care. Drawing from the definitions used by the fields of medicine and psychology, the American Music Therapy Association states that, "Evidence-based music therapy practice integrates

- the best available research,
- the music therapists' expertise, and
- the needs, values, and preferences of the individual(s) served" (2016b, para. 1).

This definition also closely resembles that of the field of early childhood: "A decision-making process that integrates the best available research evidence with family and professional wisdom and values" (Buysse & Wesley, 2006, p. 12). As the field of music therapy continues to grow and more music therapists are serving students with disabilities, it is important that music therapy researchers create and widely disseminate more synthesis studies. In addition, practitioners should familiarize themselves with the latest research and critically appraise the material to better serve their clients and families (Kern, 2010).

The following section provides an introduction to commonly used evidence-based music therapy practices in school settings with children with disabilities. This is not a comprehensive list of practices, nor does it cover every disability a therapist may encounter in the school setting. However, because of the similarities in certain behaviors across disabilities, some generalizations may be made about music therapy practices. All practices described in this section are supported by empirical evidence and meet the criteria in Box 3.10.

BOX 3.10
Description of Criteria Used to Select the Evidence-Based Music Therapy Practices Described in This Section

INFORMING EVIDENCE-BASED MUSIC THERAPY PRACTICE
- Peer-reviewed, published study
- Experimental treatment design
- Music used as a separate, independent variable contrasted with a no-music control condition
- A certified music therapist facilitated the intervention
- Used rigorous data analyses that were adequate to test the stated hypotheses
- Study design, procedures, and results were reported in sufficient detail and clarity to allow for replication

---

Transition Songs (Kern, Wolery, & Aldridge, 2007)

Children in educational settings experience multiple transitions each day. These transitions occur between activities as well as to and from the classroom. Transitions often involve routines that are designed to promote compliance and independence. Most students experience challenges during transitions, especially those with disabilities, who may have difficulties with anxiety, receptive language, attention, hearing, or vision. These difficulties affect their ability to follow directions, remain behaviorally regulated, adapt to new environments, and successfully attend to the subsequent task. Children who struggle with transitions may present behaviors including crying, screaming, lying on the floor, disengaging from the task at hand, clinging to their caregiver, or ignoring those who are trying to secure their attention. Caregivers, school staff, and peers may not know how to handle challenging behaviors in extreme cases. When other people are unsure of how to help a child experiencing difficulty with a transition, this can lead to frustration, further perpetuating the inability to help the child successfully transition. Teachers and music therapists regularly use songs that are specifically designed and implemented in a systematic way to aid students during transitions. These transition songs (1) provide structure and cues to indicate what is coming next, (2) are predictable because of the inherent qualities of the music, and (3) can be paired with visual cues, all of which are the primary components of a successful transition strategy (Kern et al., 2007).

Transition songs or greeting songs can be individually composed for students to target a specific need (e.g., leaving a parent at morning drop-off) or can be signature songs used with the entire classroom (e.g., walking from the lunchroom back to the classroom). The lyrics of the song can be embedded as directives to complete a task (e.g., "put your coat away for the day") and can be paired with visual cues such as images or symbolic gestures (e.g., waving "hello") or physical prompts such as a gentle tap on the hand or hand-over-hand assistance (e.g., physically assisting the student to turn off the water after grabbing a paper towel in the restroom). The song may involve active music participation of the students by either singing or playing along on instruments and may be sung a cappella or with guitar accompaniment by the music therapist. The music therapist can also teach these greeting or transition songs to family members, school staff, and other students in the classroom to ensure consistency in this supportive strategy and maximize the learning potential of all students.

Social Stories With Music (Brownell, 2002)

Social Stories are frequently used with students with disabilities to teach and reinforce pertinent social information. They were first described by Carol Gray in 1993 (Gray & Garrand, 1993) as a tool designed for students with ASD, but they have since been adapted for others with disabilities. Brownell (2012) pointed out that Social Stories have been effective in teaching appropriate play skills, decreasing disruptive behavior, improving physical activity, reducing precursors to temper tantrums, improving mealtime skills, and increasing appropriate social skills. Many adaptations to Social Stories have been made, including setting them to music, which is now considered an evidence-based music therapy practice (Brownell, 2012). Brownell (2002) found that sung social stories help students remember the rules of social and emotional interaction and are at least as effective as, if not more effective than, their traditionally read counterparts in modifying problem behaviors.

After identifying and defining a student's target behavior, a Social Story with music should (1) be individualized to the student, (2) be written at their reading and cognitive level, and (3) use photographs, hand-drawn pictures, or pictorial icons (Brownell, 2012). The story should include the four basic sentence types of a Social Story (Gray, 1998):

1. Descriptive sentences, which are the most important type and objectively describe the context in which the target behavior occurs. These sentences typically answer *who, where, when,* and *why* questions.
2. Directive sentences, which define expectations of the student. They are stated positively and should be used sparingly.
3. Perspective sentences, which describe how others may feel, act, or respond in a given situation.
4. Control sentences, which may not be used in every story, but function as a mnemonic to recall the content of the story.

Brownell (2012) suggested the music set to a Social Story should (1) use melodies that are simple and memorable, (2) use harmonies that are straightforward and match the mood of the story, (3) always be sung in the same key, and (4) encourage student engagement and active participation. Both original music compositions and "piggyback" songs (e.g., rewriting lyrics to a familiar tune such as "Twinkle Twinkle Little Star") may be effective. The decision whether to use a familiar melody or compose a new song should be based on the musician's comfort level, the ease in adapting the lyrics to fit within a familiar melody, the music preference of the student, and the length of the time the

story will be used (e.g., a short-term intervention may be better suited using a familiar melody to the student) (Brownell, 2012). If consistency in the music presentation (i.e., singing it the same way) is possible between the music therapist, teachers, and caregivers who use the song, then a live performance is recommended, because the tempo can be adjusted to encourage participation and allow for responses and questions from the student. The song should be accompanied with the printed version of the story and should be presented to the student immediately before the targeted behavior is to occur (Brownell, 2012).

Music to Enhance Reading Skills (Register, Darrow, Standley, & Swedberg, 2007)

Literacy acquisition and learning is a top priority for educators. Schools commonly screen for early reading failure and begin remediation, if necessary, with the intent of avoiding or minimizing later developmental delays. It is widely believed that music participation can enhance academic skills, including reading. In fact, Standley's (2008) meta-analysis revealed that the use of music interventions designed to teach reading activities resulted in a moderately strong, significant, overall effect size ($d = 0.32$), indicating that the use of music can improve reading ability. When the interventions incorporate specific reading skills matched to the individual needs of children, or when contingent music (e.g., music as a reward) is used, the benefits for literacy acquisition are much more extensive (Standley, 2008).

Of concern to many educators and parents is the fact that 30% of children have reading difficulties; furthermore, in 2014, over 40% of students in grades 3 to 12 with any disability served under IDEA required accommodations in reading on the state assessment (U.S. Department of Education, 2016). Although no one strategy has been accepted to remediate reading difficulties, the use of music, which is easily accessible, preferred by children, and can be a multimodal sensory experience, is an effective and evidence-based intervention strategy to improve reading difficulties in students with and without disabilities (Register et al., 2007). Music/reading lessons can use both passive and active music activities, including listening, singing, playing instruments, and movement. Using a variety of activities to address literacy helps create a sensory rich experience. Multiple activities planned during a lesson promote a more inclusive environment and provide opportunities for the student to participate and excel in various ways. Print material and two-dimensional puppets and props can provide further opportunities for the student to engage with the reading material. There are a plethora of options for embedding music to enhance reading lessons; the following are summaries of some that are described by Register et al. (2007):

- To practice pairing graphemes and their corresponding phonemes (phonics), design and teach an original song focused on building words. After students demonstrate mastery of the song, hand each student a card containing a single letter (e.g., b, f, t) or a sound blend (e.g., -at). During the next round of singing, instruct students to find a partner with an appropriate letter or sound by the end of the song, after which they are to pronounce their word to the class.
- To increase word knowledge (vocabulary), teach a familiar song and have students participate in singing. After the song, ask students to define preselected challenging words in the song. The therapist can assist the students in arriving at a definition by pointing out context clues within the song.
- To practice sequencing skills to enhance comprehension, give students story cards in a random order. Invite the students to join in singing the song, which tells the story of the book, and instruct them to place the story cards in the correct order. An extension of this intervention would be to have the students write subsequent verses of the song, which allows them to practice making predictions.
- To practice joint attention and help with comprehension, give each student an instrument and instruct them to play it each time they hear a specific vocabulary word or a character's name in the story.

Orff-Based Music Therapy (Hilliard, 2007)

Orff-based music therapy derives from Orff Schulwerk (German for "schoolwork"), a common international approach to music education developed by composer Carl Orff (1895–1982) in the 1920s that is founded in the philosophy of learning by doing (Colwell, Achey Pehotsky, Gillmeister, & Woolrich, 2008). The Orff Schulwerk music and movement pedagogy extends far beyond the development of artistic skill. This wider development encompasses intellectual, social, emotional, and aesthetic skill building and uniquely prepares students to solve problems in many other contexts outside of music (American Orff-Schulwerk Association, 2014a). Rhythm, the foundation of the elemental music used in Orff Schulwerk, allows everyone—regardless of ability or disability—to participate (Colwell et al., 2008). Furthermore,

active music making is central to the Orff approach, which incorporates singing, chanting, playing instruments, movement, and dance in a process-oriented method. Since 1962 (and probably earlier than this), music educators have recognized the benefits of using the Orff Schulwerk approach in reaching functional goals with many populations for whom music therapists also serve. These include individuals with Down syndrome, ASD, behavioral challenges, physical disabilities, and neurologic disorders (Colwell et al., 2008). Colwell (2005) summarizes the aspects of the Orff Schulwerk approach that naturally support music therapy, including:

- allowing everyone to participate in the music;
- beginning where the individual is developmentally;
- using a multisensory approach;
- moving from the experiential (sound) to the conceptual (symbol);
- designing experiences that are success oriented;
- using culturally specific material;
- using rhythm as the underlying foundation of elemental music; and
- focusing on the process rather than the musical product.

Research demonstrates Orff-based music therapy interventions can be used to address a variety of goals. Hilliard (2007) investigated the effects of Orff-based music therapy with grieving children and documented significant benefits in their behaviors, including anger issues, physical aggression, lying, and grief symptoms. A later study by Colwell, Edwards, Hernandez, and Brees (2013) with hospitalized children revealed improvements in facial affect, on-task behavior, and anxiety, among other areas. Within the population of students with disabilities, the clinical use of Orff-based music therapy interventions extends beyond these areas to address goals across multiple domains, including socialization, behavioral regulation, impulse control, greetings, sequencing, emotional expression, choice making, movement, and memory (Detmer, 2015).

Orff-based music therapy interventions are individualized and designed to address a specific target behavior; however, they all follow a process and include Orff media. The Orff process refers to the series of steps through which the teacher/therapist guides the student to reach the short- or long-term goal (Shamrock, 1986). This often includes the gradual layering of musical lines to increase complexity. The process may be developed from a small germ of an idea or by taking a larger idea and breaking it down into manageable steps (Scott, 2010). In a true Orff pedagogic ideal, the

Orff-based Music Therapy Intervention Planning Tool
Created by Michael R. Detmer, MME, MT-BC

Client: _____   **Name of intervention:** _____

Domain(s):   ☐Cognitive   ☐Communicative   ☐Emotional   ☐Physiological   ☐Psychosocial   ☐Sensorimotor

Goal: _____

Objective: _____

Technique(s):   ☐Exploration   ☐Imitation   ☐Improvisation   ☐Expression

Media: ☐Chanting   ☐Poetry   ☐Singing   ☐Call and response   ☐Body Percussion
        ☐Improvisational dance   ☐Folk dance   ☐Choreographed dance   ☐Interpretive dance
        ☐Xylophone   ☐Metallophone   ☐Glockenspiel   ☐Recorder
        ☐Percussion: _____   ☐Other: _____

Description of Therapeutic Function of Music/Media: _____

_____

Step-by-step Process:

Potential adaptations: _____

Potential extensions: _____

Data Collection: _____

Notes:

FIG. 3.1 Orff-based music therapy intervention planning tool.

teacher/therapist strives to be a facilitator of the process rather than a director (Shamrock, 1986). The Orff media consists of speech, movement, singing, and playing instruments (American Orff-Schulwerk Association, 2014b; Colwell et al., 2008). Speech may include chants or poetry, and singing may include call and response, singing games, folk songs, or composed songs. Movement includes body percussion and dance: interpretive, improvisational, folk, or choreographed. Instruments include xylophones, metallophones, glockenspiels, unpitched percussion, and recorders (Colwell et al., 2008). See case study #1 for an example of how the Orff process and media are applied within a therapeutic context. In addition, Fig. 3.1 is a tool that may be used by music therapists to design quality Orff-based music therapy interventions.

CASE EXAMPLE #1

Lily is a bright, sweet, conversational, and funny 10-year-old with ASD. Her IEP addresses many target behaviors, including appropriately responding to questions, solving/answering addition and subtraction problems, verbally identifying the main idea of a text passage, and independently brushing her teeth. Her IEP team is primarily concerned with her sensory overstimulation related to unexpected noises (e.g., alarms) and her difficulty with transitions and changes in routine. For example, if changes occur to the schedule of events during a class, the bus is late picking her up from school, or her class has a substitute teacher, Lily becomes very anxious and agitated as evidenced by inconsolable high-pitched screaming, a bright red face, and moving away from all people. Because she is highly motivated by music and demonstrates increased sustained attention during music-oriented tasks, her IEP team has added music therapy as a related service to help Lily with her ability to calm down after becoming upset. After Lily's initial music therapy session in which the board-certified music therapist (MT-BC) completed a full assessment, a primary goal was identified: to decrease the time to recover from dysregulation. In the second session, a week later, the MT-BC began working toward the first objective under this goal: Given a prompt by the MT-BC, Lily will verbally identify and physically demonstrate a minimum of one coping strategy to calm herself down, by the end of a 30-min session, across three consecutive sessions by Dec. 16, 2016. The MT-BC used an original Orff-based music therapy intervention to teach Lily a song, which included embedded instructions for her to engage in music (a preferred activity) when upset rather than scream and run away. The MT-BC used the following Orff process:

1. Model chant: "When I need a break, I know just what to do; I'll find an instrument and play a tune or two."

2. Invite Lily to chant along with the MT-BC.

3. Repeat chant and prompt Lily pat to the half-note beat, alternating between her left and right knees.

4. Give Lily mallets and instruct her to play the "C" and "G" on the xylophone, mirroring the pats on her knees (i.e., a bordun), while the MT-BC supports with the chant.

5. Instruct Lily to speak the chant while continuing to play the bordun.

6. After Lily demonstrates integration of the chant while playing, invite her to improvise on the xylophone at the end of the next chant.

7. Repeat the chant, followed by a cue for Lily to improvise on the xylophone, when the MT-BC counts down from 10 and cues Lily to "stop" after "1."

Following the introduction of this song, the MT-BC then engaged Lily in a conversation about what she could do when she gets upset at school. Lily quickly answered, "Find an instrument!" In the following sessions, the MT-BC and Lily reviewed the strategy and practiced it during periods of agitation. Because music therapy is also listed under "Supplementary Aides and Services" on Lily's IEP to consult and provide resources to staff and parents, the MT-BC taught Lily's parents, teachers, and occupational therapist the chant and encouraged them to cue Lily with it when she became upset. Within 2 weeks, Lily's mom came to the music therapy room at her school and told the MT-BC that Lily now consistently goes to her room, without the need for a prompt, to play her mini drum set when she gets agitated.

CASE EXAMPLE #2

Dylan is an energetic and affectionate 8-year-old diagnosed with attention-deficit hyperactivity disorder. He often needs reminders to stay on task and fluctuates between extreme behavior states of very quiet and disengaged to actively running around and talking in a loud voice while perseverating on a topic, usually superheroes. Dylan has fallen behind in all academic areas and is on an IEP to address his sustained attention, interactions with peers and adults, and early academic skills. In addition to speech therapy, Dylan receives music therapy once per week for 30 min. Dylan's music therapist (MT-BC) designed a treatment plan focusing on three goal areas: successful transitions between activities, joint attention, and academic skills. Dylan loves music and has a strong rapport with his music therapist. Every week, he comes barreling into the room and runs around to touch all of the instruments. The MT-BC uses the iso-principle technique, in which music stimuli is matched to the client's behavior/mood/physiologic state and slowly adjusted in complexity, volume, and tempo to produce a change in the client. In Dylan's case, the MT-BC starts the session with a guitar strapped around his neck and a small handheld shaker in his right hand. The MT-BC also gives Dylan two small shakers to occupy each hand and begins playing a very fast version of an originally composed song, "Move and Groove to the Music." Dylan quickly engages by shaking his instruments, singing along, and following embedded cues in the music ("jump," "spin," "tip toe"). Over the next 1 to 2 min, the MT-BC starts to slow the tempo of the song

and uses more relaxed lyrical cues ("sway," "rock," "sit") to eventually help Dylan transition to quietly sitting in his chair on the floor mat. The MT-BC then welcomes Dylan, gives him verbal praise for assuming his "listening position," and begins playing and singing the "Hello" song, which includes prompts for Dylan to wave and greet the MT-BC and a listing of activities for the day. Following the "Hello" song, Dylan moves the pictorial image of a boy waving to the right side of his schedule board as the MT-BC sings "All done with hello, all done with hello, all done with hello, now it's time for counting." At this point, Dylan automatically stands up and walks across the room to the desk and chair. Per Dylan's IEP, the MT-BC is working with Dylan on counting by 2s, 5s, and 10s. One intervention used for the 2s counting task begins with an original, musical mnemonic song, "2s, 2s, up by 2s, if I can do it, so can you: 2, 4, 6, 8….!" This prepares Dylan for the next task of writing a 2s number sequence (2, 4, 6, 8…) up to 20. This intervention is designed as a music contingency, where after each number Dylan writes, he reaches to the MT-BC's guitar to strum the strings with his left (nonwriting) hand. If Dylan writes the correct number, the MT-BC allows the guitar to sound and sings the correct number as a form of praise. If Dylan writes the incorrect number, the MT-BC mutes the guitar strings, preventing Dylan's strum from sounding, which cues Dylan to recheck his work and try again. Because Dylan is engaged by music and wants to play the guitar, he is motivated to attend to the counting/writing task for a sustained period and to do quality work to receive the music reward.

FUNDING, INITIATION, AND SUSTAINING SERVICES

If music therapy is warranted as a related service on a student's IEP as determined by the IEP team, the U.S. Department of Education (2006) states it must be provided at no cost to the parents. Schools may contract with an independent music therapist or hire a staff therapist, depending on the size of the population requiring services. If parents/caregivers are seeking music therapy outside of the school, private pay is an option, or some music therapists will bill insurance or work with a local agency or the state to offset costs with a waiver. Many music therapists also provide services on a sliding fee scale to assist families with limited resources. If a school is interested in providing music therapy as an enrichment or programmatic service for a wider range of the student population, including those not covered under IDEA (e.g., a free parent-and-child after-school music therapy drumming group targeting socialization and anger management), there may be special education state/county funding or grants for which they can apply. The school may also elect to independently cover the cost for parents/caregivers or partner with other schools within the district to increase funding options.

The first step to initiating music therapy services is for a parent or school staff member to make a referral to a music therapist. If there is no music therapist on staff, the school or family can find a music therapist in the community by searching the database on the Certification Board for Music Therapists (www.cbmt.org) or the American Music Therapy Association (www.musictherapy.org) Web site. Another option is to reach out to the local or regional music therapy association or a nearby university that has an approved music therapy training program.

Music therapists may create a referral questionnaire or checklist to assist the IEP team in determining if a student would be appropriate for a music therapy assessment. If the student is indeed eligible for an assessment, the music therapist must receive a formal permission-to-assess form signed by the students' guardians, after which the music therapist has 60 days to complete the eligibility assessment and present the data to the IEP team. The music therapist may create an original assessment tool or use formal tools that can be applied with children in educational settings, such as the Special Education Music Therapy Assessment Process (Coleman & Brunk, 2003), the Music Therapy Special Education Assessment Scale (Bradfield, Carlenius, Gold, & White, 2007), the Individualized Music Therapy Assessment Profile (Baxter et al., 2007), the Individual Music-Centered Assessment Profile for Neurodevelopmental Disorders (Carpente, 2013), or the SCERTS Model (Walworth, Register, & Engel, 2009). If the student is deemed eligible for services based on the eligibility assessment, a music therapist (often different from the music therapist who assessed the student for eligibility, to avoid conflict of interest) then sets goals and objectives for the student, in consultation with the IEP team. These goals should follow the same framework as other practitioners' goals by ensuring they are SMART: specific, measurable, attainable, realistic, and have a time frame (Ritter-Cantesanu, 2014). Following the design of a music therapy treatment plan, the IEP team may discuss whether the student would benefit more from individual or group services. Several considerations should be made when choosing the best treatment format, including EBP; specific needs of the student; commonality of goal areas among potential students in the group; scheduling; developmental age; and logistics such as location, instrument availability, and staff assistance/support.

A sustainable music therapy practice includes three primary components:
1. a highly competent, sensitive, and certified music therapist with knowledge of the latest EBP;
2. clear, articulate, precise, and unbiased documentation of student progress; and
3. professional and successful relationships with the IEP team.

A successful IEP team requires the stakeholders have not only knowledge of their own disciplines but also a strong understanding of and appreciation for their colleagues' disciplines as well. To help educate other team members about music therapy, which some professionals may not have heard of, music therapists often provide regular staff education and in-services on the benefits of music therapy for students with disabilities. Also, it is important that music therapists understand concepts and initiatives in the field of special education and use one shared core vocabulary when interacting with educators, therapists, families, and administrators (Adamek, Darrow, & Jellison, 2014). Using common vocabulary will allow for more efficient and productive interactions, thus providing the most well-informed services to students with special needs. Finally, the IEP team should aim to operate from a transdisciplinary model, in which the disciplinary lines become blurred or eliminated because of members' strong understanding of and collaboration with each discipline and an emphasis placed on the student rather than professional identities (DeLoach & Detmer, 2015).

A LOOK AHEAD: AREAS FOR FUTURE RESEARCH

Music therapy is a highly effective tool to improve a range of goal areas with students with disabilities across a variety of domains. However, relative to other helping professions, music therapy is a young profession. Along with this youth come a relatively limited number of studies and many gaps in the literature. Based on the information presented in this chapter, the author's clinical and research experience, and recommendations made by music therapy researchers in the special education field, the following is a list of considerations for future research initiatives:

- Create research teams that are interdisciplinary and include clinical music therapists as investigators to find the answers to the most relevant questions.
- Replicate existing studies, particularly in various settings, with other demographics, and with larger samples to confirm previous findings.
- Conduct more meta-analyses and systematic reviews in an effort to synthesize the current literature, generalize results, and develop sound research initiatives.
- Improve scientific integrity of research designs and data analyses to increase validity and application of results.
- Include larger sample sizes to increase the power of studies, thus producing more conclusive outcomes.
- Submit manuscripts with study methods and data analyses reported with sufficient detail to allow for replication and successful clinical application.
- Disseminate research results more widely, including via continuing education, online platforms, fact sheets, podcasts, and social media.
- Further investigate the effect of music therapy on those with physical disabilities or limited motor skills.
- Conduct research in inclusive classroom environments to explore the mutual benefits for those with and without disabilities.

Music therapists work among multiple disciplinary teams serving students with disabilities in schools across the United States. Music therapy is federally supported, as it is recognized as a related service in the IEP (U.S. Department of Education, 2010a), and research over the past several decades suggests music therapy can help students reach their IEP goals (Brown & Jellison, 2012). As researchers, therapists, teachers, parents, and administrators aim to improve the educational outcomes in students with disabilities, music therapy services should be considered. MT-BCs commonly serve as consultants to the IEP team or provide direct services to students who are eligible for music therapy. Information on how to find a music therapist or how music therapy may benefit staff, students, and families can be found by visiting the Web sites of the Certification Board for Music Therapists (www.cbmt.org) and the American Music Therapy Association (www.musictherapy.org).

REFERENCES

Adamek, M. S., & Darrow, A. A. (2005). *Music in special education*. Silver Spring, MD: American Music Therapy Association, Inc.

Adamek, M., Darrow, A. A., & Jellison, J. (2014). Successful interdisciplinary communication in schools: Understanding important special education concepts and initiatives. *Imagine, 5*, 28–37.

American Music Therapy Association. (2016a). *AMTA member survey & workforce analysis*. Retrieved from https://netforum.avectra.com/eweb/Shopping/Shopping.aspx?Cart=0&Site=AMTA2&.

American Music Therapy Association. (2016b). *Strategic priority on research*. Retrieved from http://www.musictherapy.org/research/strategic_priority_on_research/overview/.

American Orff-Schulwerk Association. (2014a). *More on Orff Schulwerk*. Retrieved from http://aosa.org/about/more-on-orff-schulwerk/.

American Orff-Schulwerk Association. (2014b). *The teaching process*. Retrieved from http://aosa.org/about/what-is-orff-schulwerk/the-teaching-process/.

American Psychological Association. (2013). *Diagnostic and statistical manual of mental disorders* (5th ed.). Arlington, VA: American Psychiatric Publishing.

Baxter, H., Berghofer, J., MacEwan, L., Nelson, J., Peters, K., & Roberts, P. (2007). *The individualized music therapy assessment profile IMTAP*. Philadelphia, PA: Jessica Kingsley Press.

Bradfield, C., Carlenius, J., Gold, C., & White, M. (2007). *MT-SEAS: Music therapy special education assessment scale manual (a supplement to the SEMTAP)*. Grapevine, TX: Prelude Music Therapy.

Brownell, M. D. (2002). Musically adapted social stories to modify behaviors in students with autism: Four case studies. *Journal of Music Therapy, 39*, 117–144 http://dx.doi.org/10.1093/jmt/39.2.117.

Brownell, M. D. (2012). Social Stories™: Pairing the story with music. In P. Kern, & M. Humpal (Eds.), *Early childhood music therapy and autism spectrum disorders: Developing potential in young children and their families*. London and Philadelphia: Jessica Kingsley Publishers.

Brown, L. S., & Jellison, J. A. (2012). Music research with children and youth with disabilities and typically developing peers: A systematic review. *Journal of Music Therapy, 49*, 335–364 http://dx.doi.org/10.1093/jmt/49.3.335.

Buysse, V., & Wesley, P. W. (2006). *Evidence-based practice in the early childhood field*. Washington, DC: ZERO TO THREE.

Carpente, J. (2013). *IMCAP-ND a clinical manual: Individual music-centered assessment profile for neurodevelopmental disorders.* North Baldwin, NY: Regina Publishers.

Cohen, J. (1988). *Statistical power analysis for the behavioral sciences* (2nd ed.). Hillsdale, NJ: Lawrence Earlbaum Associates.

Coleman, K. A., & Brunk, B. K. (2003). *SEMTAP: Special education music therapy assessment process handbook* (2nd ed.). Grapevine, TX: Prelude Music Therapy.

Colwell, C. (2005). An Orff approach to music therapy. *The Orff Echo, 38*(1), 19–21.

Colwell, C. M., Achey Pehotsky, C., Gillmeister, G., & Woolrich, J. (2008). The Orff approach to music therapy. In A. A. Darrow (Ed.), *Introduction to approaches in music therapy* (2nd ed.). Silver Spring, MD: American Music Therapy Association, Inc.

Colwell, C. M., Edwards, R., Hernandez, E., & Brees, K. (2013). Impact of music therapy interventions (listening, composition, Orff-based) on the physiological and psychosocial behaviors of hospitalized children: A feasibility study. *Journal of Pediatric Nursing, 28*, 249–257. http://dx.doi.org/10.1016/j.pedn.2012.08.008.

DeLoach, D., & Detmer, M. R. (September 1, 2015). *Interdisciplinary versus transdisciplinary integrative care within music therapy for children with ASD.* Retrieved from http://imagine.musictherapy.biz/Imagine/podcasts/podcasts.html.

Detmer, M. R. (November 13, 2015). *Orff-based music therapy: Addressing anxiety and beyond.* Paper presented at the American Music Therapy Association conference, Kansas City, MO.

Doren, G. A. (1879). The status of the work- Ohio. In *Proceedings of the association of medical officers of the American institutions for idiotic and feebleminded persons. Sessions: Syracuse, June 8-12, 1878* (pp. 103-104). Philadelphia: J. B. Lippincott & Co.

Gooding, L. F. (2011). The effect of a music therapy social skills training program on improving social competence in children and adolescents with social skills deficits. *Journal of Music Therapy, 48*, 440–462. http://dx.doi.org/10.1093/jmt/48.4.440.

Gray, C. A. (1998). Social Stories™ and comic book conversations with students with Asperger syndrome and high-functioning autism. In E. Schopler, G. V. Mesibov, & L. J. Kunce (Eds.), *Asperger syndrome or high functioning autism?* (pp. 167–198). New York: Plenum Press.

Gray, C. A., & Garrand, J. (1993). Social Stories™: Improving responses of individuals with autism with accurate social information. *Focus on Autistic Behavior, 8*, 1–10.

Hilliard, R. E. (2007). The effects of Orff-based music therapy and social work groups on childhood grief symptoms and behaviors. *Journal of Music Therapy, 44*, 123–138. http://dx.doi.org/10.1093/jmt/44.2.123.

Humpal, M. E., & Colwell, C. (2006). *Effective clinical practice in music therapy: Early childhood and school age educational settings.* Silver Spring, MD: American Music Therapy Association.

Kern, P. (2010). Evidence-based practice in early childhood music therapy: A decision making process. *Music Therapy Perspectives, 29*, 91–98. http://dx.doi.org/10.1093/mtp/28.2.116.

Kern, P., Wolery, M., & Aldridge, D. (2007). Use of songs to promote independence in morning greeting routines for young children with autism. *Journal of Autism & Developmental Disorders, 37*, 1264–1271 http://dx.doi.org/10.1007/s10803-006-0271-1.

Klein, S. B., (2010). *Music therapy for school-aged individuals with varying exceptionalities: A content analysis (1975-2009).* (Unpublished doctoral dissertation). The Florida State University. Tallahassee, FL.

Montello, L. M., & Coons, E. E. (1998). Effect of active versus passive group music therapy on preadolescents with emotional, learning, and behavioral disorders. *Journal of Music Therapy, 35*, 49–67. http://dx.doi.org/10.1093/jmt/35.1.49.

Register, D. (2001). The effects of an early intervention music curriculum on pre-reading/writing. *Journal of Music Therapy, 38*, 239–248. http://dx.doi.org/10.1093/jmt/38.3.239.

Register, D., Darrow, A. A., Standley, J., & Swedberg, O. (2007). The use of music to enhance reading skills of second grade students and students with reading disabilities. *Journal of Music Therapy, 44*, 23–37. http://dx.doi.org/10.1093/jmt/44.1.23.

Rickson, D. J. (2006). Instructional and improvisational models of music therapy with adolescents who have attention deficit hyperactivity disorder (ADHD): A comparison of the effect on motor impulsivity. *Journal of Music Therapy, 48*, 39–62. http://dx.doi.org/10.1093/jmt/43.1.39.

Ritter-Cantesanu, G. (2014). Music therapy and the IEP process. *Music Therapy Perspectives, 32*, 142–152. http://dx.doi.org/10.1093/mtp/miu018.

Robb, S. (2003). Music interventions and group participation skills of preschoolers with visual impairments: Raising questions about music, arousal, and attention. *Journal of Music Therapy, 40*, 266–282. http://dx.doi.org/10.1093/jmt/40.4.266.

Scott, J. K. (2010). *Orff Schulwerk teacher educators' beliefs about singing* (Doctoral dissertation) University of Rochester. Retrieved from http://hdl.handle.net/1802/19349.

Shamrock, M. (1986). Orff Schulwerk: an integrated foundation. *Music Educators Journal, 72*(6), 51–55.

Snell, A. M. (2006). Definitions and characteristics of individuals served in early childhood and school age settings. In M. E. Humpal, & C. Colwell (Eds.), *Effective clinical practice in music therapy: Early childhood and school age educational settings.* (pp. 8–25). Silver Spring, MD: American Music Therapy Association.

Standley, J. M. (1996). A meta-analysis on the effects of music as reinforcement for education/therapy objectives. *Journal of Research in Music Education, 44*, 105–133. http://dx.doi.org/10.2307/3345665.

Standley, J. M. (2008). Does music instruction help children learn to read? Evidence of a meta-analysis. *Update:*

Applications of Research in Music Education, 27, 17–32. http://dx.doi.org/10.1177/8755123308322270.

Sussman, J. E. (2009). The effect of music on peer awareness in preschool age children with developmental disabilities. *Journal of Music Therapy, 46,* 53–68. http://dx.doi.org/10.1093/jmt/46.1.53.

U.S. Department of Education. (2006). *Individuals with disabilities education improvement act of 2004. Federal register. Rules and regulations.* Retrieved from https://www.gpo.gov/fdsys/pkg/FR-2006-08-14/pdf/06-6656.pdf.

U.S. Department of Education. (2010a). *Questions and answers on individualized education programs (IEPs), evaluations, and reevaluations [Brochure].* Retrieved from https://www2.ed.gov/policy/speced/guid/idea/iep-qa-2010.pdf.

U.S. Department of Education. (2010b). *Thirty-five years of progress in educating children with disabilities through IDEA.* Retrieved from. https://www2.ed.gov/about/offices/list/osers/idea-35-history/idea-35-history.pdf.

U.S. Department of Education. (2015). *The IDEA 40th anniversary.* Retrieved from https://www2.ed.gov/about/offices/list/osers/idea40/index.html.

U.S. Department of Education. (2016). *38th annual report to congress on the implementation of the Individuals with Disabilities Education Act.* Retrieved from. https://www2.ed.gov/about/reports/annual/osep/2016/parts-b-c/38th-arc-for-Idea.pdf.

Walworth, D., Register, D., & Engel, J. N. (2009). Using the SCERTS® Model assessment tool to identify music therapy goals for clients with autism spectrum disorder. *Journal of Music Therapy, 46,* 204–216. http://dx.doi.org/10.1093/jmt/46.3.204.

Whipple, J. (2012). Music therapy as an effective treatment with autism spectrum disorders in early childhood: A meta-analysis. In P. Kern, & M. Humpal (Eds.), *Early childhood music therapy and autism spectrum disorders: Developing potential in young children and their families* (pp. 59–76). London and Philadelphia: Jessica Kingsley Publishers.

Wolfe, D., & Hom, C. (1993). Use of melodies as structural prompts for learning and retention of sequential verbal information by preschool students. *Journal of Music Therapy, 30,* 100–118. http://dx.doi.org/10.1093/jmt/30.2.100.

CHAPTER 4

Music Therapy in Mental Health Treatment

LORI F. GOODING, PHD, MT-BC

Music therapy is an evidence-based discipline in which credentialed music therapists apply music interventions to facilitate individualized health and educational goals (American Music Therapy Association, 2014, 2016a). References to music as therapy first appeared in the 18th and 19th centuries, with much of the work focused on the use of music to alleviate mental distress (McCaffrey, 2015). Initially, music was provided for patients in asylums and hospitals across Germany, England, and the United States. By the mid-19th century, systematic uses of music had emerged, and interest in music as a form of therapy grew. During this period, music was promoted as a form of moral therapy, and the first systematic research and government-sponsored music programs were developed (American Music Therapy Association, 2016b; McCaffrey, 2015).

As interest in music as therapy grew, the term "music therapy" began to emerge in healthcare contexts. During the early 20th century, large-scale group music therapy programs for persons with mental illness were established in the United States, and by 1940 nearly 850 patients were involved in group music therapy sessions at Detroit's Eloise Hospital, a leading facility for mental healthcare in the United States (Davis, 2003). It was here at Eloise Hospital that psychiatrist Ira Altshuler, Director of Group Therapy, developed the first patient interaction guidelines for musicians working in institutional settings (Davis, 2003; McCaffrey, 2015). Music therapy continued to develop as a profession into the 1940s, as it was increasingly used to treat World War II GIs suffering from both physical and psychological injuries (Carroll, 2011; Davis, 2003; McCaffrey, 2015).

Early music therapy practice was closely connected with mental health treatment and guided by the medical model. Training for musicians was often provided by psychiatrists and included study of psychopathology, psychiatry, psychotherapies, and other therapies (McCaffrey, 2015). Relevant theories from psychotherapy were adopted into music therapy practice, and physiologic, psychological, and sociologic theoretic constructs

were used to explain the influence of music on human behavior (Choi, 2008). The term "music therapist" was adopted by individuals who applied these theories and principles (McCaffrey, 2015). It quickly became apparent, however, that more training was needed, and the demand for a college curriculum grew (American Music Therapy Association, 2016b; McCaffrey, 2015). This led to the establishment of the first music therapy degree programs in the 1940s, which was followed by the development of national certification standards in the 1980s (American Music Therapy Association, 2016b; Davis, 2003; McCaffrey, 2015). Today music therapy is defined as the "clinical and evidence-based use of music interventions to accomplish individualized goals within a therapeutic relationship by a credentialed professional who has completed an approved music therapy program" (American Music Therapy Association, 2016a, para. 1). Over 70 colleges and universities have music therapy degree programs, and the Certification Board for Music Therapists maintains accountability standards via national certification for approximately 7000 music therapists (American Music Therapy Association, 1998; Certification Board for Music Therapists, 2011). These music therapists work in a wide range of settings, including hospitals, hospices, rehabilitation facilities, skilled nursing, schools, and private practice, but individuals with mental healthcare needs remain the largest specific population served by music therapists (American Music Therapy Association, 2015; Certification Board for Music Therapists, 2011).

CHAPTER OVERVIEW

Many helping professionals use music experiences within the confines of their scope of practice, but clinical music therapy is a distinct, professional discipline in which credentialed music therapists actively apply supportive science to the use of music experiences for health treatment and educational goals (American Music Therapy Association, 2014). Because the distinction between therapeutic uses of music and music therapy is not always well known or understood, it is important to identify what music therapy is, the qualifications and competencies required for music therapy practice, and music therapy protocols that best meet the needs of the individuals served. The purpose of this chapter is to provide an overview of music therapy practices specific to mental health treatment. Populations served are identified, a summary of the research is provided, and descriptions of evidence-based practices (EBPs) are given. Information on provision of services is also included, as are considerations for future research. Finally, case examples are provided to illustrate these concepts.

OVERVIEW OF POPULATIONS SERVED

Children and Adolescents

Music therapists work with individuals from all age groups, although patients' diagnoses vary by age. Services for infants and young children are typically provided for individuals considered to be at risk for poor health, mental health, and academic outcomes (Abad & Williams, 2007; Oldfield & Bunce, 2001), whereas school-aged children and adolescents who receive music therapy as part of their mental health treatment present with a variety of disorders. Past data have suggested that children and adolescents with conduct disorder are most commonly referred to music therapy services, followed by children with adjustment and anxiety disorders (Cassity & Cassity, 1994; Goldbeck & Ellerkamp, 2012; Shuman, Kennedy, DeWitt, Edelblute, & Wamboldt, 2016). Other diagnoses and/or conditions found among children who receive music therapy services include eating disorders such as anorexia nervosa (McFerran, Baker, Patton, & Sawyer, 2006; Robarts & Sloboda, 1994), children identified as at risk (Gooding, 2011), mood disorders (Patterson et al., 2015; Shuman et al., 2016), personality disorders (Shuman et al., 2016), posttraumatic stress disorder (PTSD) (Gooding, 2011), psychotic disorders (Patterson et al., 2015), severe emotional disturbances (Layman, Hussey, & Laing, 2002; Montello & Coons, 1998), and substance use (Aletraris, Paino, Edmond, Roman, & Bride, 2014). Individuals with attention-deficit hyperactivity disorder (ADHD) and other neurodevelopmental disorders, such as autism spectrum disorder or intellectual disabilities, are also commonly seen in music therapy, although some of this work occurs in educational settings (Gooding, 2011; Jackson, 2003; McLaughlin & Adler, 2015; Reschke-Hernandez, 2011; Rickson & Watkins, 2003).

Adults

Adults served in music therapy typically present with severe and enduring mental illnesses (SEMIs) such as schizophrenia, other psychotic disorders, and/or bipolar disorder (Carr, Odell-Miller, & Priebe, 2013; Cassity & Cassity, 1994; Grocke, Bloch, & Castle, 2009). Individuals with other diagnoses are also served by music therapists, and those diagnoses may include anorexia nervosa (Robarts & Sloboda, 1994), anxiety (Zarate, 2016), depression (Maratos, Gold, Wang, & Crawford, 2008), dissociative disorders (Gleadhill & Ferris, 2010), personality disorders (Odell-Miller, 2011), PTSD (Bensimon, Amir, & Wolf, 2008), and substance use disorder or co-occurring substance use disorders and mental illness (Gardstrom, Bartkowski, Willenbrink, & Diestelkamp, 2013; Silverman, 2011). It should also be noted that individuals with conditions typically diagnosed in childhood (i.e., neurodevelopmental disorders) often receive or continue to receive services into adulthood (Clarkson & Killick, 2016).

Older Adults and Mixed-Age Populations

Older adults served in music therapy have diagnoses similar to those of adults, although some diagnoses appear to be more common among older adults (Hanser, 1990). Common diagnoses include depression (Ashida, 2000; Hanser & Thompson, 1994; Gold, Solli, Krüger, & Lie, 2009; Maratos et al., 2008) and neurocognitive disorders, such as Alzheimer disease and Parkinson disease (PD) (Elefant, Baker, Lotan, Lagesem, & Skeie, 2012; Hanser, Butterfield-Whitcomb, & Kawata, 2011; Raglio et al., 2008). Additional populations with mental health needs served by music therapists include individuals in forensic psychiatric facilities (Hakvoort, Bogaerts, Thaut, & Spreen, 2015), caregivers (Hanser et al., 2011), and medical patients with concomitant mental health issues (Rafieyan & Ries, 2007). Research has suggested that music therapists working in correctional psychiatry primarily serve adults of all ages (Codding, 2002) and that caregivers served include individuals who care for both children and adults (Hanser et al., 2011; Jacobsen, McKinney, & Holck, 2014). The literature concerning medical patients with concomitant mental illness is limited and has focused on adult examples, but there is a wide range of studies that address the use of music therapy to reduce anxiety in patients of all ages (Yinger & Gooding, 2015). For an overview of the diagnoses of individuals served by age, see Table 4.1.

SUMMARY OF THE RESEARCH

The music therapy research base in mental health is small, and the need for more high-quality research

TABLE 4.1
Overview of Common Diagnoses by Age Among Individuals Who Have Received Music Therapy Services in Mental Health Settings

	Young Children	Children	Adolescents	Adults	Older Adults
Adjustment disorders		X	X		
Anorexia nervosa		X	X	X	
Anxiety disorders		X	X	X	X
At risk	X	X			
Conduct disorder		X	X		
Dissociative disorder				X	
Mood disorders			X	X	X
Neurocognitive disorders (e.g., Alzheimer disease, PD)				X	X
Neurodevelopmental disorders (e.g., ADHD, ID)		X	X	X	
Personality disorders			X	X	X
PTSD		X	X	X	X
Psychotic disorders			X	X	X
Substance use/dual diagnosis/ co-occurring disorders			X	X	X

ADHD, attention-deficit hyperactivity disorder; *ID*, intellectual disabilities; *PD*, Parkinson disease; *PTSD*, posttraumatic stress disorder.

exists (Silverman, 2010a). However, emerging research has shown music therapy to be a promising intervention and has provided insight into both the efficacy and effectiveness of music therapy treatment. Neuroscientific and clinical studies have suggested that music can modulate a wide range of behavioral, cognitive, emotional, and psychophysiologic responses (Lin et al., 2011). In fact, research has suggested that (1) music training can be a strong stimulant for neuroplastic changes in both developing and adult brains; (2) music making couples perception and action; and (3) listening to and making music can provoke motion and emotion, increase communication and interaction, mediate emotion, and engage brain regions that might otherwise not be linked (Altenmüller & Schlaug, 2013). Nevertheless, it is not just the music itself that potentiates music therapy's effectiveness. Data have suggested that the purposeful and professional design in delivering music interventions combined with patient engagement (i.e., active music making) and therapist-patient interaction (i.e., the therapeutic relationship) contribute to music therapy's effectiveness (see Fig. 4.1). Simply listening to music does not appear to have the same benefits (Lin et al., 2011).

Music therapy has been recognized as a nonpharmacologic intervention with strong support (Jung & Newton, 2009), and previous research suggests that music therapy results in clinical improvement in individuals with various mental health needs (Lin et al., 2011). Music therapy has also been shown to be well tolerated in individuals with mental health needs (Lin et al., 2011; Kamioka et al., 2014) and has been shown to provide benefits for individuals when added to standard care. Music therapy has further been identified as a cost-effective treatment for patients with mental health needs (Gold et al., 2009; Lin et al., 2011; Ulrich, Houtmans, & Gold, 2007). Perhaps most importantly, at least one systematic review found no evidence of adverse effects with music therapy treatment (Kamioka et al., 2014).

Music therapy researchers have explored several outcome variables for patients with mental health needs. Music therapy has been shown to facilitate symptom management, increase the quality of life, and provide opportunities for emotional expression (Yinger & Gooding, 2014; Silverman, 2015). Data have suggested that music therapy can improve engagement, improve compliance, increase motivation, and improve

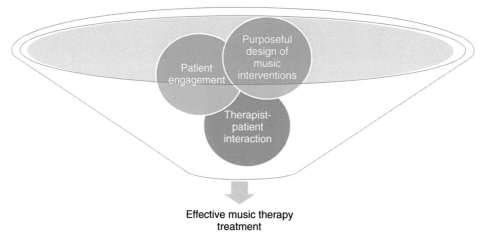

FIG. 4.1 Components of effective music therapy treatment in mental health.

attendance (Dingle, Gleadhill, & Baker, 2008; Silverman, 2015; Yinger & Gooding, 2014). Mood has been shown to be affected by music therapy, and this impact appears to be present regardless of gender, ethnicity, or diagnosis (Shuman et al., 2016). Likewise, global state and symptoms have been shown to improve among individuals participating in music therapy (Lin et al., 2011). Furthermore, patients have been shown to be receptive to music therapy services and view music therapy services as helpful (Goldberg, McNeil, & Binder, 1988; Silverman, 2015; Yinger & Gooding, 2014). Previous research has even indicated that group music therapy experiences in mental healthcare settings create an environment in which individuals' goals for recovery can be identified, explored, and practiced (MacDonald, 2015). Adherence to music therapy also appears to be high (Carr et al., 2013), and the data have suggested that patients are able to engage in music therapy regardless of the level of severity of their illness. Thus, a wide range of patients may benefit from music therapy services (Ross et al., 2008).

Music Therapy and Adult Consumers
Much of the music therapy research in mental healthcare is focused on adults. Systematic reviews and meta-analyses of adult populations have shown that music therapy is effective in reducing the symptoms of psychosis (Silverman, 2003a); improving the global state, mental state, and social functioning in individuals with schizophrenia and schizophrenia-like illnesses (Lin et al., 2011; Mössler, Chen, Heldal, & Gold, 2011); and reducing depressive symptoms (Maratos et al., 2008; Zhao, Bai, Bo, & Chi, 2016). Music therapy treatment has also been shown to be effective in promoting

self-esteem and social functioning among adult offenders in correctional facilities (Chen, Leith, Aarø, Manger, & Gold, 2016) and in improving the quality of life of individuals with severe mental illness (Grocke et al., 2014). Previous research has further suggested that music therapy is an effective treatment in substance use disorder treatment programs, particularly in terms of engaging and motivating clients. Some data have even indicated that music therapy is perceived as less threatening and intrusive than traditional therapies (Silverman, 2003b). Music therapy interventions have likewise been used with military personnel suffering from PTSD, with results showing reductions in PTSD symptoms (Bensimon et al., 2008; Bensimon, Amir, & Wolf, 2012; Blake & Bishop, 1994) and that music therapy techniques have been accepted by veterans (Garrison, 2016). Finally, music therapy has been shown to counteract isolation, facilitate positive mood changes, decrease stress and anxiety, and decrease impulsivity (Baker, Gleadhill, & Dingle, 2007).

Music Therapy and Older Adult Consumers
Much of the literature on music therapy with adults includes adults of varying ages, but there are some data specific to conditions primarily associated with older adults. For example, music therapy techniques have been shown to be effective in managing agitation and other behavioral and psychological symptoms in older adults with dementia (Livingston et al., 2014; Ueda, Suzukamo, Sato, & Izumi, 2013). Music therapy has further resulted in an improved quality of life, improved mood and anxiety, and improved emotional functions in individuals with PD (Raglio, 2015). Older adults with depression have also been shown to benefit from music

therapy services when added to standard care (Kun, Bai, Bo, & Chi, 2016), and older adults with symptoms of depression, distress, and anxiety who participated in a music-facilitated psychoeducation strategy performed significantly better than control group participants on standardized tests of depression, distress, self-esteem, and mood. Equally as important, these clinically significant improvements were maintained over a 9-month follow-up period (Hanser & Thompson, 1994).

Music Therapy and Child/Adolescent Consumers

Research on music therapy with children and adolescents with mental health needs is somewhat limited; however, this is consistent with treatment effectiveness data for this population in general (Porter et al., 2017). A systematic review of children and adolescents with psychopathology revealed a medium to large effect for music therapy on clinically relevant outcomes (Gold, Voracek, & Wigram, 2004). Results of this review also indicated that music therapy was equally effective for both children and adolescents. Modest improvements have also been found in terms of self-esteem among children and adolescents participating in music therapy (Porter et al., 2017). Likewise, improvements in social functioning have been found among children and adolescents with a variety of diagnoses who participated in music therapy (Gooding, 2011). Music therapy has contributed to improvements in joint attention among children with autism spectrum disorders (Kim, Wigram, & Gold, 2008), as well as improvements in depression symptoms (Hendricks, Robinson, Bradley, & Davis, 1999; Porter et al., 2017). In addition, music therapy treatment for children with ADHD has been perceived as favorable (Jackson, 2003), and boys diagnosed with behavioral and/or emotional disorders who participated in music therapy showed gains in social interaction, self-regulation, attitude toward school/work, academic progress, and self-awareness (McIntyre, 2007).

Music Therapy and Well-Being/Wellness

Music therapy techniques for well-being and wellness constitute another area in the mental health research literature, and perhaps one of the largest areas addressed is the use of music to manage stress and facilitate relaxation. Music listening has been promoted as a way to facilitate stress management and relaxation (Krout, 2007), and music added to relaxation techniques has been shown to be a highly effective tool for promoting relaxation. In fact, one study examined a range of relaxation techniques and found that music-assisted relaxation resulted in the largest improvements (Robb, 2000). Furthermore,

a meta-analysis conducted by Pelletier (2004) found that music was effective in decreasing arousal caused by stress. Another study found that cognitive-behavioral music therapy groups significantly impacted burnout among teachers, with the authors concluding that music therapy was an effective strategy for dealing with stress (Cheek, Bradley, Parr, & Lan, 2003). Recreational music making, particularly in the form of group drumming, has also been shown to affect the stress response and reduce burnout when led by music therapists or trained facilitators (Bittman et al., 2001; Bittman, Bruhn, Stevens, Westengard, & Umbach, 2003). Finally, older adults who participated in a music therapy-informed piano-based group music program gained both cognitive and stress reduction benefits, which may contribute to successful aging (Yinger, McVay, & Gooding, 2016).

Music Therapy Approaches/Techniques

Individuals using music therapy for well-being do not necessarily have a diagnosable mental illness but do face situations in which stress, depression, anxiety, or other factors negatively affect their quality of life and well-being (Grocke, 2009). For many of these individuals, music therapy techniques have been shown to help them find balance and/or lead more fulfilling lives. For example, the Bonny Method of Guided Imagery and Music (GIM), a process or approach of music-centered psychotherapy in which music experiences are used to bring about therapeutic change, has been used to address disenfranchised grief (Grocke, 2009). Likewise, music therapy interventions or techniques, such as music listening, singing, music-based life review, music-assisted relaxation, active music making, lyric analysis, composition, and music discussion, have been provided for patient/family emotional support for individuals and their families receiving hospice care (Gallagher, Huston, Nelson, Walsh, & Steele, 2001; Liu, Burns, Hilliard, Stump, & Unroe, 2015). In addition, music may serve as a tool to relieve occupational stress. According to a study conducted by Smith (2008), a single session of music-assisted relaxation resulted in significant reductions in anxiety levels. The author concluded that music-assisted relaxation may be used effectively in occupational environments where employees experience high anxiety levels to prevent stress and associated medical complications.

DESCRIPTION OF EVIDENCE-BASED PRACTICES

EBP enables clinicians to provide the highest quality of care by basing treatment decisions on the best available research, clinical expertise, and patients' values (Duke University Medical Center Library & UNC Health Sciences Library, 2016). The use of EBP in mental healthcare has grown, as has the need for and development of EBPs in music therapy. This has led to calls for both improved research and the further development of EBP within the field of music therapy (Silverman, 2012). Strategies for adopting EBP specifically within mental health treatment have also been generated.

Music Therapy–Specific Evidence-Based Practices

Evidence-based music therapy practice aims to provide quality music therapy services responsibly and responsively (Abrams, 2010). To do this, music therapists use the best available scientific evidence integrated with clinical expertise and patient values to select and implement music interventions that promote health in the individuals that they serve. A growing body of research has identified a variety of music therapy practices that have been deemed effective in meeting the needs of those with a mental illness.

When using music therapy to combat the symptoms of psychosis, both live and recorded music have been found to be effective, as have structured music activities and music as a form of distraction. Likewise, both active (patients actively participate, usually by playing or singing) and passive (patients listen to music) music therapy interventions have been found to be effective (Mössler, Chen, Heldal, & Gold, 2011). Patient-preferred and therapist-selected music have both been found to be helpful (Silverman, 2003a), although the data have suggested that nonclassical music is more effective than classical music. Patients with SEMIs, such as schizophrenia, also appear to benefit from greater doses of music therapy treatment, indicating a dose-response relationship (Mössler et al., 2011). Furthermore, those with severe mental illnesses seem to benefit from structured music therapy approaches (Gold et al., 2009).

For patients with low motivation, reproductive music therapy techniques have been identified as effective. Reproductive techniques involve the client and therapist playing or singing precomposed pieces of music and learning or practicing musical skills (Mössler, Assmus, Heldal, Fuchs, & Gold, 2012). For individuals with dementia, singing appears to be an effective intervention for reducing anxiety (Ueda et al., 2013). For children with emotional or behavioral disorders, active music therapy interventions have been found to be effective, particularly in terms of developing focused, sustained attention (Gold et al., 2004).

Finally, preferred music has been shown to reduce agitation in adults with dementia and may provide a cost-effective alternative to chemical and physical restraints (Sung & Chang, 2005).

Specific techniques

In addition to the broad guidance provided in the literature, there are also data to support more specific music therapy practices. As mentioned previously, music therapy interventions and techniques can be broadly divided into *active* and *passive* strategies. From there, the interventions can be further divided based on the type of musical and relational experience they create between the therapist and consumer. *Production techniques* focus on emotional expression and musical improvisation. *Reproduction techniques* focus on playing or singing precomposed music. *Reception techniques* (also known as receptive techniques) include listening to live or recorded music; these techniques are used to increase awareness or promote relaxation (Carr et al., 2013; Mössler et al., 2012). These music therapy techniques are applied systematically and integrated with psychotherapeutic techniques to facilitate change (Gooding, 2017; Mössler et al., 2012).

Specific interventions

Songwriting is a common intervention found in the psychiatric music therapy literature (Baker, Wigram, Stott, & McFerran, 2009), with both unstructured (e.g., brainstorming) and structured (e.g., fill-in-the-blank) formats used. Songwriting is the "process of creating, notating and/or recording lyrics and music by the client or clients and therapist within a therapeutic relationship to address psychosocial, emotional, cognitive, and communication needs of the client" (Wigram & Baker, 2005, p. 16). Songwriting in music therapy is frequently accompanied by verbal processing (Carr et al., 2013), and data suggest that the verbal processing plays an essential therapeutic role (Gooding, 2017). In fact, Carr et al. (2013) conducted a systematic review of music therapy practice and outcomes with acute adult psychiatric inpatients and found that verbal processing was used in the majority of studies reviewed.

Lyric analysis is another commonly used intervention in mental health settings. Lyric analysis, also known as song discussion, involves a detailed examination of the elements or structure of a song as the basis for discussion or interpretation (Dvorak, 2016). Although musical elements are included, the focus of the discussion is on the lyrics themselves with the purpose of promoting changes in thinking, increasing awareness, or facilitating insight. Like songwriting, lyric analysis incorporates verbal processing (Gooding, 2017).

TABLE 4.2	Music Therapy Interventions/Techniques Commonly Used in Mental Health Treatment	
Intervention	**Description**	**Related Literature**
Drum circles	Playing percussion instruments in a group format	Gallagher and Steele (2002) and Lipe et al. (2011)
Improvisation	Client makes up her/his own music spontaneously using voice or instruments. Improvisation can be alone, with the therapist, or with other clients. The structure may be free or structured by the therapist	Sabbatella (2004) and Erkkilä et al. (2011)
Lyric analysis	Detailed examination of the elements or structure of a song as the basis for discussion or interpretation	Dvorak (2016) and Jones (2005)
Music and art	Music paired with drawing, painting, and making collages. Making musical instruments may also be included	Lipe et al. (2011)
Music-assisted relaxation	Music paired with relaxation techniques, such as verbal suggestion, breathing exercises, and imagery	Pelletier (2004)
Music games/ recreational music therapy	Music-based games and recreational activities	Silverman and Leonard (2012) and Silverman and Rosenow (2013)
Songwriting	Creating, notating, and/or recording lyrics and music by the client or clients and therapist	Baker et al. (2009) and Grocke et al. (2009)
Sing-along	Live singing of patient-preferred music	Silverman and Leonard (2012)

Other interventions cited in the music therapy literature include improvisation, drum circles, sing-alongs, Bonny Method of GIM, music games/recreational music therapy, music and movement, music and art, music and dance, and music-assisted relaxation (Silverman, 2007). Results from a 2007 survey conducted by Silverman indicated that the three most utilized music therapy interventions in mental health treatment were improvisation, sing-alongs, and lyric analysis. Likewise, the three most used interventions in the treatment of individuals with substance use disorders were lyric analysis, music-assisted relaxation, and improvisation/music and art (tied) (Silverman, 2009). Therapist orientation, setting characteristics (e.g., model, facility type), and patient functioning level all appear to mediate music therapists' choices about service delivery, including interventions or techniques implemented (Carr et al., 2013; Silverman, 2007). So too does patient length of stay and group structure (open, semiclosed, or closed) (Carr et al., 2013). It should be noted, however, that contraindications do occur for some interventions in relation to specific diagnoses. For example, music-assisted imagery (a type of music-assisted relaxation) should not be used when clients demonstrate active psychotic symptoms (Gallagher & Steele, 2002).

As with songwriting and lyric analysis, the music interventions mentioned earlier are selected to address specific patient needs, and one intervention may serve to address multiple needs. For example, instrument play (e.g., drum circle) may be used to develop leadership skills, create group cohesiveness, or promote interaction. Likewise, music games may be used to increase engagement and motivation (Gallagher & Steele, 2002). Common objectives found in the music therapy literature include increased socialization, increased communication skills, emotional expression, decision making, development of coping skills, stress management, and self-esteem development (Silverman, 2007, 2009). For more information on the most commonly used music therapy interventions in mental health treatment, see Table 4.2. The related literature for each intervention/ technique is provided, and the reader is encouraged to consult the texts for additional information. In addition, readers are encouraged to consult Gallagher and Steele (2002) for clear and concise descriptions of many of the music therapy interventions listed previously.

Integrating Music Therapy Into Evidence-Based Mental Health Treatments

Silverman (2010b, 2015), a leading researcher in psychiatric music therapy, outlined six evidence-based treatments for individuals with severe mental illnesses (assertive community treatment, integrated dual-disorder treatment [IDDT], family-based psychoeducation, illness management and recovery, medication management, and supported employment). He then identified ways in which music therapy could be integrated into the models. Suggestions included (1) use of music therapy as a diagnostic tool, (2) use of music therapy to identify triggers among individuals who use substances, (3) use of music therapy to address employment-related skills such as interpersonal skills, (4) use of music therapy to teach illness information or coping skills, (5) use of music therapy in family treatment to reduce stigma, and (6) use of music therapy to address medication management. Because of its flexibility, music therapy may be effectively integrated into the above-mentioned models, especially when collaboration occurs (Silverman, 2010b). However, current data suggest music therapy has most often been applied to illness management and recovery and IDDT (Silverman, 2010b). In fact, one survey found that 76% of music therapists focused on coping skills, a component of illness management and recovery, whereas 42% of music therapists who work in mental health addressed substance use, a component of IDDT (Silverman, 2007).

CASE EXAMPLES

The following clinical case examples illustrate music therapy services provided for individuals who had been admitted to inpatient acute care settings for crisis stabilization or detoxification. All services were provided in an open group format and were age or unit based. (Open groups are groups in which members can join at any time; age- and unit-based groups are formed based on patients' age or treatment unit, respectively.) Child and adolescent groups were further divided by the level of functioning. Patients' diagnoses varied but were consistent with the diagnoses presented in Table 4.1. Music therapy services were integrated into an illness management and recovery model, otherwise known as psychosocial rehabilitation, psychoeducation, or psychiatric rehabilitation. This model focuses on:

- psychoeducation,
- strategies for addressing medication nonadherence,
- relapse prevention training to reduce symptoms and hospitalizations, and
- coping skills training to reduce distress and/or symptom severity using cognitive-behavioral techniques (Silverman, 2010b).

Data collected from music therapists working in mental health settings appear to suggest that the illness management and recovery model is compatible with music therapy practice. In fact, many music therapists report the implementation of psychoeducation and coping skills training (Eyre & Lee, 2015; Silverman, 2010b). However, it is important to remember that music therapy implementation varies based on therapist orientation, facility models, and patients' needs and level of functioning; thus, these examples are meant to be representative of the author's own practice. Examples are based on actual cases, but names and other identifying information have been changed to protect individuals' privacy.

Example 1: Coping Skills Development for Adolescents Aged 11 to 15 Years

Adolescents with depression, anxiety, conduct disorder, and other mental illnesses were admitted to a hospital-based inpatient unit for stabilization. Patient stays were typically brief (3 to 5 days), so sessions functioned as single units. Given the brief timeline, music games, songwriting, psychoeducation, and coping skills training were typically implemented within an illness management and recovery model. This approach and the interventions selected are consistent with the literature on music therapy in acute care settings (Eyre & Lee, 2015).

At the start of the session, the music therapist (MT) introduced herself and explained what music therapy was. Each group member then shared their name and one type of music/musical artist they liked. The patients' preferred music was then incorporated into a musical game in which group members passed a ball while music played. When the music stopped, the individual holding the ball identified one thing she or he did well and one thing she or he wanted to work on during their admission.

After completing the introductory activity, the therapist led a brief discussion about coping skills. Coping skills were defined, and the group discussed why and when they were used. Group members were encouraged to provide examples of skills that they had used in the past. The group then discussed deep breathing as a coping skill to manage anger and/or anxiety. The therapist led the group members through deep breathing exercises, first breathing only and then breathing while playing a steady beat on tubano drums. (Tubano drums are tube shaped drums with feet that can be comfortably played while seated.) Following the breathing exercises, group members were asked to identify situations in which they might use the breathing strategy. One group member shared that she could use the breathing when she was "angry at her mom," whereas another shared that it might help when trying to sleep.

After the breathing exercises, group members were given the opportunity to provide self-statements for cognitive coping. Group members were asked to recall the things that they stated that they did well at the beginning of the group and turn them into statements designed to reinforce their ability to cope. Alternatively, they could create statements about other positive coping skills or phrases that would help them focus on coping. Each person then wrote their statement on a note card and volunteers chanted the statement while keeping a steady beat on the drum. The group then joined in, repeating each self-statement while playing the drums. Patients' statement included "I can ask for help," "I am valuable," and "I'm in charge of me." Group members were encouraged to use the self-statements independently or in conjunction with deep breathing and asked to practice the skills outside of the session.

At the completion of the session, the therapist summarized the discussion and encouraged the group members to put their cards where they could read them. The session concluded with the therapist again playing patient-preferred music.

Example 2: Coping Skills Development for Adults Aged 18 Years and Up

Adults with varying diagnoses were admitted to a hospital-based inpatient unit for stabilization. This unit offered services for adults with affective, anxiety, personality, or thought disorders and/or addictive diseases. Short-term crisis stabilization was the primary goal of treatment, and patients often had coexisting medical and/or surgical needs. Treatment approaches included recreational therapy, music therapy, and group therapy. Family and individual sessions were also available. Like the adolescent example, an illness management and recovery model served as the foundation for music therapy services. Patients were generally admitted for short-term stays, thereby limiting access to music therapy services. Thus, treatment engagement and coping skills training were the focus of most sessions. Techniques and/or interventions used included music-assisted relaxation, song writing, lyric analysis, singing, and instrument play, among others. This approach and the interventions selected are consistent with the literature on music therapy in acute care settings (Eyre & Lee, 2015), as well as with services provided for substance use disorders (Silverman, 2003b).

At the start of the session, the MT introduced herself and explained what music therapy was. Group members then introduced themselves, shared one unique thing about themselves, and shared what they wanted to work on during their hospital admission. Following the introductions, the therapist played a recording of the song "I'm Movin' On" written by White and Williams and recorded by Rascal Flatts in 2000. Group members were provided with lyric sheets and asked to mark passages that stood out to them as they listened to the recording. Once the recording was completed, group members participated in lyric analysis, discussing passages that were relevant to their own lives. The therapist used song lyrics to facilitate open-ended questions and linked group members' comments to encourage discussion. One group member, a young mother-to-be who was admitted for detoxification, shared that the line "I know there's no guarantees, but I'm not alone" was meaningful for her. She shared that now that she was going to be a mother she needed to "move on" in order to make healthy choices for herself and her baby. Another group member, an older male, stated that he, like the songwriter, felt "trapped in the past" and "burdened with blame." The therapist then pointed out the line "for once I'm at peace with myself" and asked the group what changes the songwriter made to find this peace. This was followed by asking the group members what changes they would need to make to "move on" in terms of recovery from their illness. Group members were given worksheets and asked to identify at least one specific item or behavior and one positive coping skill that could support their journey. After being given the chance to share their thoughts, members were again directed to the song and reminded that the songwriter packed his bags and moved "down this road." Recovery and/or illness management were then compared to a road, and one group member stated that hospitalization was, for him, the first step to moving "down this road." The therapist then reminded the members what they had shared at the beginning of the session in terms of what they were working on while hospitalized and asked them how that would help them move on.

After completing the discussion, the therapist summarized the discussion and encouraged the group members to put their worksheets where they could read them. The session concluded with the therapist again playing the recording.

PROVISION OF SERVICES

Music therapy is an adjunct therapy, often embedded within the therapeutic milieu and offered in combination with traditional psychotherapies and psychopharmacologic interventions (Shuman et al., 2016). In the United States, music therapists must, at a minimum, complete a bachelor's degree or its equivalent in music therapy, although previous research has shown that most music therapists who work in mental health settings have advanced degrees (Silverman, 2007, 2012). Services are provided in a variety of mental or behavioral health settings, including hospitals, inpatient or residential facilities, community health centers, substance use rehabilitation programs, forensic facilities, and private practice (American Music Therapy Association, 2006; Silverman, 2007). Group music therapy is the predominant modality, with music therapy services generally provided in mixed group formats (Carr et al., 2013; Codding, 2002), although individual sessions are not uncommon (Carr et al., 2013; Silverman, 2007). Both group and individual sessions typically last 30 to 45+ min, which is consistent with the 45- to 50-min therapy hour (Silverman, 2007).

According to a survey conducted by Silverman (2007), the majority (~62%) of music therapists lead sessions independently, with fewer than 30% cofacilitating with other therapists. Patients can be referred to music therapy services via several different ways, and the process is often facility or population specific. Referral avenues may include patient self-referral, music therapist referral, referral by other professional, or programmatic referrals (all patients receive services) (Codding, 2002). Music therapists commonly conduct assessments and document on participants' progress. In terms of interprofessional collaboration, music therapists have cited collaborations with other therapists (e.g., speech language pathologists, occupational therapists, physical therapists, recreation therapists), creative arts therapists, social workers, mental health professionals, medical personnel, and clergy (Register, 2002). The research has suggested that music therapists who participate in team meetings believe that participation improves the quality of care for the individuals that they serve (Eyre & Lee, 2015). Furthermore, music therapists have also found that active communication with other members of the multidisciplinary or interprofessional team maximizes patient access and staff support (Carr et al., 2013).

Music therapists practice from a variety of theoretic orientations. Eclectic, cognitive-behavioral, behavioral, and humanistic orientations have been identified as the most common in the United States, and these are often paired with music therapy approaches, such as GIM, Orff, and Neurologic Music Therapy (Codding, 2002; Silverman, 2007). Community music therapy, which integrates community, culture, and context and focuses on mobilizing resources to promote well-being (Ghetti, 2016), and resource-oriented music therapy, which focuses on strengths while also addressing problems and strives to empower individuals through collaboration (Rolvsjord, 2010), have both gained recognition in recent years, particularly outside of the United States. However, information on community music therapy and resource-oriented music therapy in the United States is somewhat

limited, perhaps because of healthcare administrators' perceptions of the role that music therapy plays in healthcare (Ghetti, 2016).

In addition to the theoretic orientations and music therapy approaches practiced by music therapists, several models or treatment approaches specific to mental health treatment are often integrated into music therapy practice; examples include recovery-oriented care, 12 Step, transdiagnostic theory, and psychoeducation (Silverman, 2009, 2015; Solli, Rolvsjord, & Borg, 2013). Dual Diagnosis Recovery Counseling, GORSKI-CENAPS Model for Recovery and Relapse Prevention, and Motivation Enhancement have also been cited among therapists who work with individuals with substance use disorders (Silverman, 2009). This typically occurs in response to the models and systems used within the institutional settings themselves as well as in response to the predominating models of training and service provision within specific countries or regions (Carr et al., 2013)

Areas for Future Research

The music therapy profession is still a developing field, both in terms of clinical work and research. Music therapy does, however, have the most developed research base of all the creative arts therapies (Stuckey & Nobel, 2010). Yet more work is still needed, and the need for higher quality research has been identified.

Music therapy research is complex and often must balance the need for diagnosis-specific outcomes with transdiagnostic applications (Pedersen, 2014; Silverman, 2010a). Music therapy research related to mental health outcomes is also complicated by the number of factors associated with service provision, e.g., group treatment. Music as an independent variable also complicates research, as do therapist demographics. Perhaps even more importantly, the limited number of professionals who conduct research in the psychiatric music therapy arena has contributed to an undersized research base (Eyre & Lee, 2015; Silverman, 2008). Like other forms of treatment, music therapy must provide evidence of effectiveness to support reimbursement for treatment. Therefore, it is imperative that we develop high-quality, scientific, replicable, and controlled studies; find ways to better train researchers; and translate this research into clinical practice (Gooding, 2016; Meadows, 2016; Silverman, 2010b).

Specific suggestions

Scholars have identified several recommendations for music therapy research in mental health. Future studies should (1) explore underlying mechanisms that result in music therapy's effectiveness, (2) expand methodologies to include mixed-methods designs, (3) incorporate theory-based research, (4) improve reporting guidelines, and (5) develop more child and adolescent studies. Studies should also (1) explore patient characteristics that may act as covariates or confounding variables, (2) explore therapists' demographic information and its impact on treatment effectiveness, (3) explore the relationship between patient variables and treatment effectiveness, (4) address issues pertinent to contemporary practice, such as dose, specific outcome measures, and service provision parameters such as group-based treatment, and (5) explore specific interventions, differences in passive versus active music therapy, and differences in the use of live versus recorded music (Silverman, 2015; Yinger & Gooding, 2015). The aforementioned elements should be addressed via randomized controlled trials with large sample sizes and longer duration (Maratos et al., 2008). By improving the music therapy research base in mental health, we can improve treatment quality and access for individuals served.

CONCLUSION

Music therapy has been successfully implemented with both children and adults in a wide range of settings. It has been shown to be a flexible treatment modality and to be able to promote wellness as well as address the needs of those with SEMIs. Music therapy appears to have limited adverse side effects, is well tolerated, and is cost-effective. Equally as important, data have suggested that music therapists can, through the use of both passive and active interventions such as improvisation and lyric analysis, improve engagement, improve compliance, increase motivation, and improve attendance. Although more research is needed on music therapy, it is a promising modality for meeting the needs of those with mental illness.

REFERENCES

Abad, V., & Williams, K. (2007). Early intervention music therapy: Reporting on a 3-year project to address needs with at-risk families. *Music Therapy Perspectives, 25,* 52–58. http://dx.doi.org/10.1093/mtp/25.1.52.

Abrams, B. (2010). Evidence-based music therapy practice: An integral understanding. *Journal of Music Therapy, 47,* 351–379. http://dx.doi.org/10.1093/jmt/47.4.351.

Aletraris, L., Paino, M., Edmond, M. B., Roman, P. M., & Bride, B. E. (2014). The use of art and music therapy in substance abuse treatment programs. *Journal of Addictions Nursing, 25,* 190–196. http://dx.doi.org/10.1097/JAN.0000000000000048.

Altenmüller, E., & Schlaug, G. (2013). Neurobiological aspects of neurologic music therapy. *Music and Medicine, 5,* 210–216. http://dx.doi.org/10.1177/1943862113505328.

American Music Therapy Association. (1998). *Organization directory search.* Retrieved from https://netforum.avectra.com/eweb/DynamicPage.aspx?Site=AMTA2&WebCode=OrgSearch&.

American Music Therapy Association. (2006). *Music therapy and mental health.* Retrieved from http://www.musictherapy.org/assets/1/7/MT_Mental_Health_2006.pdf.

American Music Therapy Association. (2014). *Setting the record straight: What music therapy is and is not.* Retrieved from http://www.musictherapy.org/amta_press_release_on_music_therapy_-_jan_2014/.

American Music Therapy Association. (2015). *2015 Member survey and workforce analysis.* Retrieved from www.musictherapy.org.

American Music Therapy Association. (2016a). *What is music therapy?* Retrieved from http://www.musictherapy.org/.

American Music Therapy Association. (2016b). *History of music therapy.* Retrieved from http://www.musictherapy.org/about/history/.

Ashida, S. (2000). The effect of reminiscence music therapy session on changes in depressive symptoms in elderly persons with dementia. *Journal of Music Therapy, 37,* 170–182. http://dx.doi.org/10.1093/jmt/37.3.170.

Baker, F. A., Gleadhill, L. M., & Dingle, G. A. (2007). Music therapy and emotional exploration: exposing substance abuse clients to the experiences of non-drug induced emotions. *The Arts in Psychotherapy, 34,* 321–330. http://dx.doi.org/10.1016/j.aip.2007.04.005.

Baker, F. A., Wigram, T., Stott, D., & McFerran, K. (2009). Therapeutic songwriting in music therapy, Part II: Comparing the literature with practice across diverse clinical populations. *Nordic Journal of Music therapy, 18,* 32–56. http://dx.doi.org/10.1080/08098130802496373.

Bensimon, M., Amir, D., & Wolf, Y. (2008). Drumming through trauma: music therapy with post-traumatic soldiers. *The Arts in Psychotherapy, 35,* 34–48. http://dx.doi.org/10.1016/j.aip.2007.09.002.

Bensimon, M., Amir, D., & Wolf, Y. (2012). A pendulum between trauma and life: group music therapy with post-traumatized soldiers. *The Arts in Psychotherapy, 39,* 223–233. http://dx.doi.org/10.1016/j.aip.2012.03.005.

Bittman, B. B., Berk, L. S., Felten, D. L., Westengard, J., Simonton, O. C., Pappas, J. & Ninehouser, M. (2001). Composite effects of group drumming music therapy on modulation of neuroendocrine-immune parameters. *Alternative Therapies in Health and Medicine, 7,* 38–47.

Bittman, B., Bruhn, K. T., Stevens, C., Westengard, J., & Umbach, P. O. (2003). Recreational music-making: a cost-effective group interdisciplinary strategy for reducing burnout and improving mood states in long-term care workers. *Advances, 19,* 4–15.

Blake, R. L., & Bishop, S. R. (1994). Special feature: The Bonny method of guided imagery (GIM) in the treatment of post-traumatic stress disorder (PTSD) with adults in the psychiatric setting. *Music Therapy Perspectives, 12,* 125–129. http://dx.doi.org/10.1093/mtp/12.2.125.

Carr, C., Odell-Miller, H., & Priebe, S. (2013). A systematic review of music therapy practice and outcomes with acute adult psychiatric in-patients. *PLoS One, 8*(8), e70252. http://dx.doi.org/10.1371/journal.pone.0070252.

Carroll, D. C. (2011). Historical roots of music therapy: a brief overview. *Revista do Núcleo de Estudos e Pesquisas Interdisciplinares em Musicoterapia, 2,* 171–178. Retrieved from http://www.fap.pr.gov.br/arquivos/File/extensao/Arquivos2011/NEPIM/NEPIM_Volume_02/Tra01_NEPIM_Vol02_Historical Roots.pdf.

Cassity, M. D., & Cassity, J. (1994). Psychiatric music therapy assessment and treatment in clinical training facilities with adults, adolescents, and children. *Journal of Music Therapy, 31,* 2–30. http://dx.doi.org/10.1093/jmt/31.1.2.

Certification Board for Music Therapists. (2011). *The certification board for music therapists.* Retrieved from http://www.cbmt.org/.

Cheek, J. R., Bradley, L., Parr, G., & Lan, W. (2003). Using music therapy techniques to treat teacher burnout. *Journal of Mental Health Counseling, 25,* 204–217. http://dx.doi.org/10.17744/mehc.25.3.ghneva55qw5xa3wm.

Chen, X. J., Leith, H., Aarø, L. E., Manger, T., & Gold, C. (2016). Music therapy for improving mental health problems of offenders in correctional settings: systematic review and meta-analysis. *Journal of Experimental Criminology, 12,* 209–228. http://dx.doi.org/10.1007/s11292-015-9250-y.

Choi, B. C. (2008). Awareness of music therapy practices and factors influencing specific theoretical approaches. *Journal of Music Therapy, 45,* 93–109. http://dx.doi.org/10.1093/jmt/45.1.93.

Clarkson, A. R., & Killick, M. (2016). A bigger picture: community music therapy groups in residential settings for people with learning disabilities. *Voices: A World Forum for Music Therapy, 16*(3). Retrieved from https://voices.no/index.php/voices/article/view/845.

Codding, P. A. (2002). A comprehensive survey of music therapists practicing in correctional psychiatry: demographics, conditions of employment, service provision, assessment, therapeutic objectives, and related values of the therapist. *Music Therapy Perspectives, 20,* 56–68. http://dx.doi.org/10.1093/mtp/20.2.56.

Davis, W. B. (2003). Ira Maximillian Altshuler: psychiatrist and pioneer music therapist. *Journal of Music Therapy, 40,* 247–263. http://dx.doi.org/10.1093/jmt/40.3.247.

Dingle, G. A., Gleadhill, L., & Baker, F. A. (2008). Can music therapy engage patients in group cognitive behavior therapy for substance abuse treatment? *Drug and Alcohol Review, 27,* 190–196. http://dx.doi.org/10.1080/09595230701829371.

Duke University Medical Center Library & UNC Health Sciences Library. (2016). *What is evidence-based practice?* Retrieved from http://guides.mclibrary.duke.edu/c.php?g=158201&p=1036021.

Dvorak, A. L. (2016). A conceptual framework for group processing of lyric analysis interventions in music therapy mental health practice. *Music Therapy Perspectives.* Advance online publication. http://dx.doi.org/10.1093/mtp/miw018.

Elefant, C., Baker, F. A., Lotan, M., Lagesem, S. K., & Skeie, G. O. (2012). The effect if group music therapy on mood, speech, and singing in individuals with Parkinson's disease—A feasibility study. *Journal of Music Therapy, 49,* 278–302. http://dx.doi.org/10.1093/jmt/49.3.278.

Erkkilä, J., Punakanen, M., Fachner, J., Ala-Ruona, E., Pöntiö, I., Tervaniemi, M., & Gold, C. (2011). Individual music therapy for depression: Randomized controlled trial. *The British Journal of Psychiatry, 199,* 132–139. http://dx.doi.org/10.1192/bjp.bp.110.085431.

Eyre, L., & Lee, J. H. (2015). Mixed-methods survey of professional perspectives of music therapy practice in mental health. *Music Therapy Perspectives, 33,* 162–181. http://dx.doi.org/10.1093/mtp/miv034.

Gallagher, L. M., Huston, M. J., Nelson, K. A., Walsh, D., & Steele, A. L. (2001). Music therapy in palliative medicine. *Supportive Care in Cancer, 9,* 156–161. http://dx.doi.org/10.1007/s005200000189.

Gallagher, L. M., & Steele, A. L. (2002). Music therapy with offenders in a substance abuse/mental illness treatment program. *Music Therapy Perspectives, 20,* 117–122. http://dx.doi.org/10.1093/mtp/20.2.117.

Gardstrom, S., Bartkowski, J., Willenbrink, J., & Diestelkamp, W. S. (2013). The impact of group music therapy on negative affect of people with co-occurring substance use disorders and mental illnesses. *Music Therapy Perspectives, 31,* 116–126. http://dx.doi.org/10.1093/mtp/31.2.116.

Garrison, D. E. (2016). *The effect of music assisted relaxation on mood perception in Vietnam veterans: A pilot study* (Unpublished thesis). Tallahassee, FL: Florida State University.

Ghetti, C. (2016). Performing a family of practices: developments in community music therapy across international contexts. *Music Therapy Perspectives, 34,* 161–170. http://dx.doi.org/10.1093/mtp/miv047.

Gleadhill, L., & Ferris, K. (2010). A theoretical music therapy framework for working with people with dissociative identity disorder. *Australian Journal of Music Therapy, 21,* 42–55.

Goldbeck, L., & Ellerkamp, T. (2012). A randomized controlled trial of multimodal music therapy for children with anxiety. *Journal of Music Therapy, 49,* 395–413. http://dx.doi.org/10.1093/jmt/49.4.395.

Goldberg, F. S., McNiel, D. E., & Binder, R. L. (1988). Therapeutic factors in two forms of inpatient group psychotherapy: Music therapy and verbal therapy. *Group, 12,* 145–156. http://dx.doi.org/10.1007/BF01456564.

Gold, C., Solli, H. P., Krüger, V., & Lie, S. A. (2009). Dose-response relationship in music therapy for people with serious mental disorders: Systematic review and meta-analysis. *Clinical Psychology Review, 29,* 193–207. http://dx.doi.org/10.1016/j.cpr.2009.01.001.

Gold, C., Voracek, M., & Wigram, T. (2004). Effects of music therapy for children and adolescents with psychopathology: A meta-analysis. *Journal of Child Psychology and Psychiatry, 45,* 1054–1063. http://dx.doi.org/10.1111/j.1469-7610.2004.t01-1-00298.x.

Gooding, L. F. (2011). The effect of a music therapy social skills training program on improving social competence in children and adolescents with social skills deficits. *Journal of Music Therapy, 48,* 440–462. http://dx.doi.org/10.1093/jmt/48.4.440.

Gooding, L. F. (2016). An educator's response. *Music Therapy Perspectives, 34,* 54–55. http://dx.doi.org/10.1093/mtp/miw002.

Gooding, L. F. (2017). Microskills training: a model for teaching verbal processing skills in music therapy. *Voices: A World Forum for Music Therapy, 17*(1). http://dx.doi.org/10.15845/voices.v17i1.894.

Grocke, D. (2009). Music therapy research and the mental health-well-being continuum. *Australian Journal of Music Therapy, 20,* 6–15.

Grocke, D., Bloch, S., & Castle, D. (2009). The effect of group music therapy on quality of life for participants living with severe and enduring mental illness. *Journal of Music Therapy, 46,* 90–104. http://dx.doi.org/10.1093/jmt/46.2.90.

Grocke, D., Bloch, S., Castle, D., Thompson, G., Newton, R., Stewart, S., & Gold, C. (2014). Group music therapy for severe mental illness: a randomized embedded-experimental mixed methods study. *Acta Psychiatrica Scandinavica, 130,* 144–153. http://dx.doi.org/10.1111/acps.12224.

Hakvoort, L., Bogaerts, S., Thaut, M. H., & Spreen, M. (2015). Influence of music therapy on coping skills and anger management in forensic psychiatric patients: an exploratory study. *International Journal of Offender Therapy and Comparative Criminology, 59,* 810–836. http://dx.doi.org/10.1177/0306624X13516787.

Hanser, S. B. (1990). A music therapy strategy for depressed older adults in the community. *Journal of Applied Gerontology, 9,* 283–298. http://dx.doi.org/10.1177/073346489000900304.

Hanser, S. B., Butterfield-Whitcomb, J., & Kawata, M. (2011). Home-based music strategies with individuals who have dementia and their family caregivers. *Journal of Music Therapy, 48,* 2–27. http://dx.doi.org/10.1093/jmt/48.1.2.

Hanser, S. B., & Thompson, L. W. (1994). Effects of a music therapy strategy on depressed older adults. *Journal of Gerontology, 49,* 265–269. http://dx.doi.org/10.1093/geronj/49.6.P265.

Hendricks, C. B., Robinson, B., Bradley, L., & Davis, K. (1999). Using music techniques to treat adolescent depression. *Journal of Humanistic Counseling, 28,* 39–46. http://dx.doi.org/10.1002/j.2164-490x.1999.tb00160.x.

Jackson, N. A. (2003). A survey of music therapy methods and their role in the treatment of children with ADHD. *Journal of Music Therapy, 40,* 302–323. http://dx.doi.org/10.1093/jmt/40.4.302.

Jacobsen, S. L., McKinney, C. H., & Holck, U. (2014). Effects of dyadic music therapy intervention on parent-child interaction, parent stress, and parent-child relationship in families with emotionally neglected children: a randomized controlled trial. *Journal of Music Therapy, 51,* 310–332. http://dx.doi.org/10.1093/jmt/thu028.

Jones, J. D. (2005). A comparison of songwriting and lyric analysis techniques to evoke emotional change in a single session with people who are chemically dependent. *Journal of Music Therapy, 42,* 94–110. http://dx.doi.org/10.1093/jmt/42.2.94.

Jung, X. T., & Newton, R. (2009). Cochrane reviews of non-medication-based psychotherapeutic and other interventions for schizophrenia, psychosis, and bipolar disorder: A systematic literature review. *International journal of Mental Health nursing, 18,* 239–249. http://dx.doi.org/10.1111/j.1447-0349.2009.00613.x.

Kamioka, H., Tsutani, K., Yamada, M., Park, H., Okuizumi, H., Tsuruoka, K., Mutoh, Y. (2014). Effectiveness of music therapy: A summary of systematic reviews based on randomized controlled trials of music interventions. *Patient Preference and Adherence, 8,* 727–754. http://dx.doi.org/10.2147/PPA.S61340.

Kim, J., Wigram, T., & Gold, C. (2008). The effects of improvisational music therapy on joint attention behaviors in autistic children: A randomized controlled study. *Journal of Autism and Developmental Disorders, 28,* 1758–1766. http://dx.doi.org/10.1007/s10803-008-0566-6.

Krout, R. E. (2007). Music listening to facilitate relaxation and promote wellness: Integrated aspects of our neurophysiological responses to music. *The Arts in Psychotherapy, 34,* 134–141. http://dx.doi.org/10.1016/j.aip.2006.11.001.

Kun, Z., Bai, Z. G., Bo, A., & Chi, I. (2016). A systematic review and meta-analysis of music therapy for the older adults with depression: Review of music therapy for elderly depression. *International Journal of Geriatric Psychiatry.* http://dx.doi.org/10.1002/gps.4494.

Layman, D. L., Hussey, D. L., & Laing, S. J. (2002). Music therapy assessment for severely emotionally disturbed children: a pilot study. *Journal of Music Therapy, 39,* 164–187. http://dx.doi.org/10.1093/jmt/39.3.164.

Lin, S. T., Yang, P., Lai, C. Y., Su, Y. Y., Yeh, Y. C., & Huang, M. F. (2011). Mental health implications of music: insight from neuroscientific and clinical studies. *Harvard Review of Psychiatry, 19,* 34–46. http://dx.doi.org/10.3109/10673229.2011.549769.

Lipe, A. W., Ward, K. C., Watson, A. T., Manley, K., Keen, R., Kelly, J., & Clemmer, J. (2011). The effects of an arts intervention program in a community mental health setting: a collaborative approach. *The Arts in Psychotherapy, 39,* 25–30. http://dx.doi.org/10.1016/j.aip.2011.11.002.

Liu, X., Burns, D. S., Hilliard, R., Stump, T. E., & Unroe, K. T. (2015). Music therapy clinical practice in hospice: differences between home and nursing home delivery. *Journal of Music Therapy, 52,* 376–393. http://dx.doi.org/10.1093/jmt/thv012.

Livingston, G., Kelly, L., Lewis-Holmes, E., Baio, G., Morris, S., Patel, N., & Cooper, C. (2014). A systematic review of the clinical effectiveness and cost-effectiveness of sensory, psychological and behavioural interventions for managing agitation in older adults with dementia. *Health Technology Assessment, 18*(39). http://dx.doi.org/10.3310/hta18390.

MacDonald, S. (2015). Client experiences in music therapy in the psychiatric inpatient milieu. *Music Therapy Perspectives, 33,* 108–117. http://dx.doi.org/10.1093/mtp/miv019.

Maratos, A., Gold, C., Wang, X., & Crawford, M. (2008). Music therapy for depression. *Cochrane Database of Systematic Reviews* (1), CD004517. http://dx.doi.org/10.1002/14651858.CD004517.pub2.

McCaffrey, T. (2015). Music therapy's development in mental healthcare: a historical consideration of early ideas and intersecting agents. *Music & Medicine, 7,* 28–33.

McFerran, K., Baker, F., Patton, G. C., & Sawyer, S. M. (2006). A retrospective lyrical analysis of songs written by adolescents with anorexia nervosa. *European Eating Disorders Review, 14,* 297–403. http://dx.doi.org/10.1002/erv.746.

McIntyre, J. (2007). Creating order out of chaos: Music therapy with adolescent boys diagnosed with a behaviour disorder and/or emotional disorder. *Music Therapy Today, 8,* 56–79.

McLaughlin, B., & Adler, R. F. (2015). Music therapy for children with intellectual disabilities. In B. Wheeler (Ed.), *Music therapy handbook* (pp. 277–289). New York: Guilford Press.

Meadows, A. (2016). An educator's response. *Music Therapy Perspectives, 34,* 52–53. http://dx.doi.org/10.1093/mtp/miw011.

Montello, L., & Coons, E. E. (1998). Effects of active versus passive group music therapy on preadolescents with emotional, learning, and behavioral disorders. *Journal of Music Therapy, 35,* 49–67. http://dx.doi.org/10.1093/jmt/35.1.49.

Mössler, K., Assmus, J., Heldal, T. O., Fuchs, K., & Gold, C. (2012). Music therapy techniques as predictors of change in mental healthcare. *The Arts in Psychotherapy, 39,* 333–341. http://dx.doi.org/10.1016/j.aip.2012.05.002.

Mössler, K., Chen, X., Heldal, T. O., & Gold, C. (2011). Music therapy for people with schizophrenia and schizophrenia-like disorders. *Cochrane Database Systematic Reviews, 12,* 1–68. http://dx.doi.org/10.1002/14651858.CD004025.pub3.

Odell-Miller, H. (2011). Value of music therapy for people with personality disorders. *Mental Health Practice, 14,* 34–35. http://dx.doi.org/10.7748/mhp2011.07.14.10.34.c8579.

Oldfield, A., & Bunce, L. (2001). 'Mummy can play too'… Short-term music therapy with mothers and young children. *British Journal of Music Therapy, 15,* 27–36. http://dx.doi.org/10.1177/135945750101500107.

Patterson, S., Duhig, M., Darbyshire, C., Counsel, R., Higgins, N., & Williams, I. (2015). Implementing music therapy on an adolescent inpatient unit: a mixed-methods evaluation of acceptability, experience of participation and perceived impact. *Australasian Psychiatry, 23,* 556–560. http://dx.doi.org/10.1177/1039856215592320.

Pedersen, I. N. (2014). Music therapy in psychiatry today–do we need specialization based on the reduction of diagnosis-specific symptoms or on the overall development of patients' resources? Or do we need both? *Nordic Journal of Music Therapy, 23,* 173–194. http://dx.doi.org/10.1080/08098131.2013.790917.

Pelletier, C. L. (2004). The effect of music on decreasing arousal due to stress: a meta-analysis. *Journal of Music Therapy, 41,* 192–214. http://dx.doi.org/10.1093/jmt/41.3.192.

Porter, S., McConnell, T., McLaughlin, K., Lynn, F., Cardwell, C., Braiden, H. J., … Music in Mind Study Group. (2017). Music therapy for children and adolescents with behavioural and emotional problems: A randomised controlled trial. *Journal of Child Psychology and Psychiatry, 58,* 586–594. http://dx.doi.org/10.1111/jcpp.12656.

Rafieyan, R., & Ries, R. (2007). A description of the use of music therapy in consultation-liaison psychiatry. *Psychiatry, 4,* 47–52.

Raglio, A. (2015). Music therapy interventions in Parkinson's disease: the state-of-the-art. *Frontiers in Neurology, 6,* 185. http://dx.doi.org/10.3389/fneur.2015.00185.

Raglio, A., Bellelli, G., Traficante, D., Gianotti, M., Ubezio, M. C., Villani, D., & Trabucchi, M. (2008). Efficacy of music therapy in the treatment of behavioral and psychiatric symptoms of dementia. *Alzheimer Disease & Associated Disorders, 22,* 158–162. http://dx.doi.org/10.1097/WAD.0b013e3181630b6f.

Register, D. (2002). Collaboration and consultation: a survey of board certified music therapists. *Journal of Music Therapy, 39,* 305–321. http://dx.doi.org/10.1093/jmt/39.4.305.

Reschke-Hernandez, A. E. (2011). History of music therapy treatment interventions for children with autism. *Journal of Music Therapy, 48,* 169–207. http://dx.doi.org/10.1093/jmt/48.2.169.

Rickson, D. J., & Watkins, W. G. (2003). Music therapy to promote prosocial behaviors in aggressive adolescent boys-A pilot study. *Journal of Music Therapy, 40,* 283–301. http://dx.doi.org/10.1093/jmt/40.4.283.

Robarts, J. Z., & Sloboda, A. (1994). Perspectives on music therapy with people suffering from anorexia nervosa. *British Journal of Music Therapy, 8,* 7–14. http://dx.doi.org/10.1177/135945759400800104.

Robb, S. L. (2000). Music assisted progressive muscle relaxation, progressive muscle relaxation, music listening, and silence: a comparison of relaxation techniques. *Journal of Music Therapy, 37,* 2–21. http://dx.doi.org/10.1093/jmt/37.1.2.

Rolvsjord, R. (2010). *Resource-oriented music therapy in mental healthcare.* Gilsum, NH: Barcelona Publishers.

Ross, S., Cidambi, I., Dermatis, H., Weinstein, J., Ziedonis, D., Roth, S., & Galanter, M. (2008). Music therapy. *Journal of Addictive Diseases, 27,* 41–53. http://dx.doi.org/10.1300/J069v27n01_05.

Sabbatella, P. (2004, October). Improvisation in music therapy. In *Improvisation in Music, European Music Council-Documentation of the Conference, The Hague, Netherlands.* Retrieved from http://www.emc-imc.org/fileadmin/user_upload/Publications/dokuAM04.pdf.

Shuman, J., Kennedy, H., DeWitt, P., Edelblute, A., & Wamboldt, M. Z. (2016). Group music therapy impacts mood states of adolescents in a psychiatric hospital setting. *The Arts in Psychotherapy, 49,* 50–56. http://dx.doi.org/10.1016/j.aip.2016.05.014.

Silverman, M. J. (2003a). The influence of music on the symptoms of psychosis: A meta-analysis. *Journal of Music Therapy, 40,* 27–40. http://dx.doi.org/10.1093/jmt/40.1.27.

Silverman, M. J. (2003b). Music therapy and clients who are chemically dependent: A review of literature and pilot study. *The Arts in Psychotherapy, 30,* 273–281. http://dx.doi.org/10.1016/j.aip.2003.08.004.

Silverman, M. J. (2007). Evaluating current trends in psychiatric music therapy: a descriptive analysis. *Journal of Music Therapy, 44,* 388–414. http://dx.doi.org/10.1093/jmt/44.4.388.

Silverman, M. J. (2008). Quantitative comparison of cognitive behavioral therapy and music therapy research: a methodological best-practices analysis to guide future investigation for adult psychiatric patients. *Journal of Music Therapy, 46,* 105–131. http://dx.doi.org/10.1093/jmt/46.2.105.

Silverman, M. J. (2009). A descriptive analysis of music therapists working with consumers in substance abuse rehabilitation: Current clinical practice to guide future research. *The Arts in Psychotherapy, 36*, 123–130. http://dx.doi.org/10.1016/j.aip.2008.10.005.

Silverman, M. J. (2010a). Applying levels of evidence to the psychiatric music therapy literature base. *The Arts in Psychotherapy, 37*, 1–7. http://dx.doi.org/10.1016/j.aip.2009.11.005.

Silverman, M. J. (2010b). Integrating music therapy into the evidence-based treatments for psychiatric consumers. *Music Therapy Perspectives, 28*, 4–10. http://dx.doi.org/10.1093/mtp/28.1.4.

Silverman, M. J. (2011). Effects of music therapy on change readiness and craving in patients on a detoxification unit. *Journal of Music Therapy, 48*, 509–531. http://dx.doi.org/10.1093/jmt/48.4.509.

Silverman, M. J. (2012). Areas of concern in psychiatric music therapy: a descriptive analysis. *The Arts in Psychotherapy, 39*, 374–378. http://dx.doi.org/10.1016/j.aip.2012.06.002.

Silverman, M. J. (2015). *Music therapy in mental health for illness management and recovery.* New York: Oxford University Press.

Silverman, M. J., & Leonard, J. (2012). Effects of active music therapy interventions on attendance in people with severe mental illnesses: Two pilot studies. *The Arts in Psychotherapy, 39*, 390–396. http://dx.doi.org/10.1016/j.aip.2012.06.005.

Silverman, M. J., & Rosenow, S. (2013). Immediate quantitative effects of recreational music therapy on mood and perceived helpfulness in acute psychiatric inpatients: An exploratory study. *The Arts in Psychotherapy, 40*, 269–274. http://dx.doi.org/10.1016/j.aip.2013.04.001.

Smith, M. (2008). The effects of a single music relaxation session on state anxiety levels of adults in a workplace environment. *Australian Journal of Music Therapy, 19*, 45–66.

Solli, H. P., Rolvsjord, R., & Borg, M. (2013). Toward understanding music therapy as a recovery-oriented practice within mental healthcare: A meta-synthesis of service users' experiences. *Journal of Music Therapy, 50*, 244–273. http://dx.doi.org/10.1093/jmt/50.4.244.

Stuckey, H. L., & Nobel, J. (2010). The connection between art, healing, and public health: A review of current literature. *American Journal of Public Health, 100*, 254–263. http://dx.doi.org/10.2105/AJPH.2008.156497.

Sung, H. C., & Chang, A. M. (2005). Use of preferred music to decrease agitated behaviors in older people with dementia: A review of the literature. *Journal of Clinical Nursing, 14*, 1133–1140. http://dx.doi.org/10.1111/j.1365-2702.2005.01218.x.

Ueda, T., Suzukamo, Y., Sato, M., & Izumi, S. I. (2013). Effects of music therapy on behavioral and psychological symptoms of dementia: A systematic review and meta-analysis. *Ageing Research Reviews, 12*, 628–641. http://dx.doi.org/10.1016/j.arr.2013.02.003.

Ulrich, G., Houtmans, T., & Gold, C. (2007). The additional therapeutic effect of group music therapy for schizophrenic patients: A randomized study. *Acta Psychiatrica Scandinavica, 116*, 362–370. http://dx.doi.org/10.1111/j.1600-0447.2007.01073.x.

White, P., & Williams, D. V. (2000). *I'm movin' on* [recorded by Rascal Flatts]. On Rascal Flatts [album]. Nashville, TN: Lyric Street Records.

Wigram, T., & Baker, F. (2005). Introduction: songwriting as therapy. In F. Baker, & T. Wigram (Eds.), *Songwriting: Methods, techniques and clinical applications for music therapy clinicians, educators and students* (pp. 11–23). London: Jessica Kingsley.

Yinger, O. S., & Gooding, L. F. (2014). Music therapy and music medicine for children and adolescents. In D. R. Simkin, & C. W. Popper (Eds.), *Child and adolescent psychiatric clinics of North America: Alternative and complementary therapies for children with psychiatric disorders, part 2 [Monograph]. Clinics reviews articles* (Vol. 23 (3)) (pp. 535–554).

Yinger, O. S., & Gooding, L. F. (2015). A systematic review of music-based interventions for procedural support. *Journal of Music Therapy, 52*, 1–77. http://dx.doi.org/10.1093/jmt/thv004.

Yinger, O. S., McVay, V., & Gooding, L. (2016, July). *Outcomes of participation in a piano-based recreational music making group for adults over 50: A retrospective study.* Poster session presented at the 14th International Conference on Music Perception and Cognition, San Francisco, CA.

Zarate, R. (2016). Clinical improvisation and its effect on anxiety: A multiple single subject design. *The Arts in Psychotherapy, 48*, 46–83. http://dx.doi.org/10.1016/j.aip.2015.11.005.

Zhao, K., Bai, Z. G., Bo, A., & Chi, I. (2016). A systematic review and meta-analysis of music therapy for the older adults with depression. *International Journal of Geriatric Psychiatry, 31*, 1188–1198, http://dx.doi.org/10.1002/gps.4494.

CHAPTER 5

Music Therapy in Medical Treatment and Rehabilitation

DARCY DELOACH, PHD, MT-BC, NICU-MT

The variability of music therapy services provides a unique challenge in a medical model, where protocols and plans of care are standardized. In a medical model, the best evidence possible is accessed to determine appropriate interventions (Shah & Mountain, 2007). Music therapists work well within a patient-centered care model, utilizing the music intervention best suited to address the patient need. This process can be determined by the music therapist a priori or at many times is decided in the moment while ongoing patient assessment is occurring. Patient-centered care values center on the involvement of patients in healthcare decisions, which includes a focus on pain management, emotional support, and alleviation of fear and anxiety (Barry & Edgman-Levitan, 2012; Institute for Patient-and Family-Centered Care, 2017). Music therapists address each of these areas when presented by patients. Although new research continues to emerge supporting the use of various music therapy interventions with diverse patient populations and need areas, it is worth noting that positive results from board-certified music therapists working in medical settings have been published consistently for at least the past three decades. The concept of music being administered as a therapeutic tool is gaining more support as the years pass and as more research is published with designs that reflect the medical model of controlled randomized studies. In addition, related professionals are increasingly investigating the effect of music listening experiences for various patient groups, which is frequently called music medicine. This chapter will focus on research conducted by board-certified music therapists who have been trained and certified to use music interventions for specific therapeutic functions. Although music has a place for various purposes in medical settings, it is the unique application by music therapists that will be explored here.

Almost all people worldwide have music experiences. This universality of music makes music a consumer-owned phenomenon in many cultures. When discussing how music can significantly affect patient experiences, it is not uncommon to hear statements of support about how music can relax a person or make someone's mood better when they are having a rough day. Past personal music experience is one factor that music therapists assess when determining the appropriate use of music for patients. There are many models used by music therapists when determining the intervention plan for patient needs. Often the theory of pain perception is discussed in relation to how music can distract from pain or interrupt the pain signal being sent to and processed by the brain (Lee, 2016). In addition, models of personal music preference that detail how people develop their music preference are utilized when determining the type of music to be used in various patient experiences (Berlyne & Crozier, 1971; Tan, Spackman, & Peaslee, 2006) One song can be heard by 10 different people who will have 10 different responses to the same music sample. This variability makes it impossible to use music prescriptively in a medical setting as a medical researcher or staff member might be inclined to do. The Optimal Complexity Theory is commonly used when discussing aesthetics and can be applied to the various reactions people have with music. Berlyne suggests that the perceived complexity of music determines the preference or rejection of the stimuli being experienced, in this case music (see Fig. 5.1).

If a person perceives a song to be too simple or too complex, their enjoyment of the song will diminish. The two extremes of the inverted U shape would denote the extremes of each music quality. For example, simple accompaniment would denote one instrument and complex accompaniment would denote a multitude of instruments. A very predictable song that is well known and has been listened to many times will not yield as much enjoyment. On the other end of the curve, a song that has never been heard may not be enjoyable because

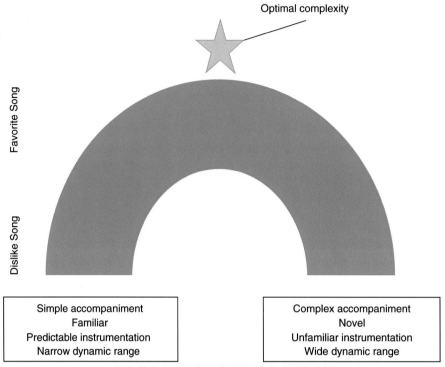

FIG. 5.1 Berlyne's optimal complexity model.

it is too unpredictable. The other consideration for music is that each of these factors layer on top of each other to yield how enjoyable a song is for a listener. It is not just the instrumentation by itself that determines how much a song is enjoyed. A song can have the same instrumentation but be covered by a different artist and not be liked by a listener. Conversely, an artist can sing one of their well-known songs a cappella without any accompaniment and a person may not like it. All of the elements of music that contribute to a song or music score combine and layer onto each other to influence how much a listener enjoys the music. Beyond the complexity of the music, LeBlanc's model (1982) of music preference highlights the emotional, environmental, and exposure factors that contribute to a person accepting or rejecting a song (see Fig. 5.2).

For patients in medical environments, the focus is drawn in LeBlanc's model to the physiologic enabling conditions, current affective state, and basic attention. For example, when patients are experiencing pain, their perception of the pain and the unfamiliar hospital environment will affect their affective mood state and their ability to attend to the music being played. The same song played in their car while driving on a leisurely day will not be perceived the same way. The combination of LeBlanc's model and Berlyne's model gives a picture of what goes on in a music therapist's brain when determining how to use music as a tool to meet a specific therapeutic function with the variety of patient needs across medical environments. The complexity of how music is consumed in different environments, with different mood states, with different presentations of instrumentation and voicing, must be understood when music therapists determine the appropriate music to be used with a specific patient need.

The complexity of patient needs and the vastness of music tools available to address patient goals and objectives contribute to the variability of music therapy service provision across the world. Music is unique to cultures, which must be considered when determining the most appropriate therapeutic application of music in medical environments. These issues will be highlighted in the case examples presented later in this chapter.

POPULATIONS SERVED

Music therapists in medical and rehabilitative settings provide intervention services to a variety of patient

Sources of Variation in Music Preference

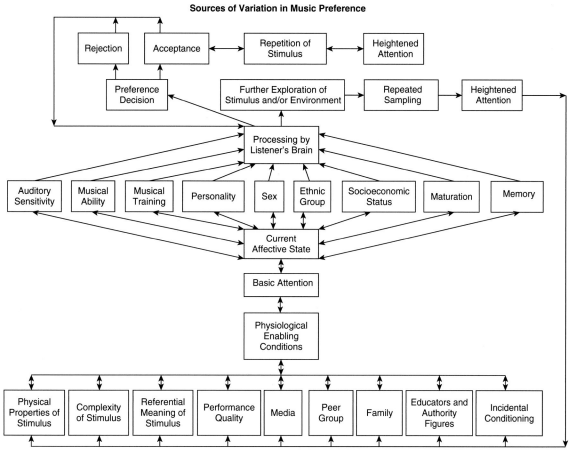

FIG. 5.2 Leblanc's model of music preference.

populations across the lifespan, both inpatient and outpatient, with a variety of diagnoses. Reasons for patient referrals cover psychosocial, physiologic, and spiritual needs, resulting in patients receiving music therapy services in a variety of units, including but not limited to intensive care, intermediate care, rehabilitation, radiology, oncology, and palliative care (see Box 5.1). When analyzing the variety of patients referred for services, common need areas emerge. Many music therapists address patient pain perception, compliance with care from other staff or procedures, coping skills, anxiety, mood, regulation, and endurance. In all music therapy interventions, music is used as a tool to address the referral need for the patient. The type of music varies based on patient music preferences, the environment where the session occurs, and the intervention structure. A thorough description of medical music therapy services is provided by Gooding (2014),

with chapters devoted to evidence-based clinical applications recommendations for the neonatal intensive care unit (NICU), pediatrics, adult medical/surgical, older adults, emergency department, end-of-life care, and psychosocial care. Although it is beyond the scope of this chapter to discuss these fully, readers are encouraged to review those chapters for more in-depth recommendations.

RESEARCH

Research on the effectiveness of music therapy interventions in medical and rehabilitation settings has been conducted over the past 30 years with increasing frequency. General outcomes will be highlighted here, with specific recommendations for patient outcomes discussed in the following section. Many hospitalized patients experience heightened anxiety about their diagnosis or the unknown future awaiting them. Patients also experience high levels of pain during their care and recovery. In addition, patients experience nausea as a side effect of treatments and medications. Music therapists working in medical environments have found significant effects for music therapy interventions in alleviating patient anxiety, pain, and nausea and in relaxation (Boldt, 1996; Robb, 2003; Standley, 1992). Meta-analyses for stress, medical/dental care, and premature infants have all yielded significant positive effects for music interactions and interventions across patient needs and ages (Pelletier, 2004; Standley, 1986, 2012). Another meta-analysis of medical settings showed significantly greater effect sizes for improvements in patients' ratings of pain, well-being, mood, and nausea/vomiting (Dileo, 2006). Table 5.1 highlights the key outcomes from several systematic reviews

of music therapy treatment within specific medical subspecialties.

Music therapy interventions have also been found to benefit both adult and pediatric patients with cancer. Music therapy and music medicine both improved mood and relaxation and decreased pain and anxiety for adult inpatients with cancer, and most patients preferred music therapy over music medicine (Bradt et al., 2015). Similarly, pediatric inpatients with cancer who received interactive music therapy experienced improved mood and positive play behaviors, as rated by self-report and parent report (Barrera, Rykov, & Doyle, 2002). Table 5.2 summarizes the results of several randomized controlled studies on the effects of music therapy with live music on adult and pediatric patients with cancer.

Transplant patients experience unique needs that can be addressed by music therapy. Table 5.3 summarizes randomized controlled trials (RCTs) on the use of music therapy with live music on patients undergoing stem cell transplantation. The importance of psychosocial interventions in medical settings is well described by Madson and Silverman (2010) who investigated the experiences of organ transplant patients. Increased patient verbalizations about the hospitalization and diagnosis are an important step in the cognitive processing necessary for homeostasis and recovery. Solid organ transplant patients who received one live music therapy session reported improved mood state, increased relaxation, and decreased pain when assessed with a Likert-type scale before and after the music therapy session. A coping-infused dialogue paired with patient-preferred music protocol with this same population resulted in more positive affect and less pain reported (Hogan & Silverman, 2015). Table 5.4 summarizes RCTs on the use of music therapy with

---

BOX 5.1
Nonexhaustive List of Medical Settings Where Music Therapists May Provide Services

Medical settings where music therapists provide services:

- Emergency care
- Intensive care
- Intermediate care
- Neurology
- Oncology
- Orthopedics
- Palliative care
- Pediatrics
- Radiology
- Rehabilitation
- Surgery

TABLE 5.1
Systematic Reviews and Meta-analyses on Music Therapy in Subspecialty Areas of Medical Treatment

Medical Specialty	Outcome	Author, Year
Medical procedures	Interactive music therapy interventions using live music may decrease pain and anxiety during adult medical procedures	Yinger and Gooding (2015)
Physical rehabilitation	Music therapy enhances physical, psychological, cognitive, and emotional functioning	Weller and Baker (2011)
Preterm birth	NICU-MT protocols that have medical and developmental benefits for preterm infants include music listening for pacification, music reinforcement of sucking, and music pacification as the basis for neurodevelopmental enhancement	Standley (2002, 2012)

MT, music therapy; *NICU*, neonatal intensive care unit.

live music on patients undergoing blood, marrow, and solid organ transplantation.

Music therapy interventions designed to address coping skills have also been shown to be effective in cardiac treatment. In one study, emotion-coping music therapy interventions were significantly more effective than talk-based emotion-coping interventions for adult patients undergoing cardiac catheterization (Ghetti, 2013). Mandel et al. (2007) found that patients who received music therapy as part of an outpatient cardiac rehabilitation program showed significant greater improvements in anxiety, general health, and social functioning 4 months after treatment compared with participants who went through cardiac rehabilitation without music therapy.

On analysis of how music therapy affects patients undergoing procedures, one of the most common causes for the administration of sedation is heightened patient anxiety, which is effectively lowered by music therapy (Yinger & Gooding, 2015). Music therapy was effective in eliminating sedation and reducing the time of procedure for echocardiograms and computed tomography scans for children under 12 years old (Walworth, 2005). In a different study, music therapy utilizing live music was more effective than chloral hydrate for inducing sleep states for infants and

TABLE 5.2
Select RCTs on the Effects of Music Therapy Incorporating Live Music in Cancer Treatment

Author, Year	Population	Outcomes
Bradt et al. (2015)	Adults receiving inpatient or outpatient cancer treatment	Both music therapy and music medicine improved mood, anxiety, relaxation, and pain; however, most patients preferred music therapy
Cook and Silverman (2013)	Adult oncology and hematology patients receiving inpatient treatment	Participants who received live music therapy showed significantly higher posttest scores in peace and faith compared with controls
Hanser et al. (2006)	Women with metastatic breast cancer	Participants who received music therapy showed significant improvements in relaxation, comfort, happiness, and heart rate compared with controls
Robb et al. (2008)	Hospitalized children receiving cancer treatment	Patients who experienced active music engagement showed significantly more coping-related behaviors, positive facial active, and active engagement than patients who listened to music or audio storybooks

RCT, randomized controlled trial.

TABLE 5.3
Select RCTS With Adolescents and Young Adults Undergoing Stem-Cell Transplantation

Author, Year	Population	Outcomes
Burns, Robb, and Haase (2009)	Adolescents and young adults with cancer undergoing stem-cell transplantation	Participants who participated in a therapeutic music video intervention showed positive trends in hope, spirituality, confidence, mastery, and self-transcendence immediately after treatment, as well as improvements in quality of life and better defensive coping after 100 days
Cassileth, Vickers, and Magill (2003)	Adults undergoing stem cell transplantation	Patients who received music therapy showed significantly less mood disturbance than patients in the control group
Robb et al. (2014)	Adolescents and young adults undergoing stem cell transplantation	Participants who took part in a therapeutic music video intervention reported significantly better courageous coping, social integration, and family environment compared with participants who experienced an audiobook control condition

RCT, randomized controlled trial.

children under 5 years old. The hospital's electroen-cephalography protocol was modified after the study for all pediatric patients, with music therapy offered as the first option for sleep induction (Loewy, Hallan, Friedman, & Martinez, 2005).

Acute pain and distress are commonly experienced by burn patients when undergoing debridement, resulting in high levels of anxiety. Pediatric burn patients who received music therapy procedural support during debridement experienced reduced pain, anxiety, and behavioral distress. The music therapists played live music utilizing both improvised melodies and patient-preferred songs (Whitehead-Pleaux, Zebrowski, Baryza,

& Sheridan, 2007). Adding music therapy interventions onto pharmacologic pain relief enhanced the patient responses in this setting. Table 5.5 summarizes RCTs on procedural support music therapy.

One question about music therapy that is commonly raised relates to how the therapeutic process is affected by therapist presence. Investigators studying music therapy within a preoperative setting found therapist effect for anxiety levels was reduced in children receiving live interactive music therapy preoperatively (Kain et al., 2004). Midazolam was more effective than music therapy in reducing patient anxiety during the administration of anesthesia. The

TABLE 5.4
Select RCTs With Adults Undergoing Blood, Bone Marrow, and Solid Organ Transplantation

Author, Year	Population	Outcomes
Fredenburg and Silverman (2014a)	Blood and marrow transplant recipients	Participants who received music therapy showed significantly more positive affect and less negative affect and pain
Fredenburg and Silverman (2014b)	Bone marrow transplant recipients	Participants who received music therapy tended to have decreases in fatigue, whereas control participants showed increased fatigue, although group differences were not significant
Ghetti (2011)	Liver and kidney transplant recipients	Participants who received active music engagement (AME) with emotional-approach coping had significant increases in positive affect, whereas participants who received only AME had significant decreases in pain. Both showed significant decreases in negative affect
Rosenow and Silverman (2014)	Blood and marrow transplant recipients	Participants who received music therapy showed decreases in fatigue, whereas controls showed increases in fatigue, although group differences were not significant

RCT, randomized controlled trial.

TABLE 5.5
RCTs on Music Therapy as Procedural Support

Author, Year	Population	Outcomes
Ferrer (2007)	Adults with cancer undergoing chemotherapy	Participants who received music therapy showed significant improvements in anxiety, fear, fatigue, relaxation, and diastolic blood pressure compared with controls
Tan, Yowler, Super, and Fratianne (2010)	Adult burn patients undergoing dressing changes	Participants who received music-based imagery before and after dressing changes and music alternate engagement during dressing changes showed significant decreases in pain and anxiety compared with controls
Yinger (2016)	Children receiving immunizations	Children who received music therapy showed significantly fewer distress behaviors and significantly more coping behaviors than controls

RCT, randomized controlled trial.

therapist effect found indicated that children interacting with one music therapist experienced significantly less anxiety than the control group, whereas children interacting with the other music therapist in the study did not. This is very interesting in considering how protocols are developed and how skill development in music therapists may result in therapists being more effective in certain patient populations than others. In other studies of music therapy during preoperative, intraoperative, or postoperative care, participants who received music therapy showed greater relaxation and reductions in anxiety than controls (Palmer, Lane, Mayo, Schluchter, & Leeming, 2015; Yates & Silverman, 2015; see Table 5.6).

Positive effects of music therapy services have also been found when studying patient satisfaction scores. When compared with patients who did not receive music therapy services, patients who were referred for and received music therapy services scored, on average, 3.4 points higher on their overall patient satisfaction score on the Press Ganey Inpatient Survey (Yinger & Standley, 2011). This is very intriguing. Patients most commonly referred for services, regardless of unit, are patients who are experiencing more severe symptoms related to their hospitalization. This study was not an RCT; rather, it analyzed retroactively patients who were referred and received music therapy services in comparison with those who were not referred. Patients not referred would not have been experiencing heightened anxiety, pain, depression, for example. Improvement of patient satisfaction for the patients who exhibited worse symptoms is worth noting.

EVIDENCE-BASED PRACTICES

The existing literature provides several best practice recommendations when using music therapy interventions in medical and rehabilitative settings. Two resources that will be summarized here are recommended for further reading on this topic: Standley (1995) and Hillmer (2014).

Standley (1995) lists seven evidence-based music therapy techniques used across patient populations. These techniques provide a comprehensive view of how music can be incorporated into medical environments (see Table 5.7) and can be used for various referrals of patient needs. For example, passive music listening can decrease anxiety for a pediatric patient waiting for a procedure or for an adult waiting for test results who focuses on biofeedback parameters while the heart rate and respiration rate are monitored. The music serves the same function of reducing anxiety and stress, even though how the music is presented, the choice of music, and the length of time needed of passive music listening before the objective is met will vary between patient populations. Similarly, the technique of pairing music with counseling can reduce distress of a patient or family member experiencing anticipatory grief or can reduce fear of the unknown for a stroke survivor with limited mobility and speech.

Hillmer (2014) discussed the evidenced-based applications of validation, empathy, reflection, and open-ended questions for music therapists to use when pairing music and counseling with medical patients. Music opens up conversations based on themes in the lyrics, memories of the music stored by the patient, and emotions evoked

TABLE 5.6		
RCTs on Music Therapy Before, During, or After Surgery		
Author, Year	**Population**	**Outcomes**
Kain et al. (2004)	Children undergoing outpatient surgery	Children who received midazolam were significantly less anxious than children who received music therapy or controls during induction of anesthesia; however, children treated by one music therapist were significantly less anxious than children treated by another music therapist and controls at separation to the operating room (OR) and entrance to the OR
Palmer et al. (2015)	Female patients undergoing surgery for diagnosis or treatment of breast cancer	Participants who heard recorded music intraoperatively with either live or recorded patient-selected music preoperatively showed significantly greater reductions in anxiety preoperatively compared with controls and the live music group had significantly shorter recovery times than the recorded music group
Yates & Silverman (2015)	Adult patients in a surgical oncology unit	Participants who received live music therapy showed significantly greater posttest relaxation and less anxiety than controls

RCT, randomized controlled trial.

TABLE 5.7 Seven Evidenced-Based Medical Music Therapy Techniques	
Passive music listening	• Music Function: Audioanalgesic, anxiolytic, or sedative • Objectives: Reduced pain, anxiety, or stress. Reduced amount of medication or length of use
Active music participation	• Music function: Focus of attention. Structure for exercise or movement • Objectives: Reduced pain, increased motor abilities, increased respiration abilities
Music and counseling	• Music function: Initiate and enhance therapist/patient/family relationships • Objectives: Reduction of fear, trauma, and distress. Acceptance of diagnosis and/or death. Enhancement of interpersonal interactions
Music and developmental or educational objectives	• Music function: Reinforce or structure learning • Objectives: Prevention of developmental regression caused by hospitalization. Increased academic learning
Music and stimulation	• Music function: Stimulate auditorily and increase awareness of other forms of stimuli • Objectives: Increased overt responses to stimuli. Reduced depression/anxiety caused by sensory deprivation
Music and biofeedback	• Music function: Reinforcer or structure for physiologic responses • Objectives: Increased awareness, self-control, and monitoring of physiologic state
Music and group activity	• Music function: Structure pleasurable and positive interpersonal interactions • Objectives: Reduction of depression/anxiety caused by isolation. Increased pleasure and feelings of well-being

From Standley, J. M. (1995). Music as a therapeutic intervention in medical and dental treatment: Research and clinical applications. In T. Wigram, B. Saperston, & R. West (Eds.), *The art and science of music therapy: A Handbook* (pp. 3–22). New York: Routledge.

by the music. In addition to Standley's evidence-based techniques, Hillmer (2014) listed guided relaxation, iso-principle, contingent music, singing, songwriting, distraction, and lyric analysis as techniques supported by the literature for adults in medical settings. In pediatric settings, many of the above-mentioned techniques are supported by the literature with the addition of music video production (Standley, Gooding, & Yinger, 2014). All of these techniques can be encompassed by the categories proposed by Standley (1995), shown in Table 5.8.

Music therapy services are not standardized but rather individualized and assessed in the moment, resulting in wide-ranging interventions that are implemented and determined by the presentation of patient mood, affect, and behavior. The description of pediatric music therapy intervention services used in the study by Barrera et al. (2002) captures this reality of service provision:

> Music therapy involved live, interactive and developmentally appropriate music-making with the child (and family) engaged in one or more activities aimed at facilitating expression of feelings, reducing distress and promoting well being. The child/family participated in the choice of the songs and/or instruments used during the sessions. Adolescents and school-age children were engaged typically by camp songs, signing, song writing, instrumental improvization [sic], and listening to prerecorded music of their choice Pre-schoolers and toddlers were engaged typically by animated play songs, rhymes, and playing instruments. Infants and toddlers participated in vocal play, play songs, lullabies, rhymes, and playing instruments. Lullabies often helped infants to sleep or they comforted children who did not feel well enough to participate more actively. Playing and/or singing together was useful in distracting the young children during medical procedures. Music therapy materials included small percussion instruments (e.g. bells, drums, pentatonic tone bars, shakers), a classical guitar, an Omnichord (electronic autoharp), an electronic keyboard, and songbooks. A small tape recorder was available to record singing and playing. Prerecorded music was sometimes included, at the patient's request (mainly adolescents), and supplied by patients (p. 381).

Although music therapists can and should use the evidence base for treatment and intervention planning, the individuality of the patient experience will determine how each session progresses. Following a strict protocol of care would not allow the variability necessary to accurately meet the patients' needs with the most appropriate intervention based on the fluid assessment as the session progresses.

CASE EXAMPLES

The following case examples have all identifying information removed.

Neonatal Intensive Care Unit

Patient. Six-day-old infant diagnosed with neonatal abstinence syndrome in the second stage of the weaning process.

Referral Source: RN referred patient for increased agitation and crying.

The music therapist waited to see the patient until the 30 min preceding the afternoon feed and medication administration, when the RN reported the patient was typically the most agitated. At the beginning of the music therapy session the patient was consistently crying and was not calming while being held by a hospital volunteer. The RN stated there was most likely nothing that would calm the patient at this point and level of agitation. The music therapist returned the patient to the crib. The Pacifier Activated Lullaby (PAL) device was used with this patient with the goal of calming the patient and eliminating crying. The PAL device uses lullabies as a reward for the desired non-nutritive sucking behavior. The PAL was set at the lowest threshold setting with only one pacifier suck required to activate the lullaby and a 10-s interval for music cutting off without a productive suck. At first presentation of the pacifier, the infant demonstrated frenzied sucking and intermittent crying. After 5 min, the patient was calmly sucking with a paced sucking pattern and whimpering intermittently. When the RN returned for the infant's scheduled feed and medication administration time, the infant was still calmly sucking the pacifier. The infant sucked within the 10-s interval to keep the music playing for the entire session, with the exception of the learning period in the first 5 min of the session.

Extended Care Unit

Patient: Seventy-two-year-old female ischemic stroke survivor with expressive aphasia.

Referral Source: Interdisciplinary team meeting for increased verbal fluency.

The patient received music therapy sessions three times per week to increase verbal fluency and comprehension. Familiar songs with accessible lyrics stored in the patient's memory were sung with the patient during each session. The patient was cued to fill in lyrics with increasing frequency as sessions progressed. Once lyrics were sung with repeated accuracy, the words were cued to be spoken instead of sung. Words were then paired together in meaningful phrases in a speech-sing format to increase the accuracy of completing words. The range of melodic prosody was then reduced over time to result in spoken phrases. At discharge, the patient had five phrases and 11 single spoken words that were intelligible.

Dementia Diagnosis

Patient: Eighty-seven-year-old male with dementia, inpatient.

Referral Source: RN verbal referral while music therapist was walking past the patient room. RN stated that the patient was extremely agitated and required restraints to prevent self-harm or harm to staff. RN requested music therapy services to reduce patient agitation.

Upon entering the patient's room, the music therapist assessed the patient agitation level. Patient was yelling and clenching both of his fists to the point of cutting his skin with his fingernails and was bleeding. The staff in the room were giving verbal instructions for calming down, which were not being followed by the patient. As the patient was not able to communicate music preference, the music therapist chose common song genres for the patient population served at that hospital. To redirect the patient's attentional focus to the music instead of the pain and confusion causing the agitation, the music therapist chose to sing a well-known older upbeat country song a cappella in close proximity to the patient's ear at a loud volume. The intervention technique used was the iso-principle, which was implemented by matching the patient's agitation level with the qualities of the music and slowly changing the music systematically to more calming music elements. Once the patient's attentional focus was on the music, this process resulted in the patient sleeping within 20 min. The restraints were removed at this time and the music therapy session ended.

Medical Surgical Intensive Care Unit

Patient: Sixty-eight-year-old male experiencing postoperative pain.

Referral Source: RN referred patient for pain reduction because of patient reporting elevated pain levels after receiving maximum pain medication dosage.

When the music therapist entered the patient room, the patient was lying in bed with toes curled, fists clenched, and grimacing. The patient's wife told the music therapist that her husband was not able to rest because of the pain. The patient was able to verbally rate his pain as a level 8 on a 10-point scale and communicate his music preference. The music therapist sang the patient's preferred music while playing guitar accompaniment and used the iso-principle technique to reduce the patient's perception of pain. The process took 25 min, and the session ended when the patient was sleeping. As the music therapist said goodbye to the wife and left the room, the patient awoke and rated his pain as a level 2.

Outpatient Surgery Unit

Patient: Five-year-old female scheduled for tonsillectomy and adenoidectomy.

Referral Source: Standing referral for preoperative anxiety reduction.

Upon entering the preoperative unit waiting room, the music therapist talked with an RN to identify which patients were exhibiting the highest levels of anxiety. The patient identified as the most anxious was seated in her mother's lap. When the music therapist approached the patient, the patient buried her face in her mother's arms. The patient's mother also showed heightened levels of anxiety in her facial expression and rapid foot tapping. The music therapist offered three different types of instruments for the child to explore and play as the music therapist sang children's songs. The child then looked in the music therapist's bag of instruments to choose what to play next and chose an instrument for her mom to play as well. The music therapist continued to let the child choose the instruments to play throughout the session to give the child more control and increase feelings of security. When it was time for the conscious sedation to be inhaled, the music therapist sang a song with the breathing instructions in the lyrics and the child complied with no resistance. The patient was then transferred to the preoperative holding area. The patient's mother thanked the music therapist for the intervention services provided, stating that it was very helpful in reducing her own concern and worry.

Inpatient Pediatrics
Patient: Thirteen-year-old diagnosed with medulloblastoma.

Referral Source: Social worker referred the patient for music therapy services because of patient's low arousal and apathy toward completing schoolwork during her extended hospitalization.

When the music therapist walked into the patient's room, the patient was lying on her bed watching television (TV). The patient greeted the music therapist verbally but did not make eye contact or turn toward the music therapist. To establish rapport, the music therapist talked with the patient about her favorite TV shows and hobbies. The patient exhibited flat affect during the entire conversation. The music therapist then asked about the patient's music preference and gave the patient a repertoire list to look through to identify songs and artists the patient liked. When a song was identified, the music therapist played part of the song to assess differences in patient responses. After music preference was identified, the music therapist led the patient through a lyric analysis to discuss feelings of isolation, sadness, and anger. The patient engaged in the lyric analysis and openly discussed feelings about her diagnosis and hospitalization. The music therapist then discussed the schoolwork needing completion while hospitalized. The patient and music therapist created a daily work plan for weekdays and scheduled music therapy sessions to occur immediately following the schoolwork time for motivation and accountability. The music therapist continued to see the patient, addressing coping skill development and improved mood state.

Chemotherapy Unit
Patient: Fifty-six-year-old female diagnosed with breast cancer.

Referral Source: RN manager identified patient as appropriate for music therapy services because of increased nausea and anxiety.

The music therapist provided intervention services in the outpatient chemotherapy room. Other patients receiving chemotherapy treatment were informed about the music therapy session and were told they could request the music to stop playing if for any reason it had a negative impact on their experience. The music therapist assessed the patient's anxiety level and preferred music verbally. The patient rated her anxiety level as extremely high and reported high levels of nausea. The music therapist immediately began singing and playing guitar to redirect the patient's attention to the music stimulus. The patient appeared to be uncomfortable as evidenced by her facial expression and fidgeting in her recliner. The music therapist played music continuously to distract the patient from the perception of the nausea and lower anxiety. The nausea was experienced in waves, which the music therapist assessed by the patient's nonverbal behaviors of discomfort. When the patient started exhibiting these behaviors, the music therapist would play a contrasting song in style and quality to redirect the patient's attention back to the music. The music therapist played for the entire chemotherapy treatment. At the end of the session, the patient stated she was able to focus on the music the entire session and rated her anxiety level as low.

Palliative Care Unit
Patient: Seventy-nine-year-old male admitted to palliative care unit.

Referral Source: Interdisciplinary team meeting. The patient was identified as restless and needing increased comfort care. Music therapy was identified as an appropriate service provision for comfort measures.

Before the first patient visit, the music therapist met with the family to determine the patient's music preferences. The patient's wife and son shared that the patient had loved music throughout his lifetime and identified favorite artists and songs. The patient received music therapy sessions three times per week until the patient died. During these sessions the music therapist timed the session based on the time of day when the patient was the most restless by nurse report. At the beginning of each session, the patient's restlessness and agitation level were assessed by the music therapist. The music therapist then chose familiar music that matched the patient's agitation level in the qualities and intensity of the music. The patient quickly entrained to the music each session, with more time needed to entrain as the weeks progressed. The patient typically first entrained with respiration rate, followed by heart rate. The music therapist then utilized the iso-principle technique to decrease restlessness and increase comfort levels. Each session ended with the patient sleeping peacefully.

TABLE 5.8
Updated Medical Music Therapy Techniques

	Passive Music Listening	Active Music Participation	Music and Counseling	Music for Developmental or Educational Needs	Music and Stimulation	Music and Biofeedback	Music and Group Activity
Patient needs	• Pain reduction • Anxiety reduction • Increased motivation	• Cognitive stimulation • Decreased isolation	• Improved coping • Acceptance • Anticipatory grief	• Academic achievement • Developmental skills across domains	• Nonverbal skills • Sensory stimulation	• Emotional regulation • Increased physical Activity • Mindfulness	• Increased physical Activity • Socialization
Examples	• Guided relaxation • Iso-priciple • Contingent music	• Music video production • Singing	• Songwriting • lyric analysis	• Contingent music • Therapeutic instrument Play • Singing	• Drumming • Therapeutic instrumental Play • Singing	• Iso-principle • Improvisation	• Executive functioning stimulation • Memory recall

PROVISION OF SERVICES

Music therapy services can be implemented in hospital settings on specific units or via referral pathways. One of the unique aspects of being a music therapist in a healthcare setting is the applicability of services for all patient areas and units. Unlike other types of therapists, there are a variety of needs that can be met through music therapy that are not unit specific. As a result, some hospitals have music therapists set up on a referral pathway that is not unit dedicated. In that model, the referrals are flagged either upon admission or as patients exhibit symptoms during their stay. Referral pathways target specific patient needs such as pain, or anxiety, depression, reality orientation, or coping. In this model music therapists triage patients throughout the hospital for the referral need and will move from unit to unit throughout each day (see Fig. 5.3).

Other hospitals hire music therapists for specific patient units such as cancer, palliative care, neurology, orthopedics, pediatrics, or pre/postoperative. In this model, music therapists address all of the patient needs on a specific unit, usually remaining in that unit for implementation of services. In this scenario, music therapists can work on a different goal/need area for each patient seen in a day (Fig. 5.4).

The area providing the funding for the music therapy position initially determines referral pathways and implementation of music therapy services. For example, private donors may fund a position specifically for pediatric oncology services. The surgical department may fund a position for pre/postoperative music therapy to decrease anxiety and length of time of recovery. On the other hand, the hospital general budget may fund a music therapy position to increase patient satisfaction hospital wide. In the case of third-party reimbursement funding streams, an NICU may fund a music therapy position to provide protocols of care covered by insurance reimbursement. In each scenario, the referral pathway must be determined for music therapists to decide patient flow of care.

AREAS OF FUTURE RESEARCH

Many patient care areas still need investigation to formalize music therapy protocols to predictably meet an improved outcome for a specific patient need. This

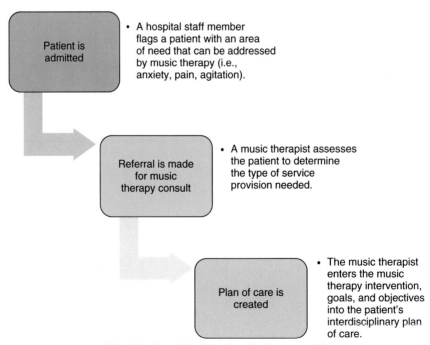

• A hospital staff member flags a patient with an area of need that can be addressed by music therapy (i.e., anxiety, pain, agitation).

Patient is admitted

• A music therapist assesses the patient to determine the type of service provision needed.

Referral is made for music therapy consult

• The music therapist enters the music therapy intervention, goals, and objectives into the patient's interdisciplinary plan of care.

Plan of care is created

FIG. 5.3 Hospital-wide referral pathway model.

would enable submission of research outcomes to third-party providers for coverage of services. Although this would be beneficial for music therapy service funding, it has not happened across patient populations for good reason. Identification of which patient populations will likely respond to a music therapy protocol of care leads researchers away from individualized patient care that makes intervention services so successful. Patients with limited previous music exposure and experiences, as in NICU patients, are more likely to respond similarly to music interventions. This allows the creation of protocols of care with predictable responses. With the high variability inherent in the interventions being investigated within the music therapy literature, it is amazing that research does yield robust effect sizes. This leads to the question of how different music interventions and types of music can be effective with such high variability in past patient experiences with music.

The techniques used by music therapists in medical settings have remained virtually unchanged and continually supported by independent researcher findings for decades. As such, it is curious why music therapy is not incorporated into all medical facilities. The variability with which music affects people with a myriad of needs in medical settings makes the application of music difficult to predict for many medical professionals. Music therapists are trained in the unique properties of music across domains: physical, psychological, emotional, and spiritual. Although music therapists will continue to investigate the effectiveness of various techniques, the individuality of how those techniques are applied in therapeutic situations will likely preclude the creation of protocols across patient needs and services provided. Each patient has his or her own history with music, which allows interventions to be successful and at the same time easily replicable. Fitting this reality into a medical model as a standard of care has proven difficult, in spite of the continued positive findings in the literature base. Interestingly, hospital administrators who have witnessed or seen their in-house reports of music therapy efficacy have continued to provide funding for services. In markets where choice of care drives administrator's funding decisions, music therapists have been hired to improve patient experiences and individualize the patient care.

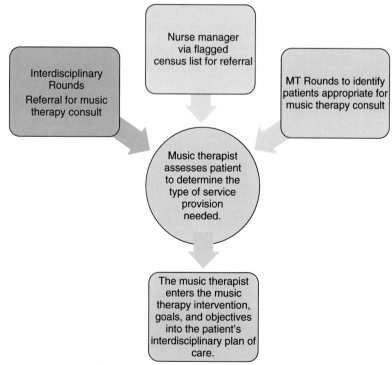

FIG. 5.4 Unit-specific referral pathway model.

REFERENCES

Barrera, M. E., Rykov, M. H., & Doyle, S. L. (2002). The effects of interactive music therapy on hospitalized children with cancer: A pilot study. *Psycho-Oncology, 11*, 379–388. http://dx.doi.org/10.1002/pon.589.

Barry, M. J., & Edgman-Levitan, S. (2012). Shared-decision making - the pinnacle of patient-centered care. *The New England Journal of Medicine, 366*, 780–781. http://dx.doi.org/10.1056/NEJMp1109283.

Berlyne, D. E., & Crozier, J. B. (1971). Effects of complexity and prochoice stimulation on exploratory choice. *Perception & Psychophysics, 10*, 242–246. http://dx.doi.org/10.3758/BF03212813.

Boldt, S. (1996). The effects of music therapy on motivation, psychological well-being, physical comfort, and exercise endurance of bone marrow transplant patients. *Journal of Music Therapy, 33*, 164–188. http://dx.doi.org/10.1093/jmt/33.3.164.

Bradt, J., Potvin, N., Kesslick, A., Shim, M., Radl, D., Schriver, E., ... Komarnicky-Kocher, L. T. (2015). The impact of music therapy versus music medicine psychological outcomes and pain in cancer patients: A mixed methods study. *Supportive Care in Cancer, 23*, 1261–1271. http://dx.doi.org/10.1007/s00520-014-2478-7.

Burns, D. S., Robb, S. L., & Haase, J. E. (2009). Exploring the feasibility of a therapeutic music video intervention in adolescents and young adults during stem-cell transplantation. *Cancer Nursing, 32*(5), E8–E16. http://dx.doi.org/10.1097/NCC.0b013e3181a4802c.

Cassileth, B. R., Vickers, A. J., & Magill, L. A. (2003). Music therapy for mood disturbance during hospitalization for autologous stem cell transplantation. *Cancer, 98*, 2723–2729. http://dx.doi.org/10.1002/cncr.11842.

Cook, E. L., & Silverman, M. J. (2013). Effects of music therapy on spirituality with patients on a medical oncology/hematology unit: a mixed-methods approach. *The Arts in Psychotherapy, 40*, 239–244. http://dx.doi.org/10.1016/j.aip.2013.02.004.

Dileo, C. (2006). Effects of music and music therapy on medical patients: A meta-analysis of the research and implications for the future. *Journal of the Society for Integrative Oncology, 4*, 67–70.

Ferrer, A. J. (2007). The effect of live music on decreasing anxiety in patients undergoing chemotherapy treatment. *Journal of Music Therapy, 44*, 242–255. http://dx.doi.org/10.1093/jmt/44.3.242.

Fredenburg, H. A., & Silverman, M. J. (2014a). Effects of music therapy on positive and negative affect and pain with hospitalized patients recovering from a blood and marrow transplant: A randomized effectiveness study. *The Arts in Psychotherapy, 41*, 174–180. http://dx.doi.org/10.1016/j.aip.2014.01.007.

Fredenburg, H. A., & Silverman, M. J. (2014b). Effects of cognitive-behavioral music therapy on fatigue in patients in a blood and marrow transplantation unit: A mixed-method pilot study. *The Arts in Psychotherapy, 41*, 433–444. http://dx.doi.org/10.1016/j.aip.2014.09.002.

Ghetti, C. M. (2011). Active music engagement with emotional-approach coping to improve well-being in liver and kidney transplant recipients. *Journal of Music Therapy, 48*, 463–485. http://dx.doi.org/10.1093/jmt/48.4.463.

Ghetti, C. M. (2013). Effect of music therapy with emotional-approach coping on preprocedural anxiety in cardiac catheterization: A randomized controlled trial. *Journal of Music Therapy, 50*, 93–122. http://dx.doi.org/10.1093/jmt/50.2.93.

Gooding, L. (2014). *Medical music therapy: Building a comprehensive program*. Silver Spring, MD: American Music Therapy Association.

Hanser, S. B., Bauer-Wu, S., Kubicek, L., Healey, M., Manola, J., Hernandez, M., & Bunnell, C. (2006). Effects of a music therapy intervention on quality of life and distress in women with metastatic breast cancer. *Journal of the Society for Integrative Oncology, 4*, 116–124. http://dx.doi.org/10.2310/7200.2006.014.

Hillmer, M. (2014). Adult medical/surgical music therapy. In L. Gooding (Ed.), *Medical music therapy: Building a comprehensive program* (pp. 135–153). Silver Spring, MD: American Music Therapy Association.

Hogan, T. J., & Silverman, M. J. (2015). Coping-infused dialogue through patient-preferred live music: A medical music therapy protocol and randomized pilot study for hospitalized transplant patients. *Journal of Music Therapy, 52*, 420–436. http://dx.doi.org/10.1093/jmt/thv008.

Institute for Patient-and Family-Centered Care. (2017). *Patient-and family-centered care*. Retrieved from http://www.ipfcc.org/about/pfcc.html.

Kain, Z. N., Caldwell-Andrews, A. A., Krivutza, D. M., Weinberg, M. E., Gaal, D., Wang, S.-M., & Mayes, L. (2004). Interactive music therapy as a treatment for preoperative anxiety in children: A randomized controlled trial. *Anesthesia & Analgesia, 98*, 1260–1266. http://dx.doi.org/10.1213/01.ANE.0000111205.82346.C1.

LeBlanc, A. (1982). An interactive theory of music preference. *Journal of Music Therapy, 19*, 28–45. http://dx.doi.org/10.1093/jmt/19.1.28.

Lee, J. H. (2016). The effects of music on pain: A meta-analysis. *Journal of Music Therapy, 53*, 430–477. http://dx.doi.org/10.1093/jmt/thw012.

Loewy, J., Hallan, C., Friedman, E., & Martinez, C. (2005). Sleep/sedation in children undergoing EEG testing: A comparison of chloral hydrate and music therapy. *Journal of PeriAnesthesia Nursing, 20*, 323–332. http://dx.doi.org/10.1016/j.jopan.2005.08.001.

Madson, A. T., & Silverman, M. J. (2010). The effect of music therapy on relaxation, anxiety, pain perception, and nausea in adult solid organ transplant patients. *Journal of Music Therapy, 47*, 220–232. http://dx.doi.org/10.1093/jmt/47.3.220.

Mandel, S. E., Hanser, S. B., Secic, M., & Davis, B. A. (2007). Effects of music therapy on health-related outcomes in cardiac rehabilitation: A randomized controlled trial. *Journal of Music Therapy, 44*, 176–197. http://dx.doi.org/10.1093/jmt/44.3.176.

Palmer, J., Lane, D., Mayo, D., Schluchter, M., & Leeming, R. (2015). Effects of music therapy on anesthesia requirements and anxiety in women undergoing ambulatory breast surgery for cancer diagnosis and treatment: a randomized controlled trial. *Journal of Clinical Oncology*, *33*, 3162–3168. http://dx.doi.org/10.1200/JCO.2014.59.6049.

Pelletier, C. L. (2004). The effect of music on decreasing arousal due to stress: A meta-analysis. *Journal of Music Therapy*, *41*, 192–214. http://dx.doi.org/10.1093/jmt/41.3.192.

Robb, S. L. (2003). Designing music therapy interventions for hospitalized children and adolescents using a contextual support model of music therapy. *Music Therapy Perspectives*, *21*, 27–40. http://dx.doi.org/10.1093/jmt/40.4.266.

Robb, S. L., Burns, D. S., Stegenga, K. A., Haut, P. R., Monahan, P. O., Meza, J., ... Haase, J. E. (2014). Randomized clinical trial of therapeutic music video intervention for resilience outcomes in adolescents/young adults undergoing hematopoietic stem cell transplant. *Cancer*, *120*, 909–917. http://dx.doi.org/10.1002/cncr.28355.

Robb, S. L., Clair, A. A., Watanabe, M., Monahan, P. O., Azzouz, F., Stouffer, J. W., ... Hannan, A. (2008). Randomized controlled trial of the active music engagement (AME) intervention on children with cancer. *Psycho-Oncology*, *17*, 699–708. http://dx.doi.org/10.1002/pon.1301.

Rosenow, S. C., & Silverman, M. J. (2014). Effects of single session music therapy on hospitalized patients recovering from a bone marrow transplant: Two studies. *The Arts in Psychotherapy*, *41*, 65–70. http://dx.doi.org/10.1016/j.aip.2013.11.003.

Shah, P., & Mountain, D. (2007). The medical model is dead – Long live the medical model. *The British Journal of Psychiatry*, *191*, 375–377. http://dx.doi.org/10.1192/bjp.bp.107.037242.

Standley, J. M. (1986). Music research in medical/dental treatment: meta-analysis and clinical applications. *Journal of Music Therapy*, *23*(2), 56–122. http://dx.doi.org/10.1093/jmt/23.2.56.

Standley, J. M. (1992). Clinical applications of music and chemotherapy: The effects on nausea and emesis. *Music Therapy Perspectives*, *10*, 27–35. https://doi.org/10.1093/mtp/10.1.27.

Standley, J. M. (1995). Music as a therapeutic intervention in medical and dental treatment: research and clinical applications. In T. Wigram, B. Saperston, & R. West (Eds.), *The art and science of music therapy: A handbook* (pp. 3–22). New York: Routledge.

Standley, J. M. (2002). A meta-analysis of the efficacy of music therapy for premature infants. *Journal of Pediatric Nursing*, *17*, 107–113. http://dx.doi.org/10.1053/jpdn.2002.124128.

Standley, J. (2012). Music therapy research in the NICU: an updated meta-analysis. *Neonatal Network: The Journal of Neonatal Nursing*, *31*, 311–316. http://dx.doi.org/10.1891/0730-0832.31.5.311.

Standley, J. M., Gooding, L., & Yinger, O. (2014). Pediatric medical music therapy. In L. Gooding (Ed.), *Medical music therapy: Building a comprehensive program* (pp. 117–133). Silver Spring, MD: American Music Therapy Association.

Tan, S.-L., Spackman, M. P., & Peaslee, C. L. (2006). The effects of repeated exposure on liking and judgments of musical unity of intact and patchwork compositions. *Music Perception: An Interdisciplinary Journal*, *23*, 407–421. http://dx.doi.org/10.1525/mp.2006.23.5.407.

Tan, X., Yowler, C. J., Super, D. M., & Fratianne (2010). The efficacy of music therapy protocols for decreasing pain, anxiety, and muscle tension levels during burn dressing changes: A prospective randomized crossover trial. *Journal of Burn Care & Research*, *31*, 590–597. http://dx.doi.org/10.1097/BCR.0b013e3181e4d71b.

Walworth, D. D. (2005). Procedural-support music therapy in the healthcare setting: A cost-effectiveness analysis. *Journal of Pediatric Nursing*, *20*, 276–284. http://dx.doi.org/10.1016/j.pedn.2005.02.016.

Weller, C. M., & Baker, F. A. (2011). The role of music therapy in physical rehabilitation: A systematic literature review. *Nordic Journal of Music Therapy*, *20*, 43–61. http://dx.doi.org/10.1080/08098131.2010.485785.

Whitehead-Pleaux, A., Zebrowski, N., Baryza, M. J., & Sheridan, R. L. (2007). Exploring the effects of music therapy on pediatric pain: Phase 1. *Journal of Music Therapy*, *44*, 217–241. http://dx.doi.org/10.1093/jmt/44.3.217.

Yates, G., & Silverman, M. N. (2015). Immediate effects of single-session music therapy on affective state inpatients on a post-surgical oncology unit: A randomized effectiveness study. *The Arts in Psychotherapy*, *44*, 57–61. http://dx.doi.org/10.1016/j.aip.2014.11.002.

Yinger, O. S. (2016). Music therapy as procedural support for young children undergoing immunizations: A randomized controlled study. *Journal of Music Therapy*, *53*, 336–363. http://dx.doi.org/10.1093/jmt/thw010.

Yinger, O. S., & Gooding, L. F. (2015). A systematic review of music-based interventions for procedural support. *Journal of Music Therapy*, *52*, 1–77. http://dx.doi.org/10.1093/jmt/thv004.

Yinger, O. S., & Standley, S. (2011). The effects of medical music therapy on patient satisfaction: As measured by the Press Ganey Inpatient Survey. *Music Therapy Perspectives*, *29*, 149–156. http://dx.doi.org/10.1093/mtp/29.2.149.

FURTHER READING

Clark, M., Isaacks-Downton, G., Wells, N., Redlin-Frazier, S., Eck, C., Hepworth, J. T., ... Chakravarthy, J. T. (2006). Use of preferred music to reduce emotional distress and symptom activity during radiation therapy. *Journal of Music Therapy*, *43*, 247–265. http://dx.doi.org/10.1093/jmt/43.3.247.

Stanczyk, M. M. (2011). Music therapy in supportive cancer care. *Reports of Practical Oncology and Radiotherapy*, *16*, 170–172. http://dx.doi.org/10.1016/j.rpor.2011.04.005.

CHAPTER 6

Music Therapy in Hospice and Palliative Care

MEGANNE K. MASKO, PHD, MT-BC/L

CHAPTER OVERVIEW

The end of life can be difficult not only for the person who is dying, but also for his or her friends, family members, and caregivers (Kübler-Ross, 1969). Music therapists frequently work within an interdisciplinary group of hospice professionals to provide compassionate care at the end of life. This chapter will provide the reader with an overview of music therapy in hospice and palliative care in the United States. The chapter begins with a broad description of hospice and palliative care, a brief history of hospice care, and a general overview of the people music therapists are most likely to encounter in this work. Next, readers will find a summary of evidence-based practice (EBP) in music therapy, including information about research, assessment, quality improvement projects, and patient preferences in clinical practice. Case examples help to illustrate the many roles served by music therapists on hospice and palliative care teams and a section on service provision highlights how those music therapists come to be in those roles. Finally, a section on areas of future research draws attention to some of the challenges and opportunities for future hospice music therapy researchers.

HOSPICE AND PALLIATIVE CARE

Hospice and palliative care are two distinct, but interconnected, clinical populations with whom music therapists work. In the strictest sense of the terms, hospice care is a philosophy of care, whereas palliative care is a model of medical care.

Hospice care is the belief that every person has the right to a pain-free and dignified death. According to the World Health Organization (WHO):

Palliative care is an approach that improves the quality of life of patients (adults and children) and their families who are facing problems associated with life-threatening illness. It prevents and relieves suffering through the early identification, correct assessment and treatment of pain and other problems, whether physical, psychosocial or spiritual.

WHO (2015, PARA. 1).

As Raffa wrote, "All hospice is palliative care, but not all palliative care is hospice" (2003, p. 1). In practice, hospice care is reserved for patients with a medical prognosis of 6 months or less if the qualifying disease was to run its typical course, whereas palliative care does not have a prognostic time constraint placed on it. Patients who receive palliative care services may still be receiving disease-focused (or curative) treatment, whereas hospice patients are not.

According to the National Cancer Institute (2012):

Hospice care focuses on controlling pain and other symptoms of illness so patients can remain as comfortable as possible near the end of life. Hospice focuses on caring, not curing. The goal is to neither hasten nor postpone death (para 1).

The focus of both hospice and palliative care is to improve quality of life for patients and their support systems, and music therapy (MT) can be a powerful nonpharmacologic way to do just that. According to Hilliard (2001), adult hospice patients receiving MT services reported an overall higher quality of life than those who did not receive MT. Likewise, MT can decrease fatigue and anxiety and increase the quality of life for hospice caregivers (Choi, 2010).

Music therapists are not specifically identified in the hospice regulations. The hospice interdisciplinary group (IDG), as defined in the Social Security Act (SSA), 42 USC § 1861 (1982), must include at least a physician, nurse, social worker, pastoral or other counselor, and volunteers. Hospice care teams may also include psychologists, clinical social workers, home health aides, physical or occupational therapists, speech-language pathologists, or other professionals such as music therapists (see Fig. 6.1).

A growing number of hospices and palliative care programs employ board-certified music therapists (MT-BCs). According to Dain, Bradley, Hurzeler, and Aldridge (2015), approximately 53% of hospices in the United States employ a music therapist. The annual

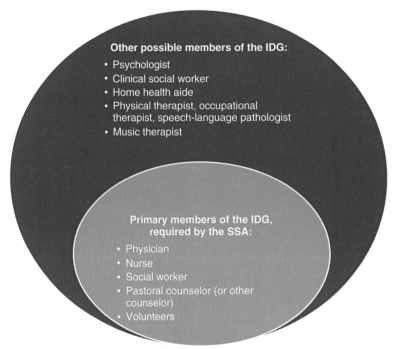

FIG. 6.1 Members of the hospice interdisciplinary group. *IDG*, interdisciplinary group; *SSA*, Social Security Act.

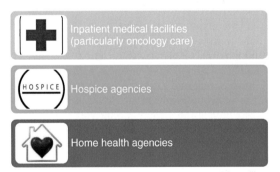

FIG. 6.2 Settings where music therapists provide palliative care.

workforce survey conducted by the American Music Therapy Association (AMTA, 2015) indicated that approximately 12% of survey respondents worked with terminally ill patients. In addition, music therapists working in oncology programs are likely to provide inpatient palliative care services. As of July 2016, the Joint Commission offered a community-based palliative care certification for home health and hospice agencies, so music therapists working with those categories of agencies may also provide services to patients receiving palliative care (see Fig. 6.2).

HISTORY OF HOSPICE CARE

Historically, hospices were places for travelers to rest, especially those suffering from illness, and were maintained according to religious custom (Marrelli, 1999). The ancient Egyptians built temples that functioned as both hospitals and hospices. Greeks, Romans, early Christians, Buddhists, and Muslims developed centers to care for the ill, poor, and disabled (Cohen, 1979). Crusaders traveling to and from the Holy Land received care from orders such as The Knights Hospitallers (Connor, 1998). Later religious orders in France, Ireland, and England made it their vocational callings to tend to the sick and dying (Siebold, 1992). It was in one of those religious hospices that Dame Cicely Saunders developed the basic concepts of the modern hospice movement (Saunders, 1981). Saunders trained as a nurse, social worker, and physician before beginning her work at St. Joseph's Hospice in London in 1958 (Siebold, 1992). Saunder's research on pain management, in conjunction with the work of psychiatrist Elizabeth Kübler-Ross, inspired Florence Wald, former dean of the Yale Graduate School of Nursing, to open the first American home-based hospice in 1974 (du Boulay, 1984; Forman, Kitzes, Anderson, & Sheehan, 2003). The use of music to provide relief from symptoms of terminal illnesses has been documented before the rise of the modern hospice movement (Davis & Gfeller, 2008), and music therapists have been working in hospice care since shortly after the movement came to North America (Gilbert, 1977; Munro & Mount, 1978).

OVERVIEW OF POPULATION

Everyone dies. The old and the young, those with and without disabilities, and people from every gender identity and sexual orientation, socioeconomic status, ethnic background, religion, and region. People die from accidents, sudden illnesses, and prolonged health conditions. The number of people in the United States dying while receiving hospice services has steadily increased over the past several years (National Hospice and Palliative Care Organization, NHPCO, 2015).

Approximately 1.3 million people received end-of-life (EOL) care via hospice services in the United States in 2013 (Centers for Disease Control and Prevention, 2016). Patients with cancer remain the largest group utilizing hospice services (36.6%), followed by patients with dementia (14.8%), heart disease (14.7%), and lung disease (9.3%). Of those patients receiving hospice services, approximately half had a length of stay (LOS; the amount of time they received services) of 17 days or less. The average LOS for hospice patients was 73 days (NHPCO, 2015). Patients receiving hospice services must be certified as hospice eligible at the time of admission and then again at intervals of 90 days for the first 6 months of care. Patients who continue to qualify for hospice services after the first 6 months of hospice admission must be recertified by a physician every 60 days (NHPCO, 2012).

The majority (58.9%, or approximately 942,000) of hospice patients died in their place of residence, be that a private home, residential facility, or nursing facility (NHPCO, 2015, p. 6). Approximately 31.8% of patients died in an inpatient hospice facility, and the remaining 9.3% of patients died in a hospital. According to a retrospective study by Liu, Burns, Hilliard, Stump, and Unroe (2015), music therapists work more with patients in nursing and residential facilities than private homes.

Regardless of the patients' residence, music therapists working in hospice enter patients' private physical and emotional spaces when providing services. When writing about work as a music therapist in pediatric palliative care in Australia, Forrest (2014) noted:

> *I am a guest in the family home; and there can be many things happening in the home that may become part of, or even prevent music therapy from happening, such as family rituals and behaviours; the presence or absence of family members, friends and pets; and other activities that are taking place at the same time as music therapy. The culture of the family also includes their beliefs, family and community supports, and the ways in which they understand and conceptualise health, illness, death and dying (p. 17).*

The vast majority of hospice patients in the United States are 65 years and older (84%), 41.1% of whom are 85 years and older. Only 0.5% of hospice admissions were children and adults younger than 24 years. This means that music therapists working in hospice and palliative care are more likely to work with adults older than 65 years, although there are certainly regional variations in provision of, and access to, pediatric hospice care (NHPCO, 2015).

There is an increasing need for high-quality and culturally competent hospice and palliative care for patients living with disabilities (NHPCO, 2009). Although major healthcare disparities still exist between people with and without disabilities, people with disabilities are living longer. This means they are more likely to develop ailments associated with older age, such as cancer, heart disease, and lung disease. In addition, some types of disabilities have health issues related specifically to the cause of the disability. For example, people with Down syndrome are at an increased risk for congenital heart defects and Alzheimer disease because of their third copy of the 21st chromosome (Bull & American Academy of Pediatrics, 2011; Down Syndrome Research Foundation, 2015). Music therapists need to be prepared to provide services that take into account the unique EOL needs of individuals with disabilities. Likewise, they need to be prepared to work with veterans and other survivors of trauma.

SUMMARY OF RESEARCH

It is important to note that, due to linguistic differences in how the terms are used around the world, it can be difficult to separate out palliative MT research from hospice MT research. The body of literature supporting the use of MT in hospice and palliative care is small but growing, and the quality of research continues to improve.

In an update to a Cochrane systematic review of MT in EOL care, McConnell, Scott, and Porter (2016) found a small amount of evidence supporting the use of MT to treat pain and overall quality of life, but there was no evidence to support treatment of social or communication symptoms in EOL care. They noted that the findings of their review, "while encouraging, demonstrate that, at present, the beneficial therapeutic effects of music therapy for the palliative care population have not been fully demonstrated" (p. 881).

There are two main types of research a person is likely to encounter when searching for external evidence about the efficacy and effectiveness of MT in palliative and hospice care: research conducted by primary

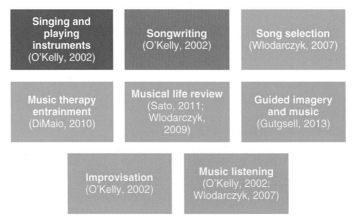

FIG. 6.3 Interventions used in hospice and palliative care music therapy.

care providers without a music therapist, and research conducted by, or with, credentialed music therapists. Research conducted by primary care providers tends to focus on music listening interventions, many of which do not require the clinical training of a credentialed music therapist, whereas music therapist–led research includes multiple types of music-based interventions (see Fig. 6.3), such as singing and playing instruments, songwriting, song selection, entrainment, musical life review, music-assisted relaxation, guided imagery and music, improvisation, and music listening (Clements-Cortés, 2016; Mramor, 2001; O'Kelly, 2002; Sato, 2011; Trauger-Querry & Haghighi, 1999; Wlodarczyk, 2009).

MT has the capacity to "meet the multidimensional needs of the terminally ill and their loved ones" (Hilliard, 2001, p. 165). The flexibility of music as a therapeutic medium means that MT interventions and sessions often address multiple goal areas simultaneously. According to a large study conducted by Burns, Perkins, Tong, Hilliard, and Cripe (2015), family members of adult hospice patients who received MT services reported lower levels of dyspnea (shortness of breath) and "higher likelihood of discussions surrounding spiritual beliefs along with adequate spiritual support" (p. 229). Family members of patients who received MT services also reported overall higher levels of satisfaction with hospice services than those of patients who did not receive MT services.

DiMaio (2010) found that MT entrainment sessions conducted from a humanistic perspective reduced reported pain and provided opportunities for adult hospice patients and caregivers to have their feelings and experiences validated by the music therapist. Likewise, in a study by Hilliard (2001), hospice patients reported that MT helped reduce pain and anxiety, facilitate life review, provide opportunities for creative and emotional expression, and address anticipatory grief.

Music therapists often have very few visits with their patients because of the short LOS of most hospice patients. As such, it is important that patients are able to see benefits from what could be considered the briefest of therapies. A number of studies have analyzed the effects of a single MT session on patient needs in both palliative and hospice care. Krout (2001) found that a single MT session improved patients' pain control, sense of relaxation, and physical comfort, according to both patient self-report and outside observer report (p. 388).

Gutgsell et al. (2013) conducted a single 20-min MT session consisting of autogenic relaxation, imagery, and music listening with adult palliative care patients. The authors found that patients in the MT group reported statistically significant lower levels of pain than did patients in the control group. It is possible that some of the benefit from MT stems from opportunities for choice and control offered during sessions (Sheridan & McFerran, 2004). Table 6.1 includes a summary of selected controlled MT studies in hospice and palliative care.

Bereavement

MT sessions also provide meaning for the families of hospice patients that can carry through the bereavement process (see Table 6.2). Parents of terminally ill children report receiving comfort from MT sessions after the deaths of their children (Lindenfelser, Grocke, & McFerran, 2008). Parents in Australia reported that MT "contributed significantly to the memory of their child, and 'gave them something to hang on to' after their child had died" (p. 339). Magill (2009) found that families of hospice patients reported receiving continued significant spiritual support even after the death of their loved ones. In a qualitative study of bereaved caregivers of hospice patients, caregivers reported feeling joy, empowerment, connections within themselves,

TABLE 6.1
Summary of Selected Controlled Music Therapy Studies in Hospice and Palliative Care

Author, Year	Setting/Population	Interventions	Outcomes
Burns et al. (2015)[a]	Patients with cancer receiving hospice care	Not specified	Less dyspnea, spiritual support for patients; greater satisfaction for family members
Gutgsell et al. (2013)[b]	Inpatients receiving palliative care	Autogenic relaxation and live music	Significantly greater decrease in pain
Hilliard (2003)[b]	Newly admitted hospice patients with terminal cancer	Various: song choice, music listening, singing, isoprinciple	Significantly better quality of life

[a]Retrospective cross-sectional analysis; propensity scores used to adjust for nonrandom assignment.
[b]Randomized controlled trial.

TABLE 6.2
Summary of Selected Music Therapy Research in Bereavement

Author, Year	Setting/Population	Interventions	Outcomes
Hilliard (2007)	Bereaved school-aged students	Orff-based music therapy: improvisation, singing, chanting, rhythm activities, and discussion/education	Significant improvement in behavioral distress and grief symptoms
Lindenfelser et al. (2008)	Parents of pediatric palliative care patients	Not specified	Music therapy enhanced remembrance, communication, and expression
Magill (2009)	Bereaved caregivers	Music-assisted life review	Themes of joy, empowerment, and reflection

connections with other people, connections with entities beyond themselves, remembrance, and hope in response to MT sessions with their loved ones.

A small study by Hilliard (2007) indicated that children can benefit from MT for bereavement. Students who participated in an Orff-based school bereavement group showed significant improvement in behavioral distress and grief symptoms as compared with students in the control group. The MT sessions included improvisation, singing, chanting, rhythm activities, and discussion and education about the grieving process.

EVIDENCE-BASED PRACTICE
The external evidence from which music therapists draw to assist in engaging in EBP was summarized earlier. That, however, is only one piece of the EBP process. MT is, by its very nature, a highly individualized treatment practice. In terms of EBP, that means that music therapists are likely to place a great deal of emphasis on internal evidence (individual assessment information and responses, quality improvement projects, etc.) and patient preference when creating and implementing MT treatment plans.

There are three types of assessment in both hospice and palliative care settings: initial, comprehensive, and ongoing. The initial assessment is typically done by a primary member of the hospice team (nurse or social worker, although the music therapist may be involved depending upon the policies and procedures of the agency) and includes gathering as much information as possible about a patient so that referrals can be made to other members of the IDG as appropriate.

Comprehensive assessments often involve two parts, one completed before an assessment session and the second completed during an assessment session with the patient (and perhaps family). The first part includes learning as much about the patient as possible from the chart and other IDG members so the second, in-person, portion of the assessment can be completed successfully. Maue-Johnson and Tanguay published an example of a comprehensive hospice MT assessment in 2006 (see Fig. 6.4). Although electronic health records are the norm, the content of the paper assessment can easily be programmed into electronic documentation systems.

Hospice Music Therapy Assessment

Name_____D.O.B. _____Date_____Time_____
Gender_____Ethnicity_____Patient residence □ home □ SNF   □ ALF   □ hospital □ inpatient
Terminal diagnoses/condition(s)_____
Referred by _____Date of referral_____
Reasons for referral to MT _____

Physical

Pain (0-10) _____ Nonverbal pain indicators Motor activity Respiration
□ self report □ VAS   □ vocal complaints   □ normal   □ normal
Location _____   □ verbal complaints   □ excessive   □ irregular
Frequency _____   □ restlessness   □ slow/lethargic □ short of breath
Sensory/Physical limitations □ rubbing   □ tense/rigid   □ shallow
□ hearing _____   □ facial grimacing   □ restless/agitated □ apneic
□ vision _____   □ bracing   □ n/a   □ labored
□ ambulation _____   □ none   □ O$_2$ in use

Cognitive/Communicative

Mental status	ST memory	LT memory	Communication	Eye contact
□ alert	□ good	□ good	□ verbal	□ usually
□ oriented x_____	□ fair	□ fair	□ fluent	□ sometimes
□ confused	□ poor	□ poor	□ impaired	□ rarely
□ lethargic	□ n/a	□ n/a	□ initiates	□ never
□ forgetful			□ responds	□ n/a
□ minimally responsive			□non-verbal (specify):_____	

Psychological/Emotional

Mood   **Anxiety**   **Coping**
□ appropriate □ observed   Pt has opportunities to express fears/concerns □ Y □ N □ n/a
□ flat/blunt   □ not observed   Pt is effectively adapting to life changes   □ Y □ N □ n/a
□ unstable   *Source of anxiety* Primary coping strategies:
□ withdrawn   □ environmental   □ engaged □ disengaged □ problem-focused □emotion-focused
□ depressed   □ physical   Primary support system:_____
□ anxious   □ emotional   **Anticipatory grieving**
□ relaxed/calm □ social   Pt verbally expresses feelings   □ Y □ N □ n/a
□ n/a   □ other (specify):____ Pt initiates discussion about illness/terminality □ Y □ N □ n/a
             _____   Pt engages in life review   □ Y □ N □ n/a

Social

Significant others	Relationship	Phone number	Contacted

Frequency of family/friend contact _____
Current involvement in social activities _____
Family coping   **Family expresses:**
Family is actively preparing for death   □ Y □ N □ n/a   □ helplessness   □ hopelessness
Family anticipatory grieving   □ Y □ N □ n/a
Family communication about pt's terminality: □ open □ mutual pretense □ suspected □ closed □ unknown
  Explain:_____
History of losses_____

FIG. 6.4 Comprehensive hospice music therapy assessment. (From Maue-Johnson, E. L., & Tanguay, C. L. (2006). Assessing the unique needs of hospice patients: A tool for music therapists. *Music Therapy Perspectives, 24,* 13–20. http://dx.doi.org/10.1093/mtp/24.1.13; used with permission.)

Spiritual

Faith tradition _____ □ practicing □ non-practicing □ unknown
Spiritual conflict/distress _____

Musical

Musical background _____
Musical preferences _____
Specific songs requested _____
Observed responses to music (Level of involvement: □ active   □ passive)
    Physical _____
_____

    Cognitive/communicative _____
_____

    Psychological/Emotional _____
_____

    Social _____
_____

    Spiritual _____
_____

Treatment Plan

□ MT will not be implemented due to _____
□ MT will be implemented _____x monthly and as needed, utilizing the following initial care plan:

Problems	Goals	Interventions

Problems
P 100—Anxiety
P 101—Breathing pattern, ineffective
P 102—Pain
P 103—Agitation/restlessness
P 104—Communication, impaired
P 105—Ineffective coping, pt
P 106—Ineffective coping, family
P 107—Anticipating grieving, pt
P 108—Anticipatory grieving, family
P 109—Depression
P 110—Loss of autonomy
P 111—Isolation
P 112—Caregiver role strain
P 113—Spiritual needs
P 114—Imminent death
P 000—Other (specify)

Goals
G 100—Increase relaxation
G 101—Enhance respiratory comfort
G 102—Increase physical comfort
G 103—Decrease pain perception
G 104—Reduce anxiety
G 105—Increase sensory stimulation
G 106—Enhance communication
    within limits of disease
G 107—Elevate mood
G 108—Increase meaningful social
    interaction
G 109—Increase social and emotional
    support
G 110—Increase self-expression
G 111—Increase non-verbal expression
G 112—Engage in life review/
    reminiscence
G 113—Increase family communication
    re: terminality
G 114—Normalize experience/
    environment
G 115—Acknowledge and process
    life changes
G 116—Process in grieving by stages
G 117—Demonstrate effective coping
G 118—Identify caregiver role strain
G 119—Identify coping strategies/resources
G 120—Increase spiritual support
G 000—Other (specify)

Interventions
I 100—Facilitatemusic-assisted relaxation
I 101—Utilize iso-rhythmic principle
I 102—Provide opportunities for socialization,
    communication, and self-expression
I 103—Provide live music for
    diversion/refocus
I 104—Provide a comforting presence
I 105—Facilitate songwriting
I 106—Facilitate lyric analysis
I 107—Validate emotional expression
I 108—Facilitate music-assisted life review
I 109—Utilize supportive counseling
    techniques
I 110—Utilize familiar, significant songs
I 111—Assist in creation of tangible legacy
I 112—Promote successful experiences
I 113—Provide means for control over
    environment
I 114—Create opportunities for positive shared
    experiences
I 115—Provide pt defined spiritual music
I 116—Conduct music-based rituals
I 117—Provide pt/family support during
    imminent death
I 118—Live music to facilitate release
I 000—Other (specify)

Music Therapist Signature _____ **Patient Name** _____

FIG. 6.4, cont'd

Ongoing assessment takes places every time a member of the hospice and/or palliative care team interacts with the patient and family. When engaging in ongoing assessment, the music therapist looks at how the patient and family are feeling and coping in the moment, as well as how they have changed since the last visit. Ongoing assessment is crucial in providing timely and appropriate care because patients can drastically change from visit to visit. Music therapists need to assess patients at every meeting and take into account assessments from other hospice team members, to meet the needs of patients and families in the moment. See Fig. 6.5 for a summary of how the three types of assessment fit within the MT treatment process.

An important aspect of EBP is incorporating patient preferences and cultural needs into care. The reality of clinical practice in hospice care, in particular, is that many patients are referred to hospice when they are already actively dying or when their physician senses they are close to EOL. Patients may not be able to tell music therapists about preferences. Credentialed music therapists are trained to look for small, observable responses to music and the environment. Many patients may not be able to verbally communicate their preferences, so the music therapist must look for changes in respiration rate, posture, body position, vocalizations, facial expression, and muscle tension to indicate positive or negative responses to the music and MT interventions.

Quality improvement projects also provide evidence from which music therapists can draw when working in hospice care. One example of a quality improvement project from Cadwalader, Orellano, Tanguay, and Roshan (2016) measured the impact of a single session of live music listening and entrainment on agitation levels in adult patients in hospice care. Agitation was measured before and after the MT session using the Overt Agitation Severity Scale (Yudofsky, Kopecky, Kunik, Silver, & Endicott, 1997). The single MT session reduced

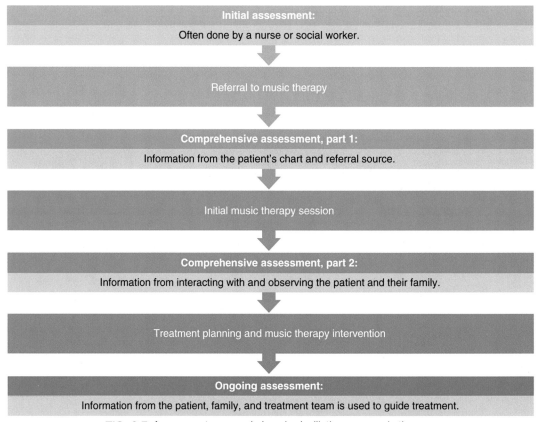

Initial assessment:

Often done by a nurse or social worker.

Referral to music therapy

Comprehensive assessment, part 1:

Information from the patient's chart and referral source.

Initial music therapy session

Comprehensive assessment, part 2:

Information from interacting with and observing the patient and their family.

Treatment planning and music therapy intervention

Ongoing assessment:

Information from the patient, family, and treatment team is used to guide treatment.

FIG. 6.5 Assessment process in hospice/palliative care music therapy.

agitation in 52 of the 73 participants included in the data analysis, with a mean decrease of 5.77 points from pretest to posttest, which was statistically significant ($t = 7.34$, $P < .0001$, $d = 0.74$). According to the authors, the results of the study indicated that MT "can be used to complement the services and treatments provided by the other team members of the interdisciplinary team to reduce agitation" (p. 872).

CASE EXAMPLES

Music therapists on hospice teams serve several important roles, including, but not limited to, communicating important information to other interdisciplinary team members, helping patients and their families achieve personal EOL goals, managing pain and anxiety, providing additional spiritual support for patients and families, creating holding spaces for patients and families during the active dying process, serving as experts in sensory processing, and assisting in the bereavement process. The following case stories highlight some of the music therapist's many roles on the hospice team.

Margaret is a 47-year-old female with a primary diagnosis of metastatic breast cancer. The cancer spread to her brain and bones, causing pain and difficulty with movement. Margaret has a 15-year-old daughter of whom she is the sole guardian. Margaret and her daughter moved in with Margaret's mother so her family could better care for both Margaret and her daughter. One of Margaret's EOL goals was to create recorded messages for her daughter to mark important milestones in the child's life, so the social worker made a referral to the hospice music therapist. Knowing little about the patient other than the information in her admission report, the music therapist scheduled a time to meet Margaret, her mother, and her daughter. Upon arrival at the house, Margaret's behaviors (furrowed brow, groaning, and shifting in her bed) indicated she was experiencing a high level of physical pain. The music therapist confirmed with Margaret that she was experiencing extreme pain, even though she had been taking her pain medication on a regular basis. The music therapist called Margaret's hospice nurse and reported the pain rating from Margaret, as well as the other observed pain indicators. Based on the assessment information provided by the music therapist, the nurse made an immediate visit to the patient's home, contacted the hospice physician, and delivered emergency medications to decrease Margaret's pain. Margaret fell asleep after receiving her emergency pain medications.

In this case, even though the music therapist did not engage in any music-based interventions with the patient or family, the MT's observations, which were quickly communicated to the hospice nurse, improved the quality of life for the patient and her caregivers.

One of the tasks music therapists often support is helping patients create legacy projects (O'Callaghan, 2013). These legacy projects often include audio or video recordings, as well as physical products associated with those recordings. Creating and sharing these products provides patients and families with opportunities for creative expression, enjoyment, emotional expression, relationship completion, and life review. Legacy projects also generate opportunities for music therapists and patients to talk about how those projects may be used in the future (Baxter & O'Callaghan, 2010).

The music therapist returned to Margaret's home a few days after the initial visit and found that Margaret's speech and energy were declining. The tumors in her brain were growing, making it difficult for her to express herself using spoken language, but she still had the goal of creating recorded messages for her daughter. Margaret's ability to communicate improved when she was singing. Rather than try to create several messages, which was no longer a realistic goal, the MT encouraged Margaret to focus on creating one recording for her daughter. Margaret played a particular song for her daughter every night as an infant, which became "their song." The music therapist helped Margaret write additional lyrics to the song to express to her daughter her hopes and dreams for her future. The music therapist recorded the accompaniment and supported Margaret in recording the lyrics to the song. Because singing was more successful than speaking, Margaret was able to convey her desired message to her daughter. The music therapist typed up the lyrics, printed them on archival paper, and added them to a package containing family photos and a recording of the song in multiple data formats for Margaret's daughter.

Music therapists can also offer a unique perspective on how people process sensory information, especially people whose sensory processing abilities may be compromised because of disease processes. This can be especially helpful to hospice patients if the hospice does not have an occupational therapist as part of the regular team. Music therapists can offer the hospice IDG information on how to create and monitor sensory environments.

George is a 92-year-old male diagnosed with end-stage dementia. He is no longer able to walk, feed, clothe, or bathe himself, nor is he able to speak. George resides in the dementia care unit of a long-term care facility. The music therapist arrives for his regularly scheduled visit and notices that George appears agitated and combative. Facility staff report that the behaviors began after they moved him into the day room following breakfast. The music therapist notices that the overhead florescent lights are on, even though there is bright sunlight coming in through the windows, a staff member is vacuuming while another staff member cleans carpets, and the volume on the large screen television is raised so it can be heard well above the noise of the vacuum and carpet cleaners. The music therapist asks the staff to turn off the lights and television, and the staff agree to complete the carpet cleaning later in the day when residents are usually in their rooms. George begins to calm down almost immediately once the lights are dimmed and the volume is reduced. The music | *therapist quietly hums George's favorite song to maintain a comforting sensory environment. After about 10 min, the music therapist adds in quiet guitar accompaniment to the singing, making sure to match George's respiration rate. George's respiration rate slows, his shoulders appear to relax, and his brow smooths as the music therapist quietly plays and sings.*

PROVISION OF SERVICES

Funding

MT is cost-effective. In a cost-benefit analysis of MT in a home hospice program, Romo and Gifford (2007) found that the total care costs of patients receiving MT in a medium-sized, for-profit home hospice were $2984 less than those of patients receiving standard care. The greatest savings could be seen in medication costs. Patients receiving MT services required $2415 less in medications than did patients receiving standard care. The total cost-benefit ratio was 0.83 but increased to 0.95 when cost per patient per day was considered. This means that MT is highly cost-effective in addressing patient needs in hospice care.

As mentioned previously, MT is not a core discipline on the hospice interdisciplinary team, which means MT is not included in the list of services directly reimbursed by Medicare or Medicaid. Hospice and palliative care services may be covered by insurance policies, but MT services are not typically directly reimbursed by those companies for services provided by hospice or palliative care agencies. MT services in hospice are usually paid for via a per diem (daily) rate of reimbursement paid to hospice agencies from insurance companies. Other options for funding MT services include grants, funds raised from community and corporate partners, and private donations. Some hospitals bill insurance for MT services, but those practices vary from facility to facility and state to state.

Referrals

Because MT is not a core discipline on the hospice interdisciplinary team (as defined by the SSA), MT services are typically provided based on referrals. Who makes referrals, and how, varies by agency, but usually anyone involved in the patient's care is able to make a referral, including the patients themselves. Music therapists receive referrals to address a variety of goal areas. In a survey of music therapists working in hospice care, participants identified anxiety, social isolation, restlessness, spirituality, and physical pain as the goal areas most frequently addressed by MT (Masko, 2013). These findings were reflective of earlier referral studies in both

the United States and Australia (Groen, 2007; Horne-Thompson, Daveson, & Hogan, 2007).

Documentation

Most music therapists are taught the mantra, "If you don't document it, then it never happened." Although this saying is true for every population with which music therapists work, it might be the most important to remember in hospice and palliative care. Keeping in mind that the majority of reimbursements for hospice services in particular come from federal (Medicare) and state (Medicaid) funds, and that the Centers for Medicare & Medicaid Services regulates hospices in the United States receiving reimbursement from them, it is especially important to make sure documentation is done correctly, promptly, and in accordance with agency, state, and federal guidelines. Agencies that do not provide appropriate and timely documentation of services and patient responses are likely to have their billing requests denied and may even be fined or lose their privilege to operate.

What does it mean that hospice MT documentation is done "correctly"? Documentation of services in hospice care must relate to the diagnosis under which the person originally qualified for hospice care. Patients may have multiple medical diagnoses, but it is the one used for the hospice admission and qualification that matters. For example, if a patient has both chronic obstructive pulmonary disease (COPD) and prostate cancer, but he was admitted to hospice because of his prostate cancer, the interventions used by the hospice team, and the documentation produced in support of those interventions, must relate to the cancer diagnosis and not the COPD.

Another criterion of "correct" hospice documentation is that it charts patient decline. Hospice care is reserved for patients for whom their disease will be life-ending in 6 months or less if the disease were to run its regular course. Negative charting documents patient decline while also showing the effectiveness of the interventions used to address patient needs. For example, a music therapist working with a patient who has dementia needs to document how the patient continues to decline cognitively and physically, while also describing how the MT

MUSIC THERAPY NARRATIVE

Patient Name: _____   Date: _____

Problem (from charting system): _____

Time in/out: _____/_____   Personal visit/Telephone contact: _____

Contact made with: Patient   Spouse   Family member(s)_____

Caregiver(s)_____   Other_____

Patient cognitive status:
☐ Alert   ☐Disoriented   ☐Confused   ☐Lethargic   ☐Sleeping   ☐Unresponsive

Patient affect:
☐Cheerful   ☐Flat   ☐Anxious   ☐ Agitated   ☐Depressed   ☐Labile

Pain behaviors observed:
☐Moaning ☐Crying ☐Rubbing ☐Shifting ☐Grimacing ☐Bracing ☐None

Does patient appear uncomfortable because of pain? ☐ Yes ☐ No ☐ Unknown

Pain rating (0-10): _____

Pain reported by: ☐ Patient   ☐ Caregiver ☐ Other_____

Primary concerns/goals identified: _____
_____
_____

Actions taken during session:

☐Developed rapport	☐Provided sensory stimulation
☐Decreased perception of pain	☐Provided outlet for creativity
☐Decreased anxiety/stress	☐Processed disease with patient/family
☐Provided interventions/instructions for relaxation	☐Provided means for family interaction
☐Decreased agitation/restlessness	☐Increased social interaction
☐Provided aural sedation	☐Provided outlet for creativity
☐Facilitated music-assisted life review	☐Processed disease with patient/family
☐Facilitated lyric analysis	☐Provided enjoyment
☐Songwriting	☐Provided additional spiritual support
☐Creation of tangible legacies	☐Reviewed progress toward EOL goals
☐Utilized iso principle	☐Actively listened to concerns

FIG. 6.6 Music therapy documentation form used in hospice and palliative care.

interventions help meet the patient's and family's goals. A clinical note might look something like this:

> Helen enjoyed the music therapy visit. She smiled and made consistent eye contact while the music therapist played and sang her preferred music, including "Que Sera, Sera." Helen was able to correctly sing 5-6 lyrics during the comprehensive assessment, but is no longer able to sing with the MT; however, she continues to regularly hum. Helen required hand-over-hand assistance to play the buffalo drum during the session as compared to previous sessions when she could hold the drum herself. Her caregiver said Helen is much less agitated after the MT visits, and that it is easier to provide personal cares when there is music present.

The value of MT is clearly delineated, as is a description of the patient's current level of functioning as compared with the assessment session. Fig. 6.6 provides an

☐Facilitated imagery   ☐Identified bereavement needs

IDG collaboration/referral: _____

Community referral: ☐ Yes _____   ☐ No

Responses to Music Therapy session:

☐ Patient demonstrated physical responses to music Pain rating at end of session (0-10): _____
_____

☐Patient demonstrates cognitive responses to music

☐Patient demonstrates communicative responses to music

☐Patient demonstrates affective responses to music

☐Patient demonstrates social responses to music

☐Patient demonstrates spiritual responses to music

☐Family/caregiver demonstrates cognitive responses to music

☐Family/caregiver demonstrates communicative responses to music

☐Family/caregiver demonstrates affective responses to music

☐Family/caregiver demonstrates social responses to music

☐Family/caregiver demonstrates spiritual responses to music

Other information: _____
_____
_____
_____
_____

FIG. 6.6, cont'd

example of a MT documentation form that can be used in hospice and palliative care.

Interdisciplinary Collaboration

Interdisciplinary collaboration and treatment is the standard in hospice and palliative care. The IDG exists to provide comprehensive and holistic care for patients and their support systems, and team members recognize that each person and discipline brings a unique perspective to the goals and needs of the patient. Assessment, treatment planning, and treatment evaluation are done by the IDG with the input of the patient and patient's family whenever possible. MT complements treatments provided by other team members (see Fig. 6.7), such as improving the effects of pain medication, increasing participation in physical therapy exercises,

and facilitating communication and spiritual expression (Horne-Thompson & Bramley, 2013; O'Kelly & Koffman, 2007).

AREAS FOR FUTURE RESEARCH

There are unique challenges when conducting research in hospice and/or palliative care. First, and foremost, research must be conducted in a way that is ethical and keeps the best interests and needs of patients and families at the forefront of everything done. This means that traditional research methodologies may not be feasible, especially when working with hospice patients. Withholding treatment to create a control condition is particularly problematic, and wait-list controls, which are often used to make

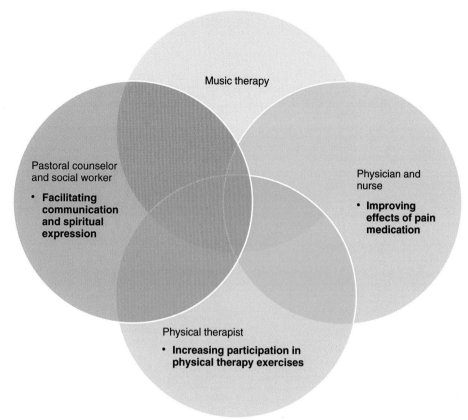

FIG. 6.7 Ways that music therapy can complement treatments provided by other team members.

sure that everyone eventually receives the treatment under investigation, are likely not acceptable or practical when working with people who are terminally ill. Second, researchers need to minimize the amount of time it takes a patient or family member to participate in clinical studies so as not to overburden them with research activities. Third, music therapists need to be flexible in meeting the often rapidly changing needs of their patients, which can make implementation of research protocols difficult. Finally, the short LOS of many hospice patients can make it difficult to measure how MT services affect clients and families over time. This is all to say that scientifically rigorous and clinically meaningful research in hospice and palliative care is possible, but it requires creativity and adaptability on the part of researchers.

Even with the challenges presented earlier, research in hospice MT is growing in both scope and quality,

a trajectory that needs to continue to move the field forward, improve outcomes for patients, and increase access to care (see Fig. 6.8). Future research can, and should, include examining the clinical preparation of music therapists for hospice and palliative care work, clinical decision making, creating theoretically sound and testable interventions to address symptom distress, addressing trauma at EOL, recognizing and attending to the unique needs of military veterans, exploring how best to meet the needs of people who have disabilities at EOL, and identifying and confronting issues of social injustice related to accessing hospice and palliative care services (Reimer-Kirkham et al., 2016). Additional research in these areas will further enhance evidence-based MT practice in hospice and palliative care, in which music therapists carefully consider the best available research, clinical expertise, and the unique needs of each individual to provide compassionate EOL care.

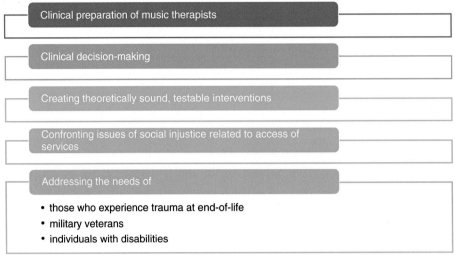

FIG. 6.8 Areas for future research in hospice and palliative care music therapy.

REFERENCES

du Boulay, S. (1984). *Cicely Saunders, founder of the modern hospice movement.* London: Hodder & Stoughton.

American Music Therapy Association. (2015). *AMTA Member Survey & Workforce Analysis.* Silver Spring, MD: AMTA.

Bull, M. J., & American Academy of Pediatrics Committee on Genetics. (2011). Clinical report- Health supervision for children with Down syndrome. *Pediatrics, 128,* 393–406. http://dx.doi.org/10.1542/peds.2011-1605.

Baxter, C., & O'Callaghan, C. (2010). Decisions about the future of music therapy: Products created by palliative care patients. *Australian Journal of Music Therapy, 21,* 2–20.

Burns, D. S., Perkins, S. M., Tong, Y., Hilliard, R. E., & Cripe, L. D. (2015). Music therapy is associated with family perception of more spiritual support and decreased breathing problems in cancer patients receiving hospice care. *Journal of Pain and Symptom Management, 50,* 225–231. http://dx.doi.org/10.1016/j.jpainsymman.2015.02.022.

Cadwalader, A., Orellano, S., Tanguay, C., & Roshan, R. (2016). The effects of a single session of music therapy on the agitated behaviors of patients receiving hospice care. *Journal of Palliative Medicine, 19,* 870–873. http://dx.doi.org/10.1098/jpm.2015.0503.

Centers for Disease Control and Prevention. (2016). *Long-term care providers and services users in the United States: Data from the national study of long-term care providers, 2013-2014.* Retrieved from http://www.cdc.gov/nchs/fastats/hospice-care.htm.

Choi, Y. K. (2010). The effect of music and muscle relaxation on anxiety, fatigue, and quality of life in family caregivers of hospice patients. *Journal of Music Therapy, 47,* 53–69. http://dx.doi.org/10.1093/jmt/47.1.53.

Clements-Cortés, A. (2016). Development and efficacy of music therapy techniques within palliative care. *Complementary Therapies in Clinical Practice, 23,* 125–129. http://dx.doi.org/10.1016/j.ctcp.2015.04.004.

Cohen, K. P. (1979). *Hospice: Prescription for terminal care.* Germantown, MD: Aspen Systems Corporation.

Connor, S. R. (1998). *Hospice: Practice, pitfalls and promise.* Washington, DC: Taylor & Francis.

Dain, A. S., Bradley, E. H., Hurzeler, R., & Aldridge, M. D. (2015). Massage, music, and art therapy in hospice: results of a national survey. *Journal of Pain and Symptom Management, 49*(6), 1035–1041. http://dx.doi.org/10.1016/j.jpainsymman.2014.11.295.

Davis, W. B., & Gfeller, K. E. (2008). Music therapy: Historical perspective. In W. B. Davis, K. E. Gfeller, & M. H. Thaut (Eds.), *An introduction to music therapy theory and practice* (3rd ed.) (pp. 17–40). Silver Springs, MD: American Music Therapy Association.

DiMaio, L. (2010). Music therapy entrainment: a humanistic music therapist's perspective of using music therapy entrainment with hospice clients experiencing pain. *Music Therapy Perspectives, 28,* 106–115. http://dx.doi.org/10.1093/mtp/28.2.106.

Down Syndrome Research Foundation. (2015). *Alzheimer's dementia.* Accessed from http://www.dsrf.org/information/down-syndrome-and-alzheimer-s/.

Forman, W., Kitzes, J., Anderson, R., & Sheehan, D. (2003). *Hospice and palliative care: Concepts and practice* (2nd ed.). Boston: Jones and Bartlett Publishers.

Forrest, L. (2014). Your song, my song, our song: developing music therapy programs for a culturally diverse community in home-based pediatric palliative care. *Australian Journal of Music Therapy, 25,* 14–25.

Gilbert, J. P. (1977). Music therapy perspectives on death and dying. *Journal of Music Therapy, 14*, 165–171. IDG = interdisciplinary group; SSA = Social Security Act.

Groen, K. (2007). Pain assessment and management in end of life care: a survey of assessment and treatment practices of hospice music therapy and nursing professionals. *Journal of Music Therapy, 44*, 90–112. http://dx.doi.org/10.1093/jmt/44.2.90.

Gutgsell, K. J., Schluchter, M., Margevicius, S., DeGolia, P. A., McLaughlin, B., Harris, M., et al. (2013). Music therapy reduces pain in palliative care patients: a randomized controlled trial. *Journal of Pain and Symptom Management, 45*(5), 822–831. http://dx.doi.org/10.1016/j.jpainsymman.2012.05.008.

Hilliard, R. (2001). The use of music therapy in meeting the multidimensional needs of hospice patients and families. *Journal of Palliative Care, 17*, 161–166.

Hilliard, R. (2003). The effects of music therapy on the quality and length of life of people diagnosed with terminal cancer. *Journal of Music Therapy, 40*, 113–137. http://dx.doi.org/10.1093/jmt/40.2.113.

Hilliard, R. (2007). The effects of Orff-based music therapy and social work groups on childhood grief systems and behaviors. *Journal of Music Therapy, 44*, 123–138. http://dx.doi.org/10.1093/jmt/44.2.123.

Horne-Thompson, A., Daveson, B., & Hogan, B. (2007). A project investigating music therapy referral trends within palliative care: An Australian perspective. *Journal of Music Therapy, 44*, 139–155. http://dx.doi.org/10.1093/jmt/44.2.139.

Horne-Thompson, A., & Bramley, R. (2013). The benefits of interdisciplinary practice in a palliative care setting: a music therapy and physiotherapy pilot project. *Progress in Palliative Care, 19*, 304–308. http://dx.doi.org/10.1179/1743291X11Y.0000000017.

Krout, R. (2001). The effects of single-session music therapy interventions on the observed and self-reported levels of pain control, physical comfort, and relaxation of hospice patients. *American Journal of Hospice and Palliative Medicine, 18*, 383–389. http://dx.doi.org/10.1177/104990910101800607.

Kübler-Ross, E. (1969). *On death and dying.* New York, NY: Macmillan.

Lindenfelser, K. J., Grocke, D., & McFerran, K. (2008). Bereaved parents' experiences of music therapy with their terminally ill child. *Journal of Music Therapy, 45*, 330–348. http://dx.doi.org/10.1093/jmt/45.3.330.

Liu, X., Burns, D., Hilliard, R., Stump, T., & Unroe, K. (2015). Music therapy clinical practice in hospice: differences between home and nursing home delivery. *Journal of Music Therapy, 52*, 376–393. http://dx.doi.org/10.1093/jmt/thv012.

Magill, L. (2009). The spiritual meaning of pre-loss music therapy to bereaved caregivers of advanced cancer patients. *Palliative and Supportive Care, 7*, 98–108. http://dx.doi.org/10.1017/S1478951509000121.

Marrelli, T. (1999). *Hospice and palliative care handbook: Quality, compliance, and reimbursement.* St. Louis: Mosby-Year Book.

Masko, M. K. (2013). *Music therapy and spiritual care in end-of-life: Ethical and training issues identified by chaplains and music therapists* (Doctoral dissertation). Retrieved from ProQuest. (3606350).

Maue-Johnson, E. L., & Tanguay, C. L. (2006). Assessing the unique needs of hospice patients: a tool for music therapists. *Music Therapy Perspectives, 24*, 13–20. http://dx.doi.org/10.1093/mtp/24.1.13.

McConnell, T., Scott, D., & Porter, S. (2016). Music therapy for end-of-life care: An updated systematic review. *Palliative Medicine, 30*, 877–883. http://dx.doi.org/10.1177/0269216316635387.

Mramor, K. (2001). Music therapy with persons who are indigent and terminally ill. *Journal of Palliative Care, 17*, 182–187.

Munro, S., & Mount, B. (1978). Music therapy in palliative care. *Canadian Medical Association Journal, 119*, 1029–1034.

National Cancer Institute. (2012). *Hospice care.* Retrieved from https://www.cancer.gov/about-cancer/advanced-cancer/care-choices/hospice-fact-sheet.

National Hospice and Palliative Care Organization. (2009). *Disabilities outreach guide.* Retrieved from https://www.nhpco.org/sites/default/files/public/Access/Outreach_Disabilities.pdf.

National Hospice and Palliative Care Organization. (2012). *Recertification of the hospice terminal illness compliance tip sheet.* Retrieved from http://www.nhpco.org/sites/default/files/public/regulatory/Recertification_Hospice_Terminal_Illness_TipSheet.pdf.

National Hospice and Palliative Care Organization. (2015). *NHPCO's facts and figures: Hospice care in America* (2015 Edition). Retrieved from https://www.nhpco.org/sites/default/files/public/Statistics_Research/2015_Facts_Figures.pdf.

O'Callaghan, C. (2013). Music therapy pre-loss care though legacy creation. *Progress in Palliative Care, 21*(2), 78–82. http://dx.doi.org/10.1179/1743291x12y.0000000044.

O'Kelly, J. (2002). Music therapy in palliative care: current perspectives. *International Journal of Palliative Nursing, 8*, 130–136. http://dx.doi.org/10.12968/ijpn.2002.8.3.10249.

O'Kelly, J., & Koffman, J. (2007). Multidisciplinary perspectives of music therapy in adult palliative care. *Palliative Medicine, 21*, 235–241. http://dx.doi.org/10.1177/0269216307077207.

Raffa, C. (2003). *Palliative care: The legal and regulatory requirements.* Retrieved from http://www.nhpco.org/sites/default/files/public/palliativecare/legal_regulatory_part1.pdf.

Reimer-Kirkham, S., Stadjuhar, K., Pauly, B., Giesbrecht, M., Mollison, A., McNeil, R., et al. (2016). Death is a social justice issue: perspectives on equity informed palliative care. *Advances in Nursing Science, 39*, 293–307. http://dx.doi.org/10.1097/ANS.0000000000000146.

Romo, R., & Gifford, L. (2007). A cost-benefit analysis of music therapy in a home hospice. *Nursing Economics, 25*, 353–358.

Sato, Y. (2011). Musical life review in hospice. *Music Therapy Perspectives, 29*, 31–38. http://dx.doi.org/10.1093/mtp/29.1.31.

Saunders, C. (1981). *Hospice: The living idea.* Philadelphia: Hodder Arnold.

Sheridan, J., & McFerran, K. (2004). Exploring the value of opportunities for choice and control in music therapy within a pediatric hospice setting. *Australian Journal of Music Therapy, 15,* 18–32.

Siebold, C. (1992). *The hospice movement: Easing death's pains.* New York: Maxwell Macmillan International.

Trauger-Querry, B., & Haghighi, K. R. (1999). Balancing the focus: art and music therapy for pain control and symptom management in hospice care. *The Hospice Journal, 14,* 25–38. http://dx.doi.org/10.1300/J01v14n01_03.

Wlodarczyk, N. (2009). The use of music and poetry in life review with hospice patients. *Journal of Poetry Therapy, 22,* 133–139. http://dx.doi.org/10.1080/08893670903198409.

World Health Organization. (2015). *Palliative care. Fact sheet No 402.* Accessed from http://www.who.int/mediacentre/factsheets/fs402/en/.

Yudofsky, S. C., Kopecky, H. J., Kunik, M., Silver, J. M., & Endicott, J. (1997). The Overt Agitation Severity Scale for the objective rating of agitation. *Journal of Neuropsychiatry and Clinical Neurosciences, 9,* 541–548. http://dx.doi.org/10.1176/jnp.9.4.541.

FURTHER READING

Salmon, D. (2005). Ultimate journeys: clinical internship in end of life care. In C. Dileo, & J. Loewy (Eds.), *Music therapy at the end of life* (pp. 251–258).

Wlodarczyk, N. (2007). The effect of music therapy on the spirituality of persons in an in-patient hospice unit as measured by self-report. *Journal of Music Therapy, 44,* 113–122. http://dx.doi.org/10.1093/jmt/44.2.113.

CHAPTER 7

Music Therapy in Gerontology

OLIVIA SWEDBERG YINGER, PHD, MT-BC

DEFINING GERONTOLOGY

There are currently more than 600 million people in the world aged 65 years and older, and this number is increasing, as is the percentage of those 65 years and older relative to the global population. In the United States, adults aged 65 years and over currently make up about 15% of the population; by 2050, they are expected to make up about 22% of the population (He, Goodkind, & Kowal, 2016). The growth of the older population is due in part to the post–World War II baby boom and the tendency for people to live longer. Increased longevity, however, leads to a number of questions, including those brought up by He, Goodkind, and Kowal in the US Census Bureau's *An Aging World: 2015*:

> *How many years can older people expect to live in good health? What are the chronic diseases that they may have to deal with? How long can they live independently? How many of them are still working? Will they have sufficient economic resources to last their lifetimes? Can they afford health care costs? The world is facing these and many more questions as population aging continues.*
>
> HE ET AL. (2016, P. 1).

There are not easy answers to all of these questions. In attempting to answer the first question, how many years can older people expect to live in good health, it is important to understand the concept of health, a state of complete physical, mental, and social well-being and not merely the absence of disease or infirmity (World Health Organization, 2017). Some people would consider themselves to be flourishing or in good health in spite of living with a chronic illness. Although music therapists may not be able to prevent aging or cure age-related disease, they often seek to help older adults maintain or improve multiple aspects of health and well-being as they age. This chapter describes how participation in music therapy can help improve well-being, potentially helping extend the number of years people can expect to live in good health.

OVERVIEW OF POPULATIONS SERVED

Although in the United States the American Association of Retired Persons provides services to adults over 50 years, in this chapter, unless otherwise noted, the term "older adult" will be used to refer to those aged 65 years and older, because this is the common full retirement age for many working Americans and the age at which Americans become eligible for Medicare. Even this narrow definition of older adulthood frequently includes individuals born across a period of three decades. In addition to differences in age, there is great diversity among older adults, as there is within a group of people of any age. Music therapists may work with older adults for the same reasons that they work with younger people or for reasons that are unique to mature age. This chapter will touch on some areas that are covered in other chapters within this book, but will focus on ways in which music therapists address concerns that are unique to older adulthood.

Music therapists work with older adults in a variety of settings (Clair & Memmott, 2008), including adult day centers (Cevasco, 2010), skilled nursing facilities (Economos, O'Keefe, & Schwantes, 2016; Mathews, Clair, & Kosloski, 2001; Suzuki, Kanamori, Nagasawa, Tokiko, & Takayuki, 2007), assisted living facilities (Cooke, Moyle, Shum, Harrison, & Murfield, 2010), retirement centers (Johnson, Otto, & Clair, 2001), senior centers (Belgrave, 2014), memory care facilities (Choi, Lee, Cheong, & Lee, 2009; McHugh, Gardstrom, Hiller, Brewer, & Diestelkamp, 2012), rehabilitation facilities (Yoo & Kim, 2016), Veteran's Affairs hospitals (Clair & Bernstein, 1990), hospitals (Kurita et al., 2006), mental health facilities (Bruer, Spitznagel, & Cloninger, 2007), in homes (Hanser, Butterfield-Whitcomb, Kawata, & Collins, 2011), and through other community-based programs such as intergenerational music groups (Belgrave, 2011) and Parkinson's disease voice programs (Yinger & LaPointe, 2012). Likewise, music therapists working within these diverse settings address an array of goals. Music therapy sessions may take place individually, with clients and their family members, or in groups (Belgrave, Darrow, Walworth, & Wlodarczyk, 2011).

Within both institutional and community settings, music therapists may address the needs of well older adults, in addition to those experiencing a variety of

TABLE 7.1
Music Therapy Outcomes in Research on Age-Related Conditions

Age-Related Condition	Outcomes
Cardiac care	Reductions in mood disturbance and tension-anxiety and increases in vigor-activity were found after participation in a music therapy support group that included music-assisted relaxation and active music therapy (Leist, 2011)
Cancer	Improvements were found in anxiety, body movement, facial expression, mood, pain, shortness of breath, and verbalizations of patients with terminal cancer who took part in individual or family music therapy (Gallagher, Lagman, Walsh, Davis, & LeGrand, 2006)
Cerebrovascular accidents (strokes)	Improvements in hand grip and pinch strength were demonstrated through keyboard playing (Chong, Han, & Kim, 2016) Improvements in drooling, respiration at rest, laryngeal pitch, and laryngeal elevation in speech were found in patients with stroke with dysphagia who took part in a music-enhanced swallowing protocol (Kim, 2010)
Emphysema	Improvements in breath management, breath support breathing mode, and quality of life were observed after group vocal instruction (Engen, 2005)
Alzheimer's disease and related dementias	Songs from individuals' past elicited memories. Group music therapy helped provide a sense of accomplishment and belonging (Dassa & Amir, 2014) and improved social, emotional, language, and musical functioning (Keough, King, & Lemmerman, 2016)
Diabetes	Relief of anxiety and pain and improvement in mood were reported by individuals with chronic kidney disease undergoing hemodialysis who received individual music therapy (Eyre, 2008)
Parkinson's disease	Participants who engaged in a music-facilitated exercise program showed improvements in movement and quality of life (Clair, Lyons, & Hamburg, 2012) Significant improvements in singing quality and voice range (Elefant, Baker, Lotan, Lagesen, & Skeie, 2012) and in intensity of conversational speech (Yinger & LaPointe, 2012) were observed in participants who took part in group singing interventions

health conditions, including age-related health conditions. Some common age-related conditions include heart disease, dementia, cancer, diabetes, stroke, and chronic obstructive pulmonary disease (COPD). When receiving medical treatment, older adults receive referrals for music therapy to address a variety of goals, including management of pain or anxiety, decreasing agitation, promoting coping skills, procedural support, family support, and end-of-life care.

SUMMARY OF THE RESEARCH

There is ample evidence to support the use of music therapy to improve wellness and quality of life as people age, as well as to ameliorate symptoms of a wide range of age-related conditions. Much of the research with older adults specifically has focused on those with dementia, particularly dementia of the Alzheimer's type. Research on the use of music therapy with individuals who have other age-related conditions, such as heart disease, cancer, or emphysema, sometimes include participants under 65 years as well, because these conditions are not limited to older adults. Some of the music therapy research that includes older adult participants focuses on hospice and palliative care; this research will not be covered in depth here because other authors have covered this area of music therapy practice in greater detail (see Chapter 6). Table 7.1 includes a summary of outcomes from recent research on music therapy for people with common age-related conditions.

Improvements in or maintenance of physical, cognitive, or psychosocial functioning are common outcomes of music therapy treatment for older adults. Decreased heart rate, respiratory rate, blood pressure, and reported pain are all examples of improvements in physical functioning, as are improvements in or maintenance of ambulation, balance, and range of motion. Psychosocial outcomes may include anxiety reduction; improved mood, self-esteem, and quality of life; and increases in positive social behaviors. Attention, memory, and reality orientation are examples of areas of cognitive functioning that may be addressed (Yinger & Cevasco, 2014).

Dementia

McDermott, Crellin, Ridder, and Orrell (2013) conducted a narrative synthesis systematic review of research on music therapy for people with dementia. Unlike authors of some other reviews, McDermott excluded research that was not considered music therapy (i.e., music medicine or music listening without intervention from a qualified therapist). After examining the 18 studies that met full inclusion criteria, the authors found consistent evidence for improvement in mood and reductions in behavioral disturbances and identified the need for high-quality longitudinal studies in the future. Table 7.2 summarizes results from randomized controlled trials (RCTs) on the use of music therapy for people with dementia published since 2006; for lists of earlier studies and studies that were not RCTs, see McDermott et al. (2013). For lists of research that include studies with music-based interventions that did not involve the presence of a music therapist, see reviews by Ueda, Suzukamo, Sato, and Izumi (2013), Vasionytė and Madison (2013), or Vink, Bruinsma, and Scholten (2004).

Cardiac Care

Research on music therapy in cardiac care has included patients recovering from acute myocardial infarction or coronary artery bypass graft, patients receiving inpatient coronary care, and patients undergoing cardiac rehabilitation (Hanser & Mandel, 2005). For a review of music therapy research in cardiac healthcare before 2005, see Hanser and Mandel (2005) or Metzger (2004). Table 7.3 summarizes results from RCTs on music therapy in cardiac care.

Cancer

A systematic review and meta-analysis by Zhang et al. (2012) found that music interventions had overall positive effects on anxiety, pain management, and quality of life of people undergoing cancer treatment. Although the authors of the review categorized music interventions as "music therapy" or "music medicine," only four studies incorporated music therapy, and the authors did not compare interventions to see which was more effective. Table 7.4 summarizes RCT research on music therapy in cancer treatment.

Stroke

Although there are several preexperimental and quasi-experimental studies on the use of music therapy in stroke treatment, only one randomized controlled study could be found on music therapy treatments for older adults who have experienced strokes (Thaut et al., 2007).

The results of this study indicate that rhythmic auditory stimulation interventions may be helpful in improving gait parameters for adults who have experienced strokes (see Table 7.5), but there is a need for more research in this area.

DESCRIPTION OF EVIDENCE-BASED PRACTICES

Music Therapy Interventions

Music therapy interventions used with older adults may include listening to and discussing music, singing, playing instruments, improvising, composing, and moving to music (Yinger & Cevasco, 2014). Table 7.6 highlights several music therapy interventions that have been used in music therapy research with older adults. Music therapists use live music whenever appropriate so that they may change the characteristics of the music in the moment to better meet the needs of the individual or group. In a study by Groene (2001), older adults with dementia applauded more and gave more compliments to the performer after hearing live singing compared with recorded singing. Participants in this study also left the room less frequently, read the lyrics more often, and showed greater attention, compliments, and applause when the music had a more complex guitar accompaniment than when it had a simple accompaniment. Although this study had a small sample size ($N = 8$), it supports previous research with other populations suggesting that, in many situations, live music may be more effective than recorded music (Standley, 2000).

One situation in which it might be more appropriate to use recorded music than live music would be when leading movement exercises, because the use of recorded music leaves the music therapist's hands free to demonstrate. In a study by Mathews et al. (2001), residents of a skilled nursing facility who had dementia showed greater participation in group exercise activities when recorded rhythmic accompaniment was present. Likewise, Cevasco and Grant (2003) found that older adults with dementia participated more in exercise activities with instrumental music accompaniment than in those with vocal music accompaniment. The authors suggested that the additional stimulus within vocal music competed with verbal cues being given by the music therapist.

During discussions about music, the music therapist may ask open-ended questions about the music to elicit reminiscence or specific questions about how the music might relate to the person's current experience to begin a discussion related to coping skills. The patient's

TABLE 7.2
RCTs on the Effects of Music Therapy on Individuals With Dementia

Author (Year), Country	Participants	Design and Interventions	Outcome Measures	Results
Bruer et al. (2007), Canada	Inpatient geriatric service ward in a government-run psychiatric hospital $N=28$ (39% female), 17 had a dementia diagnosis $M=74.1$ y (7.64 y)	8-week crossover RCT Tx. 45 min of reality orientation music therapy, once a week C. 45 min of age-appropriate movie, once a week	MMSE (measured at baseline, immediately after treatment, and the next morning)	NSD between groups in MMSE score change immediately after intervention. Tx showed significantly greater improvements in MMSE scores measured the next morning
Okada et al. (2009), Japan	Hospital patients with cerebrovascular disease and advanced dementia $N=87$ (63% female) $M=82.3$ y (9.6 y)	>10-week parallel RCT Tx. 45 minutes, singing, once a week, at least 10 times, $n=55$ C. standard care, $n=32$	1. HRV 2. Plasma cytokines and catecholamine 3. Incidence of CHF events	1. Tx showed significant increases in HRV parameters; C did not 2. Tx had significantly lower levels of plasma interleukin 6, plasma adrenaline, and nonadrenaline 3. Tx had significantly fewer CHF events
Raglio et al. (2010), Italy	Nursing home residents with severe dementia $N=60$ (92% female) Tx. $M=85.4$ y (6.5 y) C. $M=84.6$ y (6.8 y)	6-month parallel RCT Tx. 30-min group music therapy, 3 times a week for 1 month followed by 1 month of no treatment (three cycles in 6 months), $n=30$ C. 30-min educational and entertainment activities, $n=30$	NPI	Tx showed significantly greater reductions in NPI global scores and significant improvements in delusions, agitation, and apathy
Raglio et al. (2015), Italy	Nursing home residents and day care center patients with moderate to severe dementia $N=120$ (78% female) Tx1. $M=81.0$ y (7.6 y) Tx2. $M=81.7$ y (7.8 y) C. $M=82.4$ y (6.8 y)	10-week parallel RCT Tx1. 30-min individual music therapy sessions, twice a week, $n=40$ Tx2. 30-min individual recorded music-listening sessions, twice a week, $n=40$ C. educational and occupational activities, $n=40$	1. NPI 2. CSDD 3. CBS-QoL	NSD between groups

Study	Sample	Design/Treatment	Outcome measures	Results
Ridder, Stige, Qvale, and Gold (2013), Denmark & Norway	Nursing home residents with moderate to severe dementia $N=42$ (69% female) $M=81$ y (66-96y)	6-week crossover RCT Tx. individual music therapy ($M=33.8$ min, $SD=9.91$), twice a week C. standard care	1. Agitation frequency and disruptiveness (CMAI) 2. QoL (ADRQL) 3. Medication use	1. Decrease in agitation disruptiveness significantly greater for Tx; NSD between groups in agitation frequency 2. NSD between groups in QoL 3. Significantly greater increases in prescription of psychotropic medication for C
Svansdottir and Snaedal (2006), Iceland	Nursing home residents and psychogeriatric ward residents with moderate to severe dementia and AD $N=38$ 71 to 87 y	6-week parallel RCT Tx. 30 min, group music therapy, three times a week, $n=20$ C. standard care, $n=18$	BEHAVE-AD	Tx showed significant reductions in activity disturbances, aggressiveness, and anxiety, although effects were not evident at 4-week follow-up. NSD between groups in paranoid/delusional ideation, hallucination, or diurnal rhythm affective disturbances
Vink et al. (2012), Netherlands	Nursing home residents with dementia $N=77$ (70% female) $M=82.16$y (6.87 y)	4-month parallel RCT Tx. 40-min group music therapy, twice a week, $n=43$ C. 40-min group recreational activities, twice a week, $n=34$	CMAI	Both groups showed decreases in agitated behavior from 1 h before to 4 h after each session; NSD between groups

AD, Alzheimer's disease; *ADRQL*, Alzheimer's disease-related quality of life; *BEHAVE-AD*, behavior pathology in Alzheimer's disease rating scale; *C*, control; *CBS-QoL*, Cornell-Brown scale for quality of life in dementia; *CHF*, congestive heart failure; *CMAI*, Cohen-Mansfield agitation inventory; *CSDD*, Cornell scale for depression in dementia; *HRV*, heart rate variability; *MMSE*, mini-mental state examination; *NPI*, neuropsychiatric inventory; *NSD*, no significant difference; *QoL*, quality of life; *RCT*, randomized controlled trial; *Tx*, treatment.

TABLE 7.3
RCTs on the Effects of Music Therapy in Cardiac Care

Author (Year), Country	Participants	Design and Interventions	Outcome Measures	Results
Ghetti (2013), United States	Individuals awaiting outpatient heart procedures (cardiac catheterization or electrophysiologic studies) $N=37$ (35% female) $M=63.6$ y, $Mdn=67$ y	Parallel RCT Tx1. single 30-min session of individual music therapy with emotional-approach coping treatment, $n=13$ Tx2. single 30-min session of talk-based emotional approach coping treatment, $n=14$ C. standard care, $n=10$	1. PANAS 2. Pain (NRS) 3. Coping self-efficacy (VAS) 4. Patient satisfaction (VAS) 5. HR, RR, SpO_2, & BP 6. Length of procedure 7. Medications	Tx1 showed significant increases in positive affective state and systolic blood pressure, whereas other groups did not. NSD between groups for pain, coping self-efficacy, patient satisfaction, HR, RR, SpO_2, length of procedure, or amount of medications
Mandel, Hanser, Secic, and Davis (2007), United States	Patients participating in the first 3 weeks of post-hospitalization cardiac rehabilitation $N=68$ (50% female) Tx. $Mdn=65$ y C. $Mdn=64$ y	7-week parallel RCT Tx. 90-min group music therapy every other week, in addition to standard care cardiac rehabilitation, $n=35$ C. standard care 60-min cardiac rehabilitation, 3 times a week, $n=33$	1. BP 2. Anxiety (STAI) 3. Depression (CES-D) 4. Distress (BSI) 5. QoL (SF-36)	Tx showed a significantly greater decrease in SBP post treatment and improvements in STAI-State and stress from pre- to postsession. Tx had a significantly larger decrease in STAI-Trait and a significantly greater improvement in general health and social functioning (measured by SF-36) 4 months post treatment. NSD between groups in posttreatment DBP, anxiety, depression, distress, or QoL

BP, blood pressure; BSI, brief symptom inventory; C, control; CES-D, Center for Epidemiologic Studies Depression Scale; DBP, diastolic blood pressure; HR, heart rate; Mdn, median; NRS, numeric rating system; NSD, no significant difference; PANAS, positive and negative affect schedule; QoL, quality of life; RCT, randomized controlled trial; RR, respiration rate; SBP, systolic blood pressure; SF-36, medical outcomes study 36-item short-form survey; SpO_2, oxygen saturation; STAI, state trait anxiety inventory; Tx, treatment; VAS, visual analog scale.

TABLE 7.4
RCTs on the Effects of Music Therapy for Older Adults With Cancer

Author (Year), Country	Participants	Design and Interventions	Outcome Measures	Results
Ferrer (2007), United States	Patients undergoing chemotherapy $N=50$ (52% female) $M=55$ y	Parallel RCT, single session Tx. 20 min of familiar, live music during chemotherapy, $n=25$ C. standard chemotherapy, $n=25$	HR BP Anxiety Fatigue Worry Fear	Tx group showed significant decreases in anxiety, fear, fatigue, and DBP, as well as significant increases in relaxation. NSD between groups for HR and SBP
Hanser et al. (2006), United States	Women with metastatic breast cancer $N=42$ (100% female) $M=51.2$ y Tx. $Mdn=53$ y C. $Mdn=50$ y	Parallel RCT Tx. three individual music therapy sessions, $n=20$ C. standard care, $n=22$	HADS FACT-G FACIT-Sp VAS HR BP	Tx group showed significant improvements in relaxation, comfort, happiness, and HR immediately after MT. NSD between groups
Hilliard (2003), United States	Adults with terminal cancer who were receiving in-home cancer care $N=80$ (50% female) Tx. $M=66$ y C. $M=65$ y	Parallel RCT Tx. clinical music therapy, $n=40$ C. standard care, $n=40$	HQLI-R PPS Length of life	Tx group had significantly higher QOL and QOL increased over time, whereas C group's QOL decreased over time. NSD between groups for PPS or length of life
Horne-Thompson and Grocke (2008), Australia	Patients with end-stage terminal diseases in inpatient hospice, 96% had a cancer diagnosis $N=25$ (44% female) $M=73.9$ y (13.32)	Parallel RCT, single session Tx. single music therapy session, $n=13$ C. standard care, $n=12$	ESAS HR	Tx showed significant reductions in anxiety, pain, tiredness, and drowsiness measures of the ESAS. NSD between groups in HR

C, control; *BP,* blood pressure; *DBP,* diastolic blood pressure; *ESAS,* Edmonton symptom assessment system; *FACT-G,* functional assessment of cancer therapy-general; *FACIT-Sp,* functional assessment of chronic illness therapy-spiritual well-being subscale; *HADS,* hospital anxiety and depression scale; *HR,* heart rate; *HQLI-R,* hospice quality of life; *MT,* music therapy; *NSD,* no significant difference; *QOL,* quality of life; *PPS,* palliative performance scale; *RCT,* randomized controlled trial; *SBP,* systolic blood pressure; *Tx,* treatment; *VAS,* visual analog scale.

TABLE 7.5
RCTs on the Effects of Music Therapy for Individuals Who Have Experienced Strokes

Author (Year), Country	Participants	Design and Interventions	Outcome Measures	Results
Thaut et al., 2007 United States	Patients with hemiparetic stroke $N=78$ (47% female) Tx. $M=69.2$ y (11.5 y) C. $M=69.7$ y (11.2 y)	Three-week parallel RCT Tx. 30 min of RAS, five times per week, $n=43$ C. 30 min of NDT/Bobath-based training five times per week, $n=35$	1. Velocity 2. Stride length 3. Cadence 4. Symmetry	Tx group showed significantly greater improvements compared with C group for velocity, stride length, cadence, and symmetry

C, control; *NDT,* neurodevelopmental technique; *RAS,* rhythmic auditory stimulation; *RCT,* randomized controlled trial; *Tx,* treatment.

TABLE 7.6
Music Therapy Interventions Commonly Used With Older Adults

Technique	Outcomes
Listening to music	• Increases in positive social behaviors and decreases in negative behaviors related to agitation for individuals with dementia when listening to stimulative, familiar background music (Ziv, Granot, Hai, Dassa, & Haimov, 2007)
Music-assisted relaxation	• Improved sleep efficiency and lower anxiety (Ziv, Rotem, Arnon, & Haimov, 2008)
Therapeutic Instrumental Music Performance	• Decreased rate of perceived exertion and perceived fatigue level (Lim, Miller, & Fabian, 2011) • Improvements in functional wrist and hand movements (Yoo, 2009) • Decreases in arthritic discomfort; improvement in finger velocity, strength, and dexterity (Zelazny, 2001)
Active group music therapy interventions (playing instruments, singing, reminiscing, moving to music, etc.)	• Short-term improvements in cognitive functioning (Bruer et al., 2007) • Smaller long-term increases in systolic blood pressure and better long-term physical and mental health (Takahashi & Matsushita, 2006) • Improvements in behavioral and psychological symptoms in individuals with dementia (Choi et al., 2009)
Active music therapy with family members/caregivers	• Improvements in relaxation, comfort, and happiness for people with dementia and their caregivers (Hanser et al., 2011)

preferred, familiar music is used whenever possible. In Dr. Naomi Feil's book *The Validation Breakthrough* (Feil, 2002), using music that is familiar to the individual is one of 14 validation techniques listed that may be helpful for older adults in various stages of dementia.

Family members and care partners of older adults are frequently involved in music therapy sessions. For example, a music therapist working with a patient in a memory care facility might involve his wife so that she can help facilitate reminiscence based on shared memories. This helps provide the music therapist with important information that he or she might not otherwise get from the patient. In addition, singing a song that is meaningful to the patient and his wife could provide an opportunity for the couple to connect in a way in which they are not otherwise able to do, particularly if the patient is less responsive because of the progression of dementia. The music therapist might provide music to support the interaction between the patient and his wife, only intervening to continue the session.

Two studies conducted in the 1980s indicated that singing and listening activities were the music activities most preferred by older adults (Gilbert & Beal, 1982; Hylton, 1983). On the other hand, in a study by Brotons and Pickett-Cooper (1994), older adults with dementia participated more during music activities that involved moving/dancing or playing instruments. Participants in this study reported that they enjoyed playing instruments, dancing, playing musical games, and composing/improvising fairly equally, although they participated less during music activities that involved composing/improvising. More recent studies support Brotons and Pickett-Cooper's finding that adults with dementia tend to participate more in movement or rhythmic activities than in activities that solely involve singing (Cevasco & Grant, 2006; Groene, Zapchenk, Marble, & Kantar, 1998). In evidence-based music therapy practice, a music therapist would base decisions about which interventions to use not only on the best available research, but also on what they have learned through their own clinical experience and on the specific needs, strengths, abilities, and preferences of the clients with whom they work.

Music Preference
Early research showed that older adults tended to prefer popular music from their young adult years (approximately age 18 to 25 years) (Bartlett & Snelus, 1980; Gibbons, 1977; Jonas, 1991). However, recent research indicates older adults also prefer music that was popular before their young adult years (Cevasco-Trotter, VanWeelden, & Bula, 2014; VanWeelden & Cevasco, 2009, 2010). Other factors besides age also influence music preferences, including educational level, the size of the community where one grew up, and one's musical training outside of the school setting (Jonas, 1991).

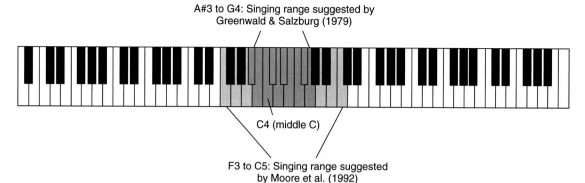

FIG. 7.1 Ideal singing range for female older adults (recommended ranges for men are one octave lower).

Because there are many factors outside of the control of older adults, particularly those who are experiencing changes in ability caused by age-related conditions, Jonas (1991) recommended that music therapists working with older adults find ways to give their clients responsibilities, offer choices, and ask for their personal opinions. Asking clients about their music preferences, either through informal conversation or through the use of a formal written questionnaire, and then incorporating preferred music within the music therapy session is an important way to offer clients a choice.

It can be challenging to determine the music preferences of adults who lack the ability to communicate because of dementia, stroke, or other conditions, particularly when there are no family members present who can provide information about the individual's preferred music. In situations such as these, music therapists and others providing music for older adults might consult one of several published song lists compiled based on music preferences of older adults reported by the adults themselves and music therapists who frequently work with older adults. One such resource is a song list published by VanWeelden and Cevasco (2007) that includes the names of songs within five genres (folk music, hymns, musicals, patriotic songs, and popular music) identified by music therapists who work with older adults. Cevasco and VanWeelden (2010) also published a list of songs from 1900 to 1969 in four popular songbook series. The songs in this resource are listed alphabetically and organized by decade. More recently, Cevasco-Trotter, VanWeelden, and Bula (2014) published a list of songs suggested by music therapists working with three sub-populations of older adults: those with Alzheimer's disease/dementia, those with other healthcare needs, and well-elderly adults.

Vocal Range

A study by Moore, Staum, and Brotons (1992) identified the singing range that was most comfortable for older adults surveyed, which was between F3 (the F below middle C) and C5 (an octave above middle C) for women and an octave lower for men. Vocal range has a tendency to decrease with age; in the study by Moore and colleagues, the range decreased from 20 semitones on average (almost two octaves) at age 60 years to 15 semitones at age 90 years (just over one octave). For 75% of the sample of older adults surveyed by Greenwald and Salzburg (1979), the comfortable singing range (that which reduces stress and strain on the vocal chords) was much narrower, extending from A# below middle C to G above middle C. This represents just less than one octave. Many popular songs have a range greater than one octave; see Yinger and Springer (2016) for a list of songs with a range less than one octave that are frequently used by music therapists working with older adults. If a song is in the higher part of the recommend range for older adults, or if the song extends beyond the recommended range, Cevasco and Grant (2006) recommend transposing the song down so that more of the pitches are in the lower part of the recommended range. Fig. 7.1 shows the recommended range for older women on a standard 88-note keyboard.

Other Considerations When Working With Older Adults

Depending on the goal of the music therapy session, a music therapist may or may not provide written lyrics to the songs being sung. A music therapist might use written lyrics if the group is preparing to sing for others, or if the goal of the session necessitates accurate enunciation of the song lyrics, and if members of the group can easily read the lyrics presented. If social interaction is an important goal for the group, having written lyrics could present an obstacle, because group members might focus more on the lyrics than on the other people in the room. Likewise, if participants are to perform movements or play instruments while singing, having written lyrics might make their tasks more challenging (Yinger, 2014). For these reasons, many music therapists attempt to choose songs that their older adult clients can, for the most part, sing from memory, because these songs are likely to be familiar, may be preferred, and enable the clients to focus on social interactions and active music making rather than reading all of the words. If no written lyrics are used, VanWeelden and Cevasco (2010) suggest that the music therapist sing multiple repetitions of the song to give ample opportunities to remember and practice the lyrics, particularly when working with clients with dementia.

Several researcher-clinicians recommend that music therapists working with older adults provide appropriate multisensory stimulation when working with adults who have dementia, in the form of auditory and visual cues (Cevasco & Grant, 2003) and by presenting a variety of activities designed to stimulate multiple senses (Brotons & Pickett-Cooper, 1994). Varying the types of activities presented (e.g., singing, moving, playing instruments) can help provide novelty and maintain clients' interest. Brotons and Pickett-Cooper (1994) emphasized the importance of adapting activities for older adults with dementia in the moment based on careful observation of clients' behavior. For example, if participants report that they enjoy singing but seem to fall asleep during activities that involve only singing, the music therapist would be wise to introduce other types of musical activities to better engage the client. Finally, Brotons and Pickett-Cooper suggest that music therapists be mindful of their expectations and that they take care not to let the therapist's low expectations limit the opportunities for clients with dementia to participate in music therapy.

CASE EXAMPLES

Group Music Therapy With Older Adults in an Assisted Living Facility

Jennifer is a music therapist who subcontracts for a private practice. Every Tuesday and Thursday, she visits an assisted living facility and provides 45-min group music therapy sessions. Her sessions take place in the cafeteria immediately after lunch. All of her participants are older than 75 years. Jennifer begins the session with a greeting song in the blues style, which she knows is a genre of music that many of her group members enjoy. When singing the greeting song, she greets each person by name and asks how they are doing. Other group members know the song, having sung it frequently in the past, and join in to greet the other group members. After greeting the group members, Jennifer puts an instrumental Big Band style recording of the song "I've Got My Love to Keep Me Warm." She has planned a sequence of movements that she demonstrates in time with the music and encourages group members to join in and move with her. The movements include toe taps, leg lifts, and seated stretches for the arms, neck, and shoulders. Some participants recognize the song and hum along; others smile and tap their toes throughout.

After getting the group "warmed up," Jennifer passes out rhythm instruments to the group. She knows that Mr. Hammond has had a stroke that limits the use of his left hand, so she makes sure to give him a maraca he can play with his right hand. Ms. Brown and Ms. Williams always sit next to each other, and Jennifer knows that when Ms. Williams forgets to play her tambourine, Ms. Brown often reaches over and taps her instrument as a reminder. After each group member has an instrument, Jennifer picks up her guitar and plays "Alexander's Ragtime Band," encouraging participants to shake their instruments and sing along. After everyone has had a chance to try out their instrument, Jennifer launches into the main activity of the day: a game she calls "Two of a Kind." Jennifer has created oversized laminated playing cards, each of which has the names of two songs written on it instead of numbers and suits. She brings the "deck" to Mr. Ewing and asks him to pick a card, any card. Mr. Ewing smiles as he selects a card in the middle. Jennifer looks at the card and begins playing and humming the first song on the card, without telling group members what it is. After two bars of hearing her hum and play guitar, Mr. Johnson joins in and sings the words to the refrain from "Shine On, Harvest Moon"; others join in as well. After the song is finished, Jennifer asks the group what that song makes them think of. After a brief period of silence, Mr. Hammond says "going out with your sweetheart" and others chuckle. Jennifer smiles and begins playing the introduction to the next song. She has only hummed 1 bar of the song when Ms. Williams joins in singing "Don't sit under the apple tree with anybody else but meeee" and tapping her tambourine vigorously. Others join in, and the entire group seems to gain momentum and energy by the time they sing "No! No! No!"

As the song winds down, Ms. Williams taps her tambourine against her hand as if she is applauding and says "I heard the Andrews Sisters sing that song live with Glenn Miller's orchestra in 1942!" Jennifer puts her guitar aside and walks over to Ms. Williams asking, "Wow! What was that like?" Ms. Williams replies "it was so exciting, especially when they started singing faster and faster. It was so amazing how they could stay perfectly together, even as they sped up." Jennifer pauses for a moment and smiles and then asks the group "Did anyone else ever hear the Andrews Sisters live?" Several in the group shake their heads, and then Mr. Ewing says "no, but I once met Bob Hope!"

Jennifer asks several questions about Mr. Ewing's experience with Bob Hope and then turns to the rest of the group and asks, "Okay, what was the name of the song we just sang? The one by the Andrews Sisters?" Ms. Williams, unsurprisingly, answers first "Don't Sit Under the Apple Tree!" "That's right," Jennifer says, "and what was the name of the song we sang before that?" There is a brief silence. Jennifer hums a few notes of the song, and Mr. Hammond says "Shine on, Harvest Moon." "Right, now here's the tricky part. What's something those two songs have in common? 'Shine On, Harvest Moon' and 'Don't Sit Under the Apple Tree': What makes them two of a kind?" There is a brief silence, after which Ms. Brown says "they're both songs about sweethearts!" "That's right," Jennifer replies, "both songs are about sweethearts."

The game continues, with group members continuing to select cards, sing songs, and then come up with ways in which the songs are similar. Sometimes the songs were sung by the same artist (e.g., "Walk the Line" and "Ring of Fire" were both made famous by Johnny Cash); sometimes the songs are from the same genre (e.g., "America the Beautiful" and "This Land is Your Land" are both patriotic songs); and sometimes songs are similar in more ways than one. On occasion, a member of the group will come up with a similarity that Jennifer had not previously considered. In between songs, Jennifer allows ample time for conversation and reminiscence. She highlights preferences or experiences that group members have in common to help further social interaction. At times, group members will engage in conversation with each other without the music therapist asking questions for several minutes.

This example highlights a group music therapy intervention that to the participants may simply seem like a musical game. However, the music therapist has carefully designed this game to engage participants in movement, cognitive stimulation, and social interaction among group members. The songs have been carefully chosen based on the group's preferences, and the questions asked by the music therapist have been selected to provide stimulation and engagement without frustration. The music therapist may adapt the music or the conversation on the spot based on responses from participants. For example, if Ms. Brown became tearful while singing a song, the music therapist might comment after the song is finished "isn't it amazing how music can stir up powerful emotions and memories? Ms. Brown, that song seems to have had an effect on you, would you like to talk about it?" This would be done gently and carefully so that Ms. Brown has the opportunity to decide whether to share more about her experience, and so that she feels supported and validated by the music therapist regardless of what she decides to share. The music therapist would then make a note of any strong responses, positive or negative, that group members have to particular songs so she can decide when or if to use those songs in future sessions.

Individual Music Therapy in the Home of a Client With Dementia

David is a music therapist working in private practice. One afternoon a week, he visits the home of Ms. Smith, an 85-year-old woman in the late stages of dementia. Ms. Smith lives with her daughter and attends an adult day facility during the week. Every afternoon, Ms. Smith's daughter, Jane, brings her mother home around 5:30. Recently, Ms. Smith has been engaging with others less and tends to sit quietly and sleep for a large portion of the time she is at the adult day facility. When she hears certain songs from her childhood, however, Ms. Smith shows signs of engagement with the music and can at times be engaged in interaction with others in music making. Jane hired David to come once a week to provide musical engagement for Ms. Smith. Recently, Jane reports that music therapy is the only time in which her mother will make eye contact and smile.

When David arrives at Ms. Smith's house, she is sitting in the living room with her eyes closed. David greets her and asks how she is doing. Although she does not reply or look at him, Ms. Smith opens her eyes. Jane sits on the couch next to her mother and tells David, "she had a bit of a rough day. Mondays are hard because she's getting back into the routine at the adult day center after two days of being at home, and lately when she's awake, she's been agitated and confused more often than not." David picks up his guitar and kneels in front of Ms. Smith. He begins picking a gentle pattern on the guitar and humming "Sentimental Journey," one of Ms. Smith's favorite songs. Ms. Smith slowly turns her gaze to David, first looking at his face and then his guitar. David begins singing the words to the song, and Ms. Smith's fingers move, tapping lightly on her knee every few beats. While continuing to sing, David holds his guitar in one hand and reaches into his bag with the other and pulls out a hand drum. He hands the drum to Jane, who carefully positions the drum under Ms. Smith's hand. At first, Ms. Smith looks confused, glancing from her daughter to the drum as David and Jane continue to sing. Jane brushes her own hand over the surface of the drum and gently guides her mother's hand to do the same. Ms. Smith rests her hand on the surface of the drum as Jane taps the beat of the song. Every few measures, Ms. Smith lightly taps the surface of the drum.

David finishes "Sentimental Journey" and moves into "Don't Fence Me In," another one of Ms. Smith's favorites. Each time the phrase "Don't fence me in" occurs in the song, David pauses and uses nonverbal cues (lifted eyebrows, a deep breath, a nod of his head) to encourage Ms. Smith to join him. Ms. Smith watches his face carefully the first two times she hears the phrase, raising her eyebrows and nodding her head along with him. The third time she hears the phrase, she takes a deep breath and smiles. David finishes the song and begins again from the beginning. This time, Ms. Smith hums along on the phrase "Don't fence me in," eliciting smiles from her daughter. After the song, Jane comments, "This is the first time all day that I've seen her awake and not upset. She loves that song!"

David continues selecting familiar, preferred songs to sing with Ms. Smith and her daughter. When Ms. Smith shows high engagement in a song by smiling, nodding, humming, or moving her hands or feet, David makes note so he can document this later. If Ms. Smith begins tapping on her lap, Jane offers the drum and mother and daughter play it together. At one point, Ms. Smith begins waving her

hand rhythmically as if she is conducting. A highlight of the session is when Ms. Smith chuckles and smiles after David sings "Roll out the Barrel." David ends the session by singing "You are My Sunshine," during which Ms. Smith hums and her daughter holds her hands. At the end of the session, Jane has tears in her eyes and a smile on her face. "Thank you," she tells David, "it means so much to be able to still have these moments of connection with my mom, when most of the time she doesn't recognize me."

For Ms. Smith, the goal of the session is to provide social interaction and stimulation, but including Ms. Smith's daughter in the session also allows the opportunity for Jane and Ms. Smith to engage in recreational intimacy, an important factor in preventing care-partner burnout.

PROVISION OF SERVICES

Funding

Funding for music therapy services for older adults varies greatly depending on the setting. Some facilities fund music therapy services through third-party reimbursement, whereas others incorporate the cost of the music therapist's salary or contract into their facility budget, occasionally using grant or donation funds to pay for music therapy services. Music therapists working with individuals in the community or through private practice may charge individuals directly for services or bill third-party payers. Still other music therapists providing services to the community do so through grants and donations, which allow individuals to receive services free of charge.

Referral Pathways

Music therapy referral pathways for older adults vary based on the setting. Many music therapists who work in assisted living facilities, skilled nursing facilities, adult day facilities, or retirement centers do so as private contractors and may work with groups once a week or every other week. In these cases, residents of the facility are often self-referred or referred by facility staff who happen to be working at the time when group music therapy occurs. In these cases, the music therapy referral process is fairly informal and there may not be a written referral document. Instead, facility staff or the music therapist may help escort interested residents into the meeting space when it is close to time for music therapy to begin. Some residents may come to music therapy on their own; this would be considered a self-referral.

In inpatient acute care facilities, music therapy sessions are often provided individually rather than in

groups. In some inpatient acute care settings, any staff member may refer patients for music therapy; in other facilities (particularly those where third-party reimbursement is sought for music therapy services), only certain healthcare staff (often physicians, physicians' assistants [PAs], and advanced registered nurse practitioners [ARNPs]) may make referrals for music therapy. Other times the referral may be initiated by any staff member, but the order requires the signature of the physician, PA, or ARNP. Settings that seek third-party reimbursement require written documentation of referrals, either in hard-copy or electronic form.

Music therapists working with older adults in community-based settings most often receive referrals from the individuals themselves, and these referrals are often informal, requiring no documentation. In lieu of a written referral, participants in community-based groups may simply complete an intake assessment form or provide information about themselves to the music therapist in conversation during the initial meeting. Music therapists working with community choirs in music wellness settings often gather less information initially and may learn about group members over time through conversation. Music therapists in rehabilitation facilities often work with other healthcare professionals, including occupation therapists, physical therapists, speech-language pathologists, and recreation therapists, and referrals often come from these sources. These referrals may also require the approval of a physician, PA, or ARNP.

Music therapists working in music education settings may receive referrals from other musicians, including music educators working in higher education or applied music instructors. Older adults with disabilities who play a musical instrument or want to study a musical instrument may seek the services of a music therapist to provide adapted music instruction. In these cases, the music therapist may work closely with the individual's family and/or other caregivers to ensure that the individual's needs are best met. Referrals in these instances may come from family members of individuals with disabilities.

Upon receiving a referral, music therapists complete an initial assessment. Several music therapy–specific assessment tools exist for use with older adults. Hintz (2000) created a geriatric music therapy clinical assessment that measures music skills and related behaviors. Norman (2012) developed an assessment tool for use by music therapists working with older adults in skilled nursing facilities. More recently, Economos et al. (2016) described a Resource-Oriented Music Therapy Assessment Tool for use with clients in skilled nursing facilities. Lipe, York, and Jensen (2007) examined the construct validity of two music-based assessments of music cognition in people with dementia, the Music-Based Evaluation of Cognitive Functioning and the Residual Music Skills Test, both of which tested some areas of general cognition (measured by the Mini-Mental State Examination) and some areas of cognition unique to music. Music therapists may use assessment tools that are not music-specific; however, these assessment tools may provide information that other standardized tools cannot.

Collaboration With Other Disciplines

Music therapists often collaborate with other healthcare professionals, including occupational therapists, physical therapists, and speech-language pathologists. Although there are numerous benefits to cotreating, it can be challenging to do so if services are paid for through third-party reimbursement, because third-party payers often deny claims for two professionals providing services simultaneously. Instead of cotreating, some music therapists work with other healthcare professionals as members of interdisciplinary, multidisciplinary, or transdisciplinary teams. Music therapists may also collaborate with other creative arts or expressive therapists, including art therapists and drama therapists. Music educators and other musicians may collaborate with music therapists when providing community-based music therapy or music wellness services.

AREAS FOR FUTURE RESEARCH

Future researchers should clearly differentiate between music medicine and music therapy treatment. Comparisons of specific intervention characteristics will help music therapists continue to implement best practices. For example, comparisons of group and individual treatment, recorded and live music, singing and playing instruments, or new and familiar music would be beneficial. Additional research on the effects of music therapy on age-related conditions, particularly strokes, heart disease, cancer, and COPD, is warranted. Although there is considerable research on the use of music therapy with older adults who have Alzheimer's disease, future research in this area will benefit from additional RCTs with greater sample sizes and clear intervention reporting.

REFERENCES

Bartlett, J. C., & Snelus, P. (1980). Lifespan memory for popular songs. *The American Journal of Psychology, 93*, 551–560. http://dx.doi.org/10.2307/1422730.

Belgrave, M. (2011). The effect of a music therapy intergenerational program on children and older adults' intergenerational interactions, cross-age attitudes, and older adults' psychosocial well-being. *Journal of Music Therapy, 48*, 486–508. http://dx.doi.org/10.1093/jmt/48.4.486.

Belgrave, M. (2014). The Piano Wizard™ project: Developing a music-based lifelong learning programme for older adults. *Approaches: Music Therapy & Special Music Education, 6*, 12–18.

Belgrave, M., Darrow, A. A., Walworth, D., & Wlodarczyk, N. (2011). *Music therapy and geriatric populations*. Silver Spring, MD: American Music Therapy Association.

Brotons, M., & Pickett-Cooper, P. (1994). Preferences of Alzheimer's disease patients for music activities: Singing, instruments, dance/movement, games, and composition/improvisation. *Journal of Music Therapy, 31*, 220–233. http://dx.doi.org/10.1093/jmt/31.3.220.

Bruer, R. A., Spitznagel, E., & Cloninger, C. R. (2007). The temporal limits of cognitive change from music therapy in elderly persons with dementia or dementia-like cognitive impairment: A randomized controlled trial. *Journal of Music Therapy, 44*, 308–328. http://dx.doi.org/10.1093/jmt/44.4.308.

Cevasco, A. M. (2010). Effects of the therapist's nonverbal behavior on participation and affect of individuals with Alzheimer's disease during group music therapy sessions. *Journal of Music Therapy, 47*, 282–299. http://dx.doi.org/10.1093/jmt/47.3.282.

Cevasco, A. M., & Grant, R. E. (2003). Comparisons of different methods for eliciting exercise-to-music for clients with Alzheimer's disease. *Journal of Music Therapy, 40*, 41–56. http://dx.doi.org/10.1093/jmt/40.1.41.

Cevasco, A. M., & Grant, R. E. (2006). Value of musical instruments used by the therapist to elicit responses from individuals in various stages of Alzheimer's disease. *Journal of Music Therapy, 43*, 226–246. http://dx.doi.org/10.1093/jmt/43.3.226.

Cevasco, A. M., & VanWeelden, K. (2010). An analysis of songbook series for older adult populations. *Music Therapy Perspectives, 28*, 37–78. http://dx.doi.org/10.1093/mtp/28.1.37.

Cevasco-Trotter, A. M., VanWeelden, K., & Bula, J. A. (2014). Music therapists' perception of top ten popular songs by decade (1900-1960s) for three subpopulations of older adults. *Music Therapy Perspectives, 32,* 165–176. http://dx.doi.org/10.1093/mtp/miu028.

Choi, A. N., Lee, M. S., Cheong, K. J., & Lee, J. S. (2009). Effects of group music intervention on behavioral and psychological symptoms in patients with dementia: A pilot-controlled trial. *The International Journal of Neuroscience, 199,* 471–481. http://dx.doi.org/10.1093/ecam/nem182.

Chong, H. J., Han, S. J., & Kim, S. J. (2016). Keyboard playing as a hand exercise for patients with subacute stroke. *Music Therapy Perspectives, advance online publication.* http://dx.doi.org/10.1093/mtp/miw023.

Clair, A. A., & Bernstein, B. (1990). A preliminary study of music therapy programming for severely regressed persons with Alzheimer's-type dementia. *Journal of Applied Gerontology, 9,* 299–311. http://dx.doi.org/10.1177/073346489000900305.

Clair, A. A., Lyons, K. E., & Hamburg, J. (2012). A feasibility study of the effects of music and movement on physical function, quality of life, depression and anxiety in patients with Parkinson disease. *Music and Medicine, 49,* 49–55. http://dx.doi.org/10.1177/1943862111425680.

Clair, A. A., & Memmott, J. (2008). *Therapeutic uses of music with older adults* (2nd ed.). Silver Spring, MD: American Music Therapy Association.

Cooke, M. L., Moyle, W., Shum, D. H. K., Harrison, S. D., & Murfield, J. E. (2010). A randomized controlled trial exploring the effect of music on agitated behaviors and anxiety in older people with dementia. *Aging & Mental Health, 14,* 905–916. http://dx.doi.org/10.1080/13607861003713190.

Dassa, A., & Amir, D. (2014). The role of singing familiar songs in encouraging conversation among people with middle to late stage Alzheimer's disease. *Journal of Music Therapy, 51,* 131–153. http://dx.doi.org/10.1093/jmt/thu007.

Economos, A. D., O'Keefe, T., & Schwantes, M. (2016). A resource-oriented music therapy assessment tool for use in a skilled nursing facility: Development and case example. *Music Therapy Perspectives, advanced online publication.* http://dx.doi.org/10.1093/mtp/miw031.

Elefant, C., Baker, F. A., Lotan, M., Lagesen, S. K., & Skeie, G. O. (2012). The effect of group music therapy on mood, speech, and singing in individuals with Parkinson's disease–A feasibility study. *Journal of Music Therapy, 49,* 278–302. http://dx.doi.org/10.1093/jmt/49.3.278.

Engen, R. L. (2005). The singer's breath: Implications for treatment of persons with emphysema. *Journal of Music Therapy, 42,* 20–48. http://dx.doi.org/10.1093/jmt/42.1.20.

Eyre, L. (2008). Medical music therapy and kidney disease: The development of a clinical method for persons receiving hemodialysis. *Canadian Journal of Music Therapy, 14,* 55–87.

Feil, N. (2002). *The validation breakthrough: Simple techniques for communicating with people with "Alzheimer's-type dementia"* (2nd ed.). Baltimore: Health Professions Press.

Ferrer, A. J. (2007). The effect of live music on decreasing anxiety in patients undergoing chemotherapy treatment. *Journal of Music Therapy, 44,* 242–255. http://dx.doi.org/10.1093/jmt/44.3.242.

Gallagher, L. M., Lagman, R., Walsh, D., Davis, M. P., & LeGrand, S. B. (2006). The clinical effects of music therapy in palliative medicine. *Support Care Cancer, 14,* 859–866. http://dx.doi.org/10.1007/s00520-005-0013-6.

Ghetti, C. M. (2013). Effect of music therapy with emotional-approach coping on preprocedural anxiety in cardiac catheterization: A randomized controlled trial. *Journal of Music Therapy, 50,* 93–122. http://dx.doi.org/10.1093/jmt/50.2.93.

Gibbons, A. C. (1977). Popular music preferences of elderly people. *Journal of Music Therapy, 14,* 180–189. http://dx.doi.org/10.1093/jmt/14.4.180.

Gilbert, J. P., & Beal, M. R. (1982). Preferences of elderly individuals for selected music education experiences. *Journal of Research in Music Education, 30,* 247–253. http://dx.doi.org/10.2307/3345298.

Greenwald, M. A., & Salzburg, R. S. (1979). Vocal range assessment of geriatric clients. *Journal of Music Therapy, 16,* 172–179. http://dx.doi.org/10.1093/jmt/16.4.172.

Groene, R. (2001). The effect of presentation and accompaniment styles on attentional and responsive behaviors of participants with dementia diagnoses. *Journal of Music Therapy, 38,* 36–50. http://dx.doi.org/10.1093/jmt/38.1.36.

Groene, R., Zapchenk, S., Marble, G., & Kantar, S. (1998). The effect of therapist and activity characteristics on the purposeful responses of probable Alzheimer's disease participants. *Journal of Music Therapy, 35,* 119–136. http://dx.doi.org/10.1093/jmt/35.2.119.

Hanser, S. B., Bauer-Wu, S., Kubicek, L., Healey, M., Manola, J., Hernandez, M., & Bunnell, C. (2006). Effects of a music therapy intervention on quality of life and distress in women with metastatic breast cancer. *Journal of the Society for Integrative Oncology, 4,* 62–66, http://dx.doi.org/10.2310/7200.2006.014.

Hanser, S. B., Butterfield-Whitcomb, J., Kawata, M., & Collins, B. E. (2011). Home-based music strategies with individuals who have dementia and their family caregivers. *Journal of Music Therapy, 48,* 2–27. http://dx.doi.org/10.1093/jmt/48.1.2.

Hanser, S. B., & Mandel, S. E. (2005). The effects of music therapy in cardiac healthcare. *Cardiology in Review, 13,* 18–23. http://dx.doi.org/10.1097/01.crd.0000126085.76415.d7.

He, W., Goodkind, D., & Kowal, P. (2016). *An aging world: 2015. U.S. Census Bureau, international population reports, P95/16-1.* Washington, DC: U.S. Government Publishing Office.

Hilliard, R. E. (2003). The effects of music therapy on the quality and length of life of people diagnosed with terminal cancer. *Journal of Music Therapy, 40,* 113–137. http://dx.doi.org/10.1093/jmt/40.2.113.

Hintz, M. R. (2000). Geriatric music therapy clinical assessment: Assessment of music skills and related behaviors. *Music Therapy Perspectives, 18,* 31–40, http://dx.doi.org/10.1093/mtp/18.1.31.

Horne-Thompson, A., & Grocke, D. (2008). The effect of music therapy on anxiety in patients who are terminally ill. *Journal of Palliative Medicine, 11*, 582–590. http://dx.doi.org/10.1089/jpm.2007.0193.

Hylton, J. (1983). Music programs for the institutionalized elderly in a Midwestern metropolitan area. *Journal of Music Therapy, 20*, 211–223. http://dx.doi.org/10.1093/jmt/20.4.211.

Johnson, G., Otto, D., & Clair, A. A. (2001). The effect of instrumental and vocal music on adherence to a physical rehabilitation exercise program with persons who are elderly. *Journal of Music Therapy, 38*, 82–96. http://dx.doi.org/10.1093/jmt/38.2.82.

Jonas, J. L. (1991). Preferences of elderly music listeners residing in nursing homes for art music, traditional jazz, popular music of today, and country music. *Journal of Music Therapy, 28*, 149–160. http://dx.doi.org/10.1093/jmt/28.3.149.

Keough, L. A., King, B., & Lemmerman, T. (2016). Assessment-based small-group music therapy programming for individuals with dementia and Alzheimer's disease: A multi-year clinical project. *Music Therapy Perspectives, advance online publication*. http://dx.doi.org/10.1093/mtp/miw021.

Kim, S. J. (2010). Music therapy protocol development to enhance swallowing training for stroke patients with dysphagia. *Journal of Music Therapy, 47*, 102–119. http://dx.doi.org/10.1093/jmt/47.2.102.

Kurita, A., Takase, B., Okada, K., Horiguchi, Y., Abe, S., Kusama, Y., & Atarasi, H. (2006). Effects of music therapy on heart rate variability in elderly patients with cerebral vascular disease and dementia. *Journal of Arrhythmia, 22*, 161–166. http://dx.doi.org/10.1016/S1880-4276(06)80014-1.

Leist, C. P. (2011). *A music therapy support group to ameliorate psychological distress in adults with coronary heart disease in a rural community*. (Unpublished doctoral dissertation). Michigan State University.

Lim, H. A., Miller, K., & Fabian, C. (2011). The effects of Therapeutic Instrumental Music Performance on endurance level, self-perceived fatigue level, and self-perceived exertion of inpatients in physical rehabilitation. *Journal of Music Therapy, 48*, 124–148. http://dx.doi.org/10.1093/jmt/48.2.124.

Lipe, A. W., York, E., & Jensen, E. (2007). Construct validation of two music-based assessments for people with dementia. *Journal of Music Therapy, 44*, 369–387. http://dx.doi.org/10.1093/jmt/44.4.369.

Mandel, S. E., Hanser, S. B., Secic, M., & Davis, B. A. (2007). Effects of music therapy on health-related outcomes in cardiac rehabilitation: A randomized controlled trial. *Journal of Music Therapy, 44*, 176–197. http://dx.doi.org/10.1093/jmt/44.3.176.

Mathews, R. M., Clair, A. A., & Kosloski, K. (2001). Keeping the beat: Use of rhythmic music during exercise activities for the elderly with dementia. *American Journal of Alzheimer's Disease and Other Dementias, 16*, 377–380. http://dx.doi.org/10.1177/153331750101600608.

McDermott, O., Crellin, N., Ridder, H. M., & Orrell, M. (2013). Music therapy in dementia: A narrative synthesis systematic review. *International Journal of Geriatric Psychiatry, 28*, 781–794. http://dx.doi.org/10.1002/gps.3895.

McHugh, L., Gardstrom, S., Hiller, J., Brewer, M., & Diestelkamp, W. S. (2012). The effect of pre-meal, vocal re-creative music therapy on nutritional intake of residents with Alzheimer's disease and related dementias: A pilot study. *Music Therapy Perspective, 30*, 32–42. http://dx.doi.org/10.1093/mtp/30.1.32.

Metzger, L. K. (2004). Heart health and music: A steady beat or irregular rhythm? *Music Therapy Perspectives, 22*, 21–25. http://dx.doi.org/10.1093/mtp/22.1.21.

Moore, R. S., Staum, M. J., & Brotons, M. (1992). Music preferences of the elderly: Repertoire, vocal ranges, tempos, and accompaniments for singing. *Journal of Music Therapy, 29*, 236–252. http://dx.doi.org/10.1093/jmt/29.4.236.

Norman, R. (2012). Music therapy assessment of older adults in nursing homes. *Music Therapy Perspectives, 30*, 8–16. http://dx.doi.org/10.1093/mtp/30.1.8.

Okada, K., Kurita, A., Takase, B., Otsuka, T., Kodani, E., Kusama, Y., … Mizuno, K. (2009). Effects of music therapy on autonomic nervous system activity, incidence of heart failure events, and plasma cytokine and catecholamine levels in elderly patients with cerebrovascular disease and dementia. *International Heart Journal, 50*, 95–110. http://dx.doi.org/10.1536/ihj.50.95.

Raglio, A., Bellandi, D., Baiardi, P., Gianotti, M., Ubezio, M. C., Zanacchi, E., … Stramba-Badiale, M. (2015). Effect of active music therapy and individualized listening to music on dementia: A multicenter randomized controlled trial. *Journal of the American Geriatrics Society, 63*, 1534–1539. http://dx.doi.org/10.1111/jgs.13558.

Raglio, A., Bellelli, G., Traficante, D., Gianotti, M., Ubezio, M. C., Gentile, S., … Trabucchi, M. (2010). Efficacy of music therapy treatment based on cycles of sessions: A randomised controlled trial. *Aging & Mental Health, 14*, 900–904. http://dx.doi.org/10.1080/13607861003713158.

Ridder, H. M. O., Stige, B., Qvale, L. G., & Gold, C. (2013). Individual music therapy for agitation in dementia: An exploratory randomized controlled trial. *Aging & Mental Health, 17*, 667–678. http://dx.doi.org/10.1080/13607863.2013.790926.

Standley, J. M. (2000). Music research in medical treatment. In C. Furman (ed.), *Effectiveness of music therapy procedures: Documentation of research and clinical practice* (3rd ed.) (pp. 199–264). Silver Spring, MD: AMTA.

Suzuki, M., Kanamori, M., Nagasawa, S., Tokiko, I., & Takayuki, S. (2007). Music therapy-induced changes in behavioral evaluations, and saliva chromogranin A and immunoglobulin A concentrations in elderly patients with senile dementia. *Geriatrics Gerontology International, 7*, 61–71. http://dx.doi.org/10.1111/j.1447-0594.2007.00374.x.

Svansdottir, H. B., & Snaedal, J. (2006). Music therapy in moderate and severe dementia of Alzheimer's type: A case-control study. *International Psychogeriatrics, 18*, 613–621. http://dx.doi.org/10.1017/S1041610206003206.

Takahashi, T., & Matsushita, H. (2006). Long-term effects of music therapy on elderly with moderate/severe dementia. *Journal of Music Therapy, 43,* 317–333. http://dx.doi.org/10.1093/jmt/43.4.317.

Thaut, M. H., Leins, A. K., Rice, R. R., Argstatter, H., Kenyon, G. P., McIntosh, G. C., … Fetter, M. (2007). Rhythmic auditory stimulation improves gait more than NDT/Bobath training in near-ambulatory patients early poststroke: A single-blind, randomized trial. *Neurorehabilitation and Neural Repair, 21,* 455–459. http://dx.doi.org/10.1177/1545968307300523.

Ueda, T., Suzukamo, Y., Sato, M., & Izumi, S. I. (2013). Effects of music therapy on behavioral and psychological symptoms of dementia: A systematic review and meta-analysis. *Ageing Research Reviews, 12,* 628–641. http://dx.doi.org/10.1016/j.arr.2013.02.003.

VanWeelden, K., & Cevasco, A. M. (2007). Repertoire recommendations by music therapists for geriatric clients during singing activities. *Music Therapy Perspectives, 25,* 4–12. http://dx.doi.org/10.1093/mtp/25.1.4.

VanWeelden, K., & Cevasco, A. M. (2009). Geriatric clients' preferences for specific popular songs to use during singing activities. *Journal of Music Therapy, 46,* 147–159. http://dx.doi.org/10.1093/jmt/46.2.147.

VanWeelden, K., & Cevasco, A. M. (2010). Recognition of geriatric popular song repertoire: A comparison of senior citizens and music therapy students. *Journal of Music Therapy, 47,* 84–99. http://dx.doi.org/10.1093/jmt/47.1.84.

Vasionytė, I., & Madison, G. (2013). Musical interventions for patients with dementia: A meta-analysis. *Journal of Clinical Nursing, 22,* 1203–1216. http://dx.doi.org/10.1111/jocn.12166.

Vink, A. C., Bruinsma, M. S., & Scholten, R. J. P. M. (2004). Music therapy for people with dementia. *Cochrane Database of Systematic Reviews,* (3):CD003477. http://dx.doi.org/10.1002/14651858.CD003477.pub2.

Vink, A. A., Zuidersma, M., Boersma, F., de Jonte, P., Zuidema, S. U., & Slaets, J. P. J. (2012). The effect of music therapy compared with general recreational activities in reducing agitation in people with dementia: A randomized controlled trial. *International Journal of Geriatric Psychiatry, 28,* 1031–1038. http://dx.doi.org/10.1002/gps.3924.

World Health Organization. (2017). *Constitution of the World Health Organization: Principles.* Retrieved from http://www.who.int/about/mission/en/.

Yinger, O. S. (2014). Adapting choral singing experiences for older adults: The implications of sensory, perceptual, and cognitive changes. *International Journal of Music Education, 32,* 203–212. http://dx.doi.org/10.1177/0255761413508064.

Yinger, O. S., & Cevasco, A. (2014). Older adults in a medical setting. In L. Gooding (Ed.), *Medical music therapy: Building a comprehensive program.* Silver Spring, MD: American Music Therapy Association.

Yinger, O. S., & LaPointe, L. L. (2012). The effects of participation in a Group Music Therapy Voice Protocol (G-MTVP) on the speech of individuals with Parkinson's disease. *Music Therapy Perspectives, 30,* 25–31. http://dx.doi.org/10.1093/mtp/30.1.25.

Yinger, O. S., & Springer, D. G. (2016). Analyzing recommended songs for older adult populations through linguistic and musical inquiry. *Music Therapy Perspectives, 34,* 116–125. http://dx.doi.org/10.1093/mtp/miu048.

Yoo, J. (2009). The role of Therapeutic Instrumental Music Performance in hemiparetic arm rehabilitation. *Journal of Music Therapy, 27,* 16–24. http://dx.doi.org/10.1093/mtp/27.1.16.

Yoo, G. E., & Kim, S. J. (2016). Rhythmic auditory cueing in motor rehabilitation for stroke patients: Systematic review and meta-analysis. *Journal of Music Therapy, 53,* 149–177. http://dx.doi.org/10.1093/jmt/thw003.

Zelazny, C. M. (2001). Therapeutic instrumental music playing in hand rehabilitation for older adults with osteoarthritis: Four case studies. *Journal of Music Therapy, 38,* 97–113. http://dx.doi.org/10.1093/jmt/38.2.97.

Zhang, J. M., Wang, P., Yao, J. X., Zhao, L., Davis, M. P., Walsh, D., & Yue, G. H. (2012). Music interventions for psychological and physical outcomes in cancer: A systematic review and meta-analysis. *Support Care Cancer, 20,* 3043–3053. http://dx.doi.org/10.1007/s00520-012-1606-5.

Ziv, N., Granot, A., Hai, S., Dassa, A., & Haimov, I. (2007). The effect of background stimulative music on behavior in Alzheimer's patients. *Journal of Music Therapy, 44,* 329–343. http://dx.doi.org/10.1093/jmt/44.4.329.

Ziv, N., Rotem, T., Arnon, Z., & Haimov, I. (2008). The effect of music relaxation versus progressive muscular relaxation on insomnia in older people and their relationship to personality traits. *Journal of Music Therapy, 45,* 360–380. http://dx.doi.org/10.1093/jmt/45.3.360.

CHAPTER 8

Music Therapy and Wellness

LORNA E. SEGALL, PHD, MT-BC

INTRODUCTION

Many of us use music daily to enhance our lives. We may subscribe to satellite radio so we can choose precisely what kind of music we listen to. At night, we might select our favorite slow music to wind down in preparation for sleep. We can download our favorite songs on an mp3 player to motivate us to go for a run and use music with certain tempi to maintain a desired pace when we exercise. We may share familiar songs to encourage friends and families to reminisce and talk about memories. These are all examples of how we incorporate music in our daily lives to benefit from music's capacity to redirect our thoughts, change our mood, keep us healthy, and help us sleep; in other words, these examples highlight music's ability to enhance wellness. Using recorded music in these ways does not necessarily require professional assistance to be beneficial. Trained music therapists, however, provide wellness services for those needing assistance with physical or psychosocial limitations or to maintain existing wellness (Krout, 2007).

Defining wellness can be challenging, because varying definitions exist and related terms such as "well-being" and "health" are often used interchangeably with "wellness," although they may describe different constructs. Saxon, Etten, and Perkins (2010, p. 301) propose that an appropriate definition of wellness must emphasize one's "...ability to live and function in society and to exercise self-reliance to the maximum extent possible." Dr. Bill Hettler, cofounder of the National Wellness Institute (NWI), proposed that there are six dimensions of wellness: emotional, occupational, physical, social, intellectual, and spiritual. In Hettler's wellness model, each wellness category affects the others. The NWI defines wellness as "...an active process through which people become aware of, and make choices toward, a more successful existence" (National Wellness Institute, 2016, para. 3). Music therapists may address all six of the components of wellness (see Fig. 8.1).

Music Therapy and Wellness

Music therapy in wellness is used to meet the needs of individuals looking to "enhance quality of life, maximize well-being and potential, and increase self-awareness" (American Music Therapy Association, 2015, para. 2). Although music itself is used extensively to encourage preventive practices that help one maintain wellness, music therapy, which involves evidence-based practices designed and implemented by a music therapist, can provide interventions to help one regain wellness. Unlike curative treatment philosophies found in hospitals, rehabilitation centers, or behavioral health centers, wellness-based music interventions function as a preventive therapy to avoid, delay, or manage symptoms that have shown to accompany a diagnosis, whether acquired or congenital, that may potentially affect an individual's state of well-being. For example, age-related decline generally involves

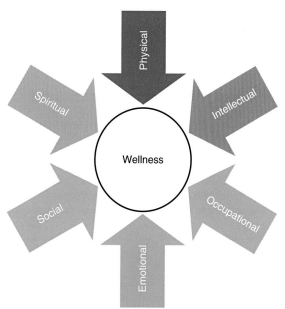

FIG. 8.1 Dimensions of wellness addressed by music therapists. (Based on the National Wellness Institute's Six Dimensions of Wellness (NWI, 2016).)

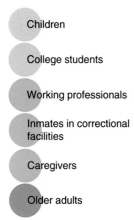

Children

College students

Working professionals

Inmates in correctional facilities

Caregivers

Older adults

FIG. 8.2 Some populations who have been shown to benefit from wellness-based music programs.

loss of muscle mass, decrease in flexibility, and respiratory weakening over time. Wellness-related goals would include maintaining a range of motion and strength and enhancing respiratory functioning. An individual starting a new job as a healthcare professional might anticipate his needs regarding coping/stress management and emotional expression and work to establish appropriate self-care practices. This chapter will describe the ways in which music therapists use evidence-based practices to enhance wellness for individuals of all ages.

OVERVIEW OF POPULATIONS SERVED

Wellness-based music therapy programs apply to all ages and populations (see Fig. 8.2). Children, through music therapy wellness interventions, can enhance social skills, establish healthy habits, and improve their focus of attention. College students and young professionals balancing school, work, and relationships often experience daily stress and high levels of anxiety. They might utilize wellness and music interventions to manage issues relating to chronic stress or to increase time spent relaxing. Correctional institutions often incorporate wellness programs for their inmates to address the chronic pressures of incarceration. In corrections, wellness programming directly benefits the inmates; indirectly, it benefits the correctional officers and staff. Having less stress in the environment can help reduce violence and create safer prisons (Kristofersson & Maas, 2013).

Another group served by wellness-based music therapy programs are today's middle-aged adults, or baby boomers, labeled as the sandwich generation. Members of this generation are providing care not only for their own children but also for aging parents (Smith-Osbourne & Felderhoff, 2014); in this way, they are

"sandwiched" between the two other generations to whom they provide care. The typical caregiver is characterized as a married, employed, 49-year-old woman providing care for her widowed 69-year-old parent who lives independently. Many of these women also have children or grandchildren living at home with them (Goyer, 2010). Individuals in this scenario benefit from stress management, emotional support, and physical activity.

Older adults participate in wellness programs to preserve cognitive functioning, physical mobility, and psychosocial engagement. Age-related diseases, such as arthritis, respiratory dysfunction, and mild cognitive impairment, can be delayed through engagement in wellness-based music interactions (Belgrave, Darrow, Walworth, & Woldarczyk, 2011; Clair & Memmott, 2008; Creech, Hallam, McQueen, & Varvarigou, 2013; Johnson, Deatrick, & Oriel, 2012). Regardless of age, place of residence, or lifestyle, wellness-based music interventions can contribute to wellness.

DESCRIPTION OF EVIDENCE-BASED PRACTICES

Children

Wellness interventions for children are important for helping establish habits that promote physical and emotional health, which may improve academic performance in the short term and help prevent illness in the long term (Ghetti, Hama, & Woolrich, 2008). Children can benefit from music therapy not only as a form of exercise, but also as a way of learning and establishing healthy habits. Mori-Inoue and Ilich (2015) explored the effects of three pilot studies including music-based exercise interventions on the healthy weight and bone health in children. Through songwriting, educational lyrics, and drumming in combination with physical exercise, the researchers met with each experimental group for three 45-min group sessions over the course of 6 weeks. Outcomes of the three studies concluded that music-based activities provided motivation and encouraged positive behavior, peer support, and elevated on-task behaviors. Little research in this area currently exists, but current outcomes warrant future exploration.

College Students

College students listen to music for many reasons, such as relaxation, distraction, or motivation. Many experience high levels of stress because of workload, academic performance expectations, work schedules, and fear of the unknown (Reed, 2015). There are many ways an individual can incorporate relaxation techniques into daily life. For many, techniques such as preferred music listening and progressive muscle relaxation (PMR) are

TABLE 8.1 Research on Music Therapy and Wellness With College Students		
Author, Year	**Music Therapy Intervention(s)**	**Outcomes**
Montello (2010)	Improvisation	Decreased levels of performance-related injuries
Bittman et al. (2001)	Group drumming	Ability to change hormonal responses to stress
Mungas and Silverman (2014)	Single-session group-based wellness drumming intervention	Reduced stress

ways in which relaxation can be found. Robb (2000) compared the outcomes of four relaxation techniques and their ability to affect anxiety and perceived relaxation. The conditions examined were music-assisted PMR (M + PMR), PMR, music listening, and silence. Outcomes of the research demonstrated that each of the techniques is effective in treating anxiety and perceived relaxation, but mean score differences of the M + PMR showed the greatest amount of change.

Music therapy can also play a role in treating the college-age musician. Often, musicians experience performance-related injuries. These injuries are often caused by high levels of stress, high expectations, leaving home for the first time, and high extracurricular demands such as homework, auditions, competitions, and relationships (Montello, 2010). Music therapy plays a unique role in addressing the needs of college-age musicians. Through improvisation, musicians become reacquainted with their initial passion for music. Improvisation also serves to encourage spontaneous creativity, auditory discrimination, meaningful expression, and staying present (Montello, 2010). Additional music therapy interventions such as musical charades, musical self-statements, and group music improvisation can help meet the wellness needs of musicians. Other group interventions such as group drumming also provide wellness benefits.

The role of group drumming was explored to determine its effect on the changes of stress-related hormones and the enrichment of particular immunologic measures for college students (Bittman et al., 2001). Inspired by evidence-based music therapy research protocols, four experimental groups received a single-session group drumming intervention. The control groups did not receive music therapy services. Results suggest that a music therapy group drumming intervention may produce neuroendocrine or immunologic effects that may play a role in the overall wellness of an individual. Future research in this area should explore the relationship between the length of intervention and duration of impact and how multiple group drumming interventions might affect those with chronic illness.

Exposure to long periods of stress can have both physiologic and psychological consequences, such as fatigue, depression, isolation, and poor nutrition (McGonigal, 2015). For students, learning methods to manage their stress can create life-long coping skills. Designing brief interventions increases the likelihood of student participation and the likelihood of increased benefit from services. Even single-session interventions can affect student levels of stress.

Mungas and Silverman (2014) implemented a single-session, group-based wellness drumming intervention to examine its effect on the affective state of college students. Fifty undergraduate and graduate students representing various majors participated in a 45-min active group drumming music making intervention (Mungas & Silverman, 2014). Students in a beginning guitar course served as the control group. Quantitative and qualitative data were collected before and after the test. Qualitative responses were collected to evaluate student perceptions of the session's impact and measured using the Quick Mood Scale. The Quick Mood Scale is used to measure affective states, such as drowsiness, anxiety, depression, aggression, confusion, and diminished coordination. Statistical between-group differences were found at posttest in the areas of awake/drowsy, relaxed/anxious, cheerful/depressed, friendly/aggressive, and clear-headed/confused. Quantitative analysis demonstrated higher posttest score means in each affect area when compared with the control condition. Qualitative results indicated that participants in the experimental group felt comfortable during the intervention and stated an overall positive experience. One participant commented that the breathing activity "...helped me to relax and focus on the stress in my body" and another participant stated, "I really liked the group drumming because we got to be creative and interact as a group. There was no pressure" (p. 290). Group drumming interventions led by music therapists facilitate creative, low-pressure experiences for students to relieve stress and encourage healthy breathing in a therapeutic environment (Mungas & Silverman, 2014). Table 8.1 summarizes research on music therapy to enhance wellness with college students.

TABLE 8.2 Research on Music Therapy and Wellness With Working Professionals		
Author, Year	**Music Therapy Intervention(s)**	**Outcomes**
Smith (2008)	Single-session music therapy intervention utilizing live music accompanied progressive muscle relaxation	Self-reported lower levels of stress and tension. Increased feelings of relaxation
Lesiuk (2010)	Preferred music listening	Work quality and employee affect

Working Professionals

Employment may be stressful regardless of responsibility, salary, and/or work environment. For many of us, occupations such as social workers, physicians, nurses, and teachers are often associated with stressful jobs (Lesiuk, 2008). Although this is true, there are other types of careers that can also be stressful. People with careers in retail, transportation, and public safety experience tremendous amounts of stress-related work. Employers and employees must remain mindful of how these elements affect work performance and job satisfaction, particularly in professions with high turnover rates and burnout (Smith, 2008). Individuals who work in call centers also experience high levels of stress related to their job (Smith, 2008). Music therapy is beginning to be explored more conscientiously in this area.

A single-session music therapy relaxation intervention was implemented to explore the anxiety levels of employees in a call center job setting (Smith, 2008). Jobs of this kind, which require extensive customer service and are sedentary in nature, can have damaging effects on emotional and physical well-being. Participants ($N = 80$) were assigned to either the music/experimental group or the discussion/control group. Participants in the music group received live music accompanied by a PMR intervention. Participants in the control group engaged in a talk-based/discussion-oriented group. Self-report data were recorded using the State Trait Anxiety Inventory. Individuals who participated in the music therapy intervention reported lower levels of stress and tension and increased feelings of relaxation. Results of the study support music interventions involving PMR to decrease anxiety levels in work environments such as the one described here.

The physiologic and psychological impacts of work-related stress can be extensive. Exposure to chronic stress can result in changes in blood pressure and sleep routines, poor nutrition habits, and a decrease in job performance (Lesiuk, 2008). Occupations characterized as highly cognitively demanding, such as working in computer information systems, can be challenging because of their high workloads, requirements to be creative and innovative problem solvers, and the need to work within the confines of short completion deadlines (Lesiuk, 2010). Mild positive affect is a term used to describe a pleasant mood response and is reported to enhance one's ability to creatively problem solve (Lesiuk, 2010). To explore how listening to preferred music might enhance affect and quality of work, Lesiuk (2010) recruited 24 participants to engage in her study. The study design consisted of a 3-week intervention, whereby weeks 1 and 3 consisted of participants listening to music of their own choice at least 30 min a day and week 2 involved no music listening. Results of the study concluded that positive affect and cognitive performance were significantly higher during the weeks when music was present. Participants in the study commented that listening to music helped to keep "…me calm and focused" and that it "…helped me concentrate" and that it helped to "…keep me in a better mood" (p. 148). See Table 8.2 for a summary of research on music therapy to enhance wellness in working professionals.

Inmates in Correctional Facilities

Chronic stress is a primary health concern for inmates. Stress can have both psychological and physiologic consequences. Stress motivates us, allows us to react quickly to situations, and improves cognitive functioning (McGonigal, 2015). Extensive periods of stress, however, can negatively affect wellness by altering our perception of reality, increasing the desire for isolation, disrupting sleep patterns, and compromising immune function (Weinstein, 2004). The corrections research literature tells us that when stress management programs are implemented in correctional facilities, inmates experience improved sleep, rates of violence decrease, and fewer inmates require utilization of health services (Kristofferson & Maas, 2013).

Daveson and Edwards (2001) explored how female inmates perceived music therapy as a method of coping and relaxation. Results of the study confirmed that music therapy in corrections is effective in helping inmates cope

TABLE 8.3 Research on Music Therapy to Enhance Wellness for Inmates in Correctional Facilities		
Author, Year	**Music Therapy Intervention(s)**	**Outcomes**
Cohen (2009)	Group singing	Elevated levels of feeling respect, making friends, family interactions, and fellow inmates
Cohen (2012)	Group singing both within the prison and in the community	Increased levels of emotional stability, sociability, happiness, and joviality
Segall (2016)	Group singing	Improvement in levels of perceived stress
Silber (2005)	Group music making	Development of interpersonal skills, self-expression, and self-control

with the unique stressors found within this environment. Participants in the study demonstrated diminished levels of stress and increased levels of relaxation and benefitted from receiving opportunities for self-expression. Group singing is another type of music therapy intervention that address wellness within this population.

To examine the effects of well-being, two inmate choirs were created (Cohen, 2009). Choir one comprised only inmates and performed within the confines of the correctional facility. Choir two consisted of inmates and community volunteers and performed outside prison walls. As measured by the *Friedman Well-Being Scale*, significant between-group differences were found in areas of emotional stability, sociability, happiness, and joviality for those inmates in choir two. Group music-making opportunities also serve to enhance interpersonal skills, self-expression, and self-control. Silber (2005) initiated a multivoice choir to present female inmates opportunities for peer relations and techniques for relating to authority and exploring self-empowerment. Group singing opportunities not only enhance inmate wellness, but can also translate to community wellness through changing perceptions.

A 12-week choral program for both inmates and community volunteers was implemented to explore community members' perceptions of inmates and inmates' perceptions of their social competency (Cohen, 2009). Inmates answered open-ended questions. Qualitative data resulted in the identification of many themes relating to feelings of self-respect, creating new relationships, enhancing familiar relationships, and improving relationships with fellow inmates. Table 8.3 summarizes research on music therapy to enhance wellness for inmates in correctional facilities.

Caregivers

Approximately 43.5 million people in the United States have provided caregiving services to an adult or child within the past year (AARP, 2015). A caregiver can be a parent tending to a child with disabilities, a nurse caring for a patient, a teacher encouraging their students, or a spouse supporting an aging spouse. Caregiving takes many different forms and include parents, spouses, teachers, neighbors, and even children. In fact, it is estimated that 1.4 million children between the ages of 8 and 18 years provide care for an adult relative (Family Caregiver Alliance, 2016). Grandparents represent most of those receiving care from children, and they often live in the same household (Family Caregiver Alliance, 2016). Although these diverse caregiving roles differ outwardly, they have similar needs relating to physical, psychosocial, and cognitive wellness.

Providing care can be such a consuming role that often the caregiver's own wellness suffers. In addition to spending time with his or her own family and job responsibilities, the average caregiver spends an additional 25 h per week providing care for the recipient (Family Caregiver Alliance, 2016). Incidence of burnout or compassion fatigue can result in poor nutrition, exhaustion, depression, and isolation. The role of the caregiver can last for 1 year or 20 years depending on the patient's needs. For members of this population, caring for oneself is imperative to maintain the physical and emotional requirements of caregiving. Many caregivers are so accustomed to putting the needs of others first that they fail to make time for themselves (Qualls & Williams, 2015). Acknowledging the importance of self-care is so important that the Web site of the American Association of Retired People (AARP) dedicated an entire section of its Web page to resources for caregivers (AARP, 2015).

One valuable method music therapists often use to teach self-care to caregivers is songwriting (Klein & Silverman, 2012). Using two groups of caregivers to explore the impact of a self-care education

TABLE 8.4
Summary of Research on Music Therapy for Wellness With Caregivers

Author, Year	Music Therapy Intervention(s)	Outcomes
Baker et al. (2012)	Active music listening, moving to music, and singing preferred songs	Improved caregiving, spousal relationships, and caregiver wellness
Klein and Silverman (2012)	Songwriting	Increased levels of fun and appreciation
O'Kelly (2008)	Songwriting	Meaningful expression, elevated levels of health, and caregiver satisfaction

intervention, Klein and Silverman created and labeled a discussion group and a songwriting group. Participants received both interventions (discussion and songwriting) and condition order was randomly assigned. Through Linguistic Inquiry and Word Count, quantitative analysis identified themes of participant responses in each group. Themes identified in the two groups included distraction from stress, fun, group cohesiveness, therapeutic insight, appreciation, comments on the presentation, and reinforcement of subject matter. Only participants in the music therapy condition reflected themes of fun and appreciation in comparison with the psychoeducational group (Klein & Silverman, 2012). Music interventions are beneficial not only for the caregiver but also for the individual receiving care.

Active music therapy interventions such as songwriting offer flexible, specific, and creative outlets for caregivers to express themselves, remain healthy, and meaningfully engage with those for whom they care (O'Kelly, 2008). Through songwriting, clients can verbalize challenging feelings, initiate therapeutic discussion, and enhance self-awareness within a therapeutic setting. Songwriting's requirement of organizing words and putting them to song reintroduces caregivers to the concepts of being creative and finding joy in life (O'Kelly, 2008). Educating caregivers on the potential wellness challenges related to their role can help them to remain healthy, happy, and meaningful contributors to their loved one's wellness.

Caregiving relationships involving couples benefit from meaningful engagement. Addressing the needs of the caregiver is important to enhance role satisfaction and to sustain a caregiver's ability to provide services (Baker, Grocke, & Pachana, 2012). Couples benefit from finding ways to continue interaction even when cognition is compromised because of dementia. Music therapists can design interventions and educate their clients

on how to use them in the therapists' absence. This allows couples the flexibility to benefit at their most ideal time without having to wait for a music therapist. Listening to music together, moving to music together, and singing songs together elevate the relationship between couples, increase satisfaction of the caregiver, and enhance the quality of life of the caregiver (Baker et al., 2012). In a study by Baker et al. (2012), couples who participated in therapist-designed treatment programs reported an improvement in spousal relationship, an increase in satisfaction with caregiving, and an increase in the well-being of the caregiver. The results of the study by Baker and colleagues reinforce the idea that music therapy interventions can address several goals simultaneously. See Table 8.4 for a summary of research on music therapy for wellness with caregivers.

Older Adults

By the year 2030, the US population of adults 65+ years will be 73 million, nearly double of what it was only 20 years earlier in 2010 (Irving & Beamish, 2014, p. xxvii). Not only is the aging population growing, but the average life expectancy has also increased over the past 50 years. Children born in 2015 are expected to live 78.8 years (Xu, Murphy, Kochanek, & Arias, 2016), an increase of 12% since 1965, when life expectancy was 70.2 years (Arias, Heron, & Xu, 2016). Longer life expectancies require individuals to work longer and remain active, meaningful contributors to their communities (Irving & Beamish, 2014, pp. 124–125). In addition, longer life spans have societal implications for financial longevity, employment, and medical care. Regardless of age, staying well is desirable and critical.

Wellness-based music therapy interventions are becoming increasingly important as the older adult population continues to grow. Wellness interventions for older adults should focus on acquiring new skills, structuring leisure time through musical development, decision making, and social engagement

TABLE 8.5
Summary of Research on Music Therapy for Wellness With Older Adults

Author, Year	Music Therapy Interventions	Outcomes
Belgrave (2014)	Intergenerational group piano lessons	Older adults: Lifelong learning, increased socialization, mastering a new skill. Students: Experiential learning, demystification of older adult stereotypes
Clements-Cortés (2014)	Group singing	Feelings of energy increased and feelings of pain and anxiety decreased as a result of participation in the intervention
Kumar et al. (1999)	Group music therapy	Older adults with Alzheimer disease showed increased melatonin after music therapy and at 6-week follow-up

(Belgrave, 2014). Through Piano Wizard technology, older adults and student music therapists work together to learn music. During this 10-week wellness-based music program, seniors come together and learn to read music and to play the piano. This program runs in partnership with music therapy students from a nearby university.

Students in the Piano Wizard project engage with the seniors as a complement to their coursework. Topics and discussions covered in the classroom are applied directly to the piano class as an experiential learning component. While seniors are given an opportunity to learn, socialize, and grow, college students can transfer their classroom knowledge into the real world. For some students, this may be their first time interacting with this population. These intergenerational experiences can be helpful in demystifying the older population and teach students how to interact with this group. After the completion of the 10-week program, the participants present a concert for each other, their friends, and family. Wellness-based interventions such as the one described earlier address a variety of goals relating to cognitive functioning, psychosocial engagement, and physical mobility (Belgrave, 2014).

In a study by Clements-Cortés (2014), 16 older adults of varying levels of cognitive functioning participated in a community choir. Led by two music therapists, choir members met once a week for 16 weeks. Participants completed Likert-style assessments regarding mood, pain, anxiety, happiness, and energy before and after each choir rehearsal. Self-report measures for happiness and mood increased at every session. Feelings of energy increased and pain decreased for 14 of 16 sessions, and anxiety decreased for 11 of

16 sessions. Through 1:1 interviews, primary themes were revealed regarding participants' experiences, including community building/making new friends; enhanced positivity; singing makes me feel well; less anxiety; and increased mood, energy, and alertness (Clements-Cortés, 2014).

In addition to addressing issues related to the psychosocial and cognitive aspects of wellness, music therapy can address issues related to sleep quality, an important aspect of wellness that affects many older adults and all areas of wellness. Sleep plays a central role in the quality of life and can be affected by many factors such as stress, lack of exercise, medications, and the natural aging process. Lack of sleep affects mood, muddies clear thinking, and affects a person's ability to manage everyday stressors. Sleep deficiencies can compromise the ability to function successfully on a daily basis. Recorded music can help induce sleep duration, quality, and efficiency. Sixty healthy older adults without cognitive impairment, medical issues, sleep medications, or caffeine were asked to listen to their preferred sedative music for 45 min at bedtime for 3 weeks (Lai & Good, 2006). Participants who listened to music demonstrated better sleep scores regarding quality of sleep, perception of better sleep, longer periods of sleep, greater sleep efficiency, shorter sleep latency, less sleep disturbance, and less daytime dysfunction (Lai & Good, 2006). Sleep is an important component of wellness for all ages, not just older adults. In a study by Kumar et al. (1999), older adults with dementia showed increased melatonin levels after music therapy, which may contribute to enhanced relaxation and sleep quality. Table 8.5 summarizes research on music therapy for wellness with older adults.

CASE EXAMPLES

Case Example #1

Population: Healthy, independent older adults.

Setting: Wellness-based music therapy singing group.

Decline in respiratory function can be managed, and respiratory function can be maintained and rehabilitated to a certain extent within the older adult population. Regardless of physical ability and disability, loss of respiratory function is age related and unavoidable. Decline in respiratory function can lead to physical challenges relating to speech, swallowing, and breath support. These issues, in turn, can exacerbate psychosocial issues relating to isolation, depression, and sleep.

For many older adults, group singing opportunities are preferable, feasible, and cost-effective interventions. They also address issues relating to physical and psychosocial issues of wellness. The following example illustrates how a group singing music therapy intervention not only focuses on maintaining respiratory function, but also addresses psychosocial issues.

All concepts discussed during the intervention emphasized how they could be applicable outside of the therapy session.

Wellness goals

- Engage in routine and novel learning experiences
- Enhance respiratory function and posture
- Provide opportunities for self-expression
- Provide peer support, interaction, and socialization

Music therapy interventions

- Singing familiar songs and learning new songs
- Stretching exercises, diaphragmatic exercises, the singing breath, vocal exercises to increase range and engage the apparatus
- Breathing exercises to reduce stress, musical expression to provide creative self-expression
- Group music making, lyric analysis, initiation of conversation as inspired by the music, reminiscence

Sample session outline

The singing intervention for this program was developed by a board-certified music therapist with a specialty in voice. Forty-five-minute group sessions included 5 min of posture instruction and alignment to emphasize the production of healthy tone, 10 min of diaphragmatic breathing instruction to acquaint participants with the anatomy and function of the diaphragmatic muscle, 10 min of vocal warm-ups to practice posture and diaphragmatic breathing, and 15 min of singing participant-preferred songs to provide an all-encompassing activity in which to engage the participant. To ensure optimal engagement of the apparatus, songs demonstrating a wide range of pitches and phrasing were incorporated. Song selection was based on participants' preferred music style and genre to ensure optimal enjoyment, engagement, and compliance. Finally, 5 min were allocated for the initiation and closure of session. The music therapist demonstrated an appropriate application of techniques and provided an encouraging and comfortable atmosphere.

Music inspired meaningful conversations between participants. "It feels so good to just talk," said one participant. "I miss having someone to talk to and I feel like my voice is stronger from using it more." After sessions concluded, comments such as "I'm so glad I came" or "I had so much fun" were frequently heard. The group singing protocol not only demonstrated benefits for voice and swallow function but also encouraged attendance, participation, and enhanced relationships between residents, caregivers, and facility staff members.

Maintaining respiratory health in an older adult is crucial for combating physiologic and psychological age-related issues, such as pneumonia, cough effectiveness, isolation, and depression (Saxon, Etten, & Perkins, 2010). In addition, reduced respiratory function may affect nutrition, exercise, and the social aspects related to living a high quality of life (Watsford, Murphy, & Pine, 2007). Maintaining or regaining respiratory well-being is possible through exercise and moderating levels of stress (Saxon, Etten, & Perkins, 2010). Music therapy programs focusing on respiratory enhancement can offer effective outcomes (Haneishi, 2001; Kim, 2010; Loewy, 2014; Yinger & LaPointe, 2012).

Interventions such as this one assist older adults who may be less active because of the use of durable medical equipment (i.e., walker or wheel chair) and transportation limitations. Often older adults who have these limitations cannot receive the routine benefits that a normally functioning person does because of their schedule. It is these individuals who must seek activity that was once a part of their daily routine.

Case Example #2

Population: Older adults with Parkinson disease and their caregivers.

Setting: Handbell choir.

The relationship between individuals with Parkinson disease and their caregivers is, perhaps, one of those most integral. Caring for a person with Parkinson disease requires adhering to a strict medication schedule and struggling with mobility issues, making transportation an exhausting and challenging task for the caregiver. Parkinson prognosis can last for many years and require extensive commitment from the caregiver, who is often a spouse or family member. The lives of the patient and caregiver can quickly be filled with doctors' visits and therapy sessions, leaving little time for caregiver self-care. In situations in which the patient and caregiver are also spouses, nurturing the relationship is also imperative for wellness.

Opportunities for socialization and relaxation may become scarce, which can easily create opportunities for stress between the patient and the caregiver. Providing support for each of these roles simultaneously is essential to enhance the wellness of both the caregiver and the patient. Wellness-based music therapy programs offer creative, effective, and rewarding opportunities for caregivers to attend with their loved ones or those they care for. These can be achieved through group handbell choirs.

The following case example shows how a handbell choir focuses on improving various aspects of wellness for both the patient and the caregiver. Examples of this kind reinforce the concept that even during illness we can have wellness-related goals.

Wellness goals for caregivers
- Relaxation, stretching/movement, stress management
- Self-expression, peer support from other caregivers, mood elevation, decrease isolation
- Meaningful interactions and socialization
- Enhanced spiritual support

Wellness goals for individuals with Parkinson disease
- Novel use of information through music reading and new instrument play
- Playing instruments, stretching, rhythmic breathing
- Song choice, lyric analysis and related discussion
- Maintain independence, develop positive relationships with caregiver
- Spiritual support

Music therapy interventions
- Learning how to read music or learning to read new songs, learning to play a new instrument, cognitive coordination of incorporating music reading and instrument playing
- Warm-ups, playing handbells (Handbells can be of various shapes and weights. The physical movement of playing a handbell requires coordination and range of motion.)
- Lyric analysis, reminiscence
- Group cooperation to make music, rapport building through collective group processing

Sample session outline
Sessions began with gentle upper body warm-ups that may be appropriately completed in either a chair or standing position. Individuals at various stages of Parkinson disease might either be independently mobile or be utilizing assistive devices such as walkers or wheelchairs. Exercises were adaptable to meet any level of ability to provide challenging exercises for a variety of abilities for caregivers and patients. Emphasis was placed on deep, diaphragmatic breathing to encourage relaxation and release of stress. Participants were reminded of how these exercises

could be incorporated outside of the music therapy group and into their daily lives.

Therapeutic discussion was facilitated by the music therapist to establish an atmosphere of sharing, support, and community. To facilitate the varying levels of music reading and cognitive functioning, the sheet music was modified to meet the reading levels of each participant.

Individuals who had difficulty raising the lower, heavier handbells were assigned higher, lighter notes. Those who could play several bells/notes simultaneously were assigned multiple handbells. Those who needed to play just one note were given one handbell. Music used in this way provides flexibility, adaptability, and opportunity for growth. With members functioning at their highest, individual level, the group could perform music.

Interactions such as these set the stage for patients and caregivers to engage in an environment of normalcy. To participate in an enjoyable activity with others who understand each other provides a sense of community, understanding, and support. Modifications made by the music therapist enabled the patients with Parkinson disease to function independently of each other. Sessions were often characterized by laughter, reminiscence as inspired by song choice and lyric analysis, feelings of accomplishment, and encouragement of others. Participants in the session became more confident of their musical skills as evidenced by their requests of increasingly difficult music from the music therapist. Those with more musical experience assisted those who needed help. One participant with advanced Parkinson disease was able to assist a group member with the rhythm of a particular piece. The participant reflected, "It makes me happy to know I'm still good for something."

Interventions such as this demonstrate that even within the experience of illness, wellness goals exist and are worthy of attention.

Case Example #3
Population: Older adults 55+ years and college students 18 to 2 years.
   Setting: Intergenerational choir.
   Intergenerational choirs provide opportunities for the young and old to work together through group singing interventions. Music choice within the settings consists of familiar and unfamiliar music to facilitate learning. Groups such as these provide wellness opportunities for both the young and the old.

Wellness goals for older adults
- Music learning and conversation
- Maintain flexibility, respiratory function
- Decrease isolation, maintain awareness of others, expand social circles
- Increase socialization, elevate mood

continued

Wellness goals for young adults
- Increase awareness of self and others, demystify the aging stereotype

Music therapy interventions for older adults
- Learn new songs, encourage memorization, engage in conversation with young adults, recall familiar songs
- Engage in movement/choreography to address issues of mobility, flexibility, posture, and fine/gross motor movement
- Encourage group participation in music making
- Lyric analysis, reminiscence

Sample session outline
Wellness sessions were conducted at an assisted living facility in a multipurpose room. One-hour sessions began with stretching and vocal warm-ups. Exercises were created to accommodate various levels of ability—those who used wheelchairs or walkers or who moved independently could participate. Group members were reminded to transfer these breathing exercises into their daily routines to optimally address levels of stress and anxiety. Students alternated sitting next to an older adult and aided if needed.

To accommodate issues relating to visual acuity, lyrics were projected onto a screen at the front of the room. This functions not only to increase eye contact between the choir and the director, but also to improve posture and nonverbal communication between singers and song leaders.

Familiar and unfamiliar songs present opportunities for each age group to learn new material and enhance cognitive functioning. Familiar music has benefits relating to reminiscence, mood elevation, and confidence of participation. Learning new material is advantageous because it requires enhanced, more complex, cognitive processing. Although some choir members expressed a distaste for learning new material at first, after the music became increasingly familiar, choir members began to like the music more.

Older adults in the intergenerational choir particularly enjoyed engaging with the young adult participants. Often, after rehearsals, group members spent time visiting as inspired by the session. Older choir members often remark how enjoyable it is to have "new life" and the presence of youth brings out the life in the older adults. New friendships are made, thereby enhancing the quality of life of both the young and the old.

Case Example #4
Population: Working professionals.
Setting: Drumming/percussion group.

Increasingly, companies are promoting health and wellness programs for their employees. Some companies make available programs offering discounts on gym memberships, create work-out facilities within their buildings,

initiate competitive step goals, and provide employee massage or yoga classes to participate in during breaks. Google, perhaps widely known for its innovative workplace atmosphere, exemplifies workplace wellness by offering high-quality food/nutrition and creative work spaces and encouraging employees to work in ways that function best for them. Some organizations are offering music therapy interventions to enhance employee mental health and wellness. Music's ability to affect physiologic measures such as heart rate and blood pressure reinforce its impact on maintaining focus of attention and problem solving, important elements of job performance. Anticipating the needs of employees can help determine the types of wellness objectives that might be most appropriate.

Work in hospice care can be challenging in several wellness-related areas. Staff members, such as social workers, chaplains, physicians, nurses, and certified nursing assistants, are at high risk for compassion fatigue, burnout, and isolation because of the solitary aspect of the field. Members of a patient team may not interact with one another outside of team meetings. This can cause hospice workers to feel isolated from their colleagues. Interdisciplinary engagement can provide support to maintain wellness in an environment at risk for stress, isolation, and job dissatisfaction. This can be a helpful exercise for corporations whose varying levels of management may have limited interaction. For example, Certified Nursing Assistants are not always in direct communication with physicians. The knowledge of both disciplines, however, is imperative to achieve optimal patient care. Interventions that allow open and productive communication between these two disciplines enhance communication and, ultimately, provide optimal care for the patient. Each discipline has a unique knowledge of the patient from two very different perspectives.

Goals in corporate settings
- Increase movement and physical relaxation/stretching
- Encourage self-expression and stress relief
- Enhance mood, professional peer interaction, team building

Sample session outline
Group drumming interventions are beneficial because they are feasible, effective, and able to accommodate various levels of skill and ability. Drum circles also allow participants to receive an immediate and satisfying music experience.

Employees sit in a circle, utilizing a relatively large space. Placed in front of each chair is a drum. Drums may be of various sizes, timbres, and shapes. Shakers, claves, and bells are also incorporated into this intervention. The music therapist/drum facilitator begins with simple rhythms and engages the group in call and response, improvisation, and fill-in-the-beat–type drumming exercises. For the participants, interventions such as this encourage group listening, leadership, creativity, and cross-discipline interaction. This also serves as an icebreaker for the group and for participants to become familiar with their instrument. Throughout the intervention, the music therapist/drum facilitator highlights the connections between drumming and the work place environment.

In an effort to enhance leadership and team building, individuals within the group may be given an opportunity to be the guest drum facilitator. This presents unique opportunities for the entry level professional to direct top-level executives. Senior executives also have a chance to show a more human side of their persona through creativity and humor. The newness of the music levels the playing field for all participants.

Drumming interventions can also facilitate learning of names and verbalizing job-related stressors/benefits and promote cross-disciplinary engagement. Drumming allows individuals to communicate through music, thereby encouraging safe self-expression and meaningful conversation.

Case Example #5

Population: Medical professionals.
   Setting: Drumming/percussion group.

Wellness goals

- Movement to address issues related to blood pressure, stress levels, and muscle tension as a result of physical requirements of job, extensive amounts of sedentary time documenting on a computer, and reviewing medical records
- Emotional support, mood elevation, self-expression
- Interaction with interdisciplinary colleagues in a unique way to strengthen professional relationships

Music therapy interventions

- PMR, movement to music, education about music's ability to encourage exercise
- Lyric analysis
- Songwriting
- Group drumming

Sample session outline

Participants sit next to a coworker from a different position. For example, a physician sits next to a certified nursing assistant, or a social worker might sit next to a nurse. Participants are paired with their neighbor and given two small percussion instruments. Using only their percussion instruments, participants are asked to play "how their job feels" for their partner. An anxious person might play a quick, repetitive beat, for example, or a tired worker might play a slow, unstructured rhythm. Based on listening and nonverbal cues, the listening partner is instructed

to observe and attempt to identify the emotion. Partners take turns. After pairs have shared their emotions with each other and discussed the accuracy of each other's guess, pairs turn inward and participate in a larger group discussion.

Participants may find that they have similar, identical, or entirely different feelings about their respective positions within the corporation. Regardless of the similarities, or lack thereof, an opportunity for discussion, rapport building, and team work is established through discussion led by the therapist. Feelings can be difficult to discuss, and rapport-building time may be required to establish an environment conducive to sharing. Through instrument play and nonverbal communication, pathways for these discussions can be built quickly and meaningfully, which allow productive sharing to happen more efficiently. Brief intervention styles such as these are important in corporate environments where time is limited and schedules are hectic. Professional interactions such as these can enhance both professional performance and patient care.

Even though such interventions are brief, they are focused and efficient, which can be an important element for professionals. Time is of the essence for many areas of therapy. Defining an objective and carrying it out efficiently provides the most meaningful results.

Case Example #6

Population: Children, ages 4 to 6 years.
   Setting: Drum circle.

Wellness goals

- Learning new concepts
- Learning about exercise, development of healthy habits
- Developing healthy self-expression as inspired by music
- Reinforce social skills (i.e., taking turns, having a conversation, having respect for others, emotional identification

Music therapy interventions

- Exploring new instruments
- Moving to music at varying tempos and dynamics
- Improvising rhythms, choosing instruments, emotional identification
- Sharing instruments with others, making music within a group environment, following directions

Sample session outline

Children, aged 4 to 6 years, are asked to sit in a circle. Within the circle is a large selection of instruments such as drums, shakers, and bells. The session begins with a hello song, which the children are taught and instructed to sing along (cognitive).

continued

Children are then asked to go into the circle and choose one instrument from the selection provided (making choices/decision making). The therapist then encourages each child to play the instrument, explore its sounds, and be creative in how it is played (improvisation, self-expression). Through nonverbal direction, the therapist instructs participants to "start" and "stop" playing their instruments (focus of attention, following directions). Through continued use of nonverbal directions, the therapist instructs participants to play loud or soft (follow directions/focus of attention). As participants continue to play, the therapist encourages one of the children to approach the front of the room and be the "conductor" (leadership, peer respect). After this has been done with two to three participants, the therapist stops the playing (self-control).

One participant in the group creates a simple rhythm (improvisation, leadership, following directions). Through eye contact only, the leader invites another group member to repeat the rhythm (improvisation, conversational skill development). Continuing with this pattern around the room, each group member is given an opportunity to participate and to observe appropriate leadership and conversational skill development. It is important throughout the intervention for the music therapist to direct participants' attention to the music objectives used to address the wellness goals.

PROVISION OF SERVICES

Funding

Many music therapy services are reimbursable through insurance or provided through programming (Simpson & Burns, 2004). For the most part, however, wellness-specific interventions are currently not reimbursable. Organizations such as hospitals, skilled nursing facilities, and assisted living facilities, however, acknowledge the value of wellness-based music therapy services and often allocate funding for this work through grants, donations, or private pay. As music therapy and wellness continue to demonstrate effective outcomes, reimbursement opportunities will likely follow.

Referral Pathways and Collaboration

Music therapy continues to establish itself as an effective treatment within many fields. Music therapists must remain vigilant in advocating for their profession and educating related fields on music therapy's benefits to patient care. Interdisciplinary team meetings occurring in medical and educational settings involving staff, teachers, parents, and academic advisors benefit from understanding how music therapy helps the patients and students in incorporating wellness goals into their care plans. When related disciplines understand how music therapy assists their patients in maintaining wellness goals, referrals increase. Not only can an understanding of the music therapy and wellness interventions enhance patient care, but an awareness of the impact of collaboration across disciplines can also enhance patient outcomes.

AREAS FOR FUTURE RESEARCH

Education and Collaboration

Education regarding what music therapy can provide remains of utmost importance. Collaboration within both the clinical and academic fields augments understanding of practice and promotes the effective use of music therapy services. Music therapists working in the field must consistently educate the public in both formal and casual settings what the discipline of music therapy offers. Ultimately, continued education regarding music therapy as a discipline enhances patient care. An understanding of music therapy's role in wellness will not only enhance patient care, but also enable related professions to understand the impact music therapy can have on the wellness of the patients.

Research

The role of research remains an important element in the incorporation of wellness-based programming. Designing meaningful experiments that can objectively reflect the impact of music therapy on wellness-based goals will further solidify the effectiveness of music therapy within this population. It also serves to substantiate the need for services. Collaboration is the key to broadening and strengthening the body of research that examines music's role within wellness. Healthcare is becoming an ensemble production, and examining music's influence within an interdisciplinary approach is especially valuable.

CONCLUSION

The development of a mind-body approach to healthcare, an evolving definition of wellness, and medical advancements affecting the life span make living a life characterized by wellness crucial. Individuals, workplaces, and service providers are recognizing the role that wellness interventions are playing and are seeking ways of making these services available. Young and old alike benefit from maintaining a wellness lifestyle and are viewing music therapy as a means to achieve that goal.

REFERENCES

AARP Public Policy Institute & National Alliance for Caregiving. (2015). *Caregiving in the U.S.: 2015 Report.* Retrieved from http://www.aarp.org/content/dam/aarp/ppi/2015/caregiving-in-the-united-states-2015-report-revised.pdf.

American Music Therapy Association. (AMTA). (2015). *AMTA standards of clinical practice: Wellness.* Retrieved from http://www.musictherapy.org/about/standards/#WELLNESS.

Arias, E., Heron, M., & Xu, J. (2016). United States life tables, 2012. *National Vital Statistics Reports, 65*(8). Hyattsville, MD: National Center for Health Statistics. Retrieved from https://www.cdc.gov/nchs/data/nvsr/nvsr65/nvsr65_08.pdf.

Baker, F. A., Grocke, D., & Pachana, N. A. (2012). Connecting through music: A study of spousal caregiver-directed music intervention designed to prolong fulfilling relationships in couples where one person has dementia. *Australian Journal of Music Therapy, 23,* 4–19.

Belgrave, M. (2014). The Piano Wizard™ Project: Developing a music-based lifelong learning program for older adults. *Approaches: Music Therapy Special Music Education, 6,* 12–18.

Belgrave, M., Darrow, A. A., Walworth, D., & Woldarczyk, N. (2011). *Music therapy and geriatric populations: A handbook for practicing music therapists and healthcare professionals.* Silver Spring, MD: AMTA.

Bittman, B. B., Berk, L. S., Felten, D. L., Westengard, J., Simonton, O. C., Pappas, J., & Ninehouser, M. (2001). Composite effects of group drumming music therapy on modulation of neuroendocrine-immune parameters in normal subjects. *Alternative Therapies in Health and Medicine, 7,* 38–47.

Clair, A. A., & Memmott, J. (2008). *Therapeutic uses of music with older adults.* Silver Spring, MD: AMTA.

Clements-Cortés, A. (2014). Buddy's glee club two: Choral singing benefits for older adults. *Canadian Journal of Music Therapy, 20*(1), 85–109.

Cohen, M. (2009). Choral singing and prison inmates: Influences of performing in a prison choir. *The Journal of Correctional Education, 60,* 52–65.

Cohen, M. (2012). Harmony within the walls: Perceptions of worthiness and competence in a community prison choir. *International Journal of Music Education, 30,* 46–56. http://dx.doi.org/10.1177/0255761411431394.

Creech, A., Hallam, S., McQueen, H., & Varvarigou, M. (2013). The power of music in the lives of older adults. *Research Studies in Music Education, 35,* 87–102. http://dx.doi.org/10.1177/1321103X13478862.

Daveson, B. A., & Edwards, J. (2001). A descriptive study exploring the role of music therapy in prisons. *The Arts in Psychotherapy, 28,* 137–141. http://doi.org/10.1016/S0197-4556(00)00089-7.

Family Caregiver Alliance. (2016). *Caregiver statistics: Demographics.* Retrieved from https://www.caregiver.org/caregiver-statistics-demographics.

Ghetti, C. M., Hama, M., & Woolrich, J. (2008). Music therapy in wellness. In A. A. Darrow (Ed.), *Introduction to approaches in music therapy* (2nd ed.) (pp. 131–151). Silver Spring, MD: American Music Therapy Association.

Goyer, A. (2010, December 10). *More grandparents raising grandkids.* Retrieved from http://www.aarp.org/relationships/grandparenting/info-12-2010/more_grandparents_raising_grandchildren.html.

Haneishi, E. (2001). Effects of a music therapy voice protocol on speech intelligibility, vocal acoustic measures, and mood of individuals with Parkinson's disease. *Journal of Music Therapy, 38,* 273–290. http://dx.doi.org/10.1093/jmt/38.4.273.

Irving, P. H., & Beamish, R. (Eds.). (2014). *The upside of aging. How long life is changing the world of health, work, innovation, policy, and purpose.* Hoboken, NJ: John Wiley & Sons, Inc.

Johnson, L., Deatrick, E. J., & Oriel, K. (2012). The use of music to improve exercise participation in people with dementia: A pilot study. *Physical & Occupational Therapy in Geriatrics, 30,* 102–108. http://dx.doi.org/10.3109/02703181.2012.680008.

Kim, S. J. (2010). Music therapy protocol development to enhance swallowing training for stroke patients with dysphagia. *Journal of Music Therapy, 47,* 102–119. http://dx.doi.org/10.1093/jmt/47.2.102.

Klein, C. M., & Silverman, M. J. (2012). With love from me to me: Using songwriting to teach coping skills to caregivers of those with Alzheimer's and other dementias. *Journal of Creativity in Mental Health, 7,* 153–164. http://dx.doi.org/10.1080/15401383.2012.685010.

Kristofersson, G. K., & Maas, M. J. (2013). Stress management techniques in the prison setting. *Journal of Forensic Nursing, 9,* 111–119. http://dx.doi.org/10.1097/JFN.0b013e31827a5a89.

Krout, R. E. (2007). Music listening to facilitate relaxation and promote wellness: Integrated aspects of our neurophysiological response to music. *The Arts in Psychotherapy, 34,* 134–141. http://dx.doi.org/10.1016/j.aip.2006.11.001.

Kumar, A. M., Tims, F., Cruess, D. G., Mintzer, M. J., Ironson, G., Loewenstein, D., ... Kumar, M. (1999). Music therapy increases serum melatonin levels in patients with Alzheimer's disease. *Alternative Therapies in Health and Medicine, 5,* 49–57.

Lai, H., & Good, M. (2006). Music improves sleep quality in older adults. *Journal of Advanced Nursing, 53,* 134–144. http://dx.doi.org/10.1111/j.1365-2648.2006.03693.x.

Lesiuk, T. (2008). The effect of preferred music listening on stress levels of air traffic controllers. *The Arts in Psychotherapy, 35,* 1–10. http://dx.doi.org/10.1016/j.aip.2007.07.003.

Lesiuk, T. (2010). The effect of preferred music on mood and performance in a high-cognitive demand occupation. *The Journal of Music Therapy, 47,* 137–154. http://dx.doi.org/10.1093/jmt/47.2.137.

Loewy, J. (2014). Integrating music, language and the voice in music therapy. *Voices, 4*(1). http://dx.doi.org/10.15845/voices.v4i1.140.

McGonigal, K. (2015). *The upside of stress: Why stress is good for you, and how to get good at it.* New York, NY: Penguin Random House.

Montello, L. (2010). The performance wellness seminar: An integrative music therapy approach to preventing performance-related disorders in college-age musicians. *Music and Medicine, 2,* 109–116. http://dx.doi.org/10.1177/1943862110364231.

Mori-Inoue, S., & Ilich, J. Z. (2015). Music therapy as an avenue to promote healthy eating, exercise and bone health in children. *Bone Abstracts*, *4*, 58. http://dx.doi.org/10.1530/boneabs.4.P58.

Mungas, R., & Silverman, M. J. (2014). Immediate effects of group-based wellness drumming on affective states in university students. *The Arts in Psychotherapy*, *41*, 287–292. http://dx.doi.org/10.1016/j.aip.2014.04.008.

National Wellness Institute. (2016). *NWI's six dimensions of wellness model*. Retrieved from http://www.nationalwellness.org.

O'Kelly, J. (2008). Saying it in song: Music therapy as a care support intervention. *International Journal of Palliative Nursing*, *14*, 281–286.

Qualls, S. H., & Williams, A. A. (2015). *Caregiver family therapy: Empowering families to meet the challenges of aging*. Washington, D.C.: American Psychological Association.

Reed, M. (2015, October 29). Stress in college: Experts provide tips to cope. *USA Today*. http://college.usatoday.com/2015/10/29/college-student-stress/.

Robb, S. L. (2000). Music assisted progressive muscle relaxation, progressive muscle relaxation, music listening, and silence: A comparison of relaxation techniques. *Journal of Music Therapy*, *37*, 2–21. http://dx.doi.org/10.1093/jmt/37.1.2.

Saxon, S. V., Etten, M. J., & Perkins, E. A. (2010). *Physical change & aging: A guide for the helping professions*. (5th ed.). New York, NY: Springer Publishing Company.

Segall, L. E. (2016). *The effect of a music therapy intervention on inmate levels of executive function and perceived stress*. (Unpublished doctoral dissertation). Tallahassee, FL: Florida State University.

Silber, L. (2005). Bars behind bars: The impact of a women's prison choir on social harmony. *Music Education Research*, *7*, 251–271. http://dx.doi.org/10.1080/14613800500169811.

Simpson, J., & Burns, D. S. (2004). *Music therapy reimbursement: Best practices and procedures*. Silver Springs, MD: AMTA.

Smith, M. (2008). The effects of a single music relaxation session on state anxiety levels of adults in a workplace environment. *The Australian Journal of Music Therapy*, *19*, 45–66.

Smith-Osbourne, A., & Felderhoff, B. (2014). Veterans' informal caregivers in the "sandwich generation": A systematic review toward a resilience model. *Journal of Gerontological Social Work*, *57*, 556–584. http://dx.doi.org/10.1080/01634372.2014.880101.

Watsford, M. L., Murphy, A. J., & Pine, M. J. (2007). The effects of ageing on respiratory muscle function and performance in older adults. *Journal of Science and Medicine in Sport*, *10*, 36–44. http://dx.doi.org/10.1016/j.jsams.2006.05.002.

Weinstein, R. (2004). *The stress effect*. New York, NY: Penguin Group.

Xu, J. Q., Murphy, S. L., Kochanek, K. D., & Arias, E. (2016). *Mortality in the United States, 2015. NCHS data brief, no 267*. Hyattsville, MD: National Center for Health Statistics. Retrieved from https://www.cdc.gov/nchs/products/databriefs/db267.htm.

Yinger, O. S., & LaPointe, L. L. (2012). The effects of participation in a group music therapy voice protocol (G-MTVP) on the speech of individuals with Parkinson's disease. *Music Therapy Perspectives*, *30*, 25–31. http://dx.doi.org/10.1093/mtp/30.1.25.

FURTHER READING

Harmat, L., Takács, J., & Bódizs, R. (2008). Music improves sleep quality in students. *The Journal of Advanced Nursing*, *62*, 327–335. http://dx.doi.org/10.1111/j.1365-2648.2008.04602.x.

Hooyman, N. R., & Kiyak, H. A. (2008). *Social gerontology: A multidisciplinary perspective* (8th ed.). New York, NY: Pearson Education, Inc.

Linnemann, A., Ditzen, B., Strahler, J., Doert, J. M., & Nater, U. N. (2015). Music listening as a means of stress reduction in daily life. *Psychoneuroendocrinology*, *60*, 82–90. http://dx.doi.org/10.1016/j.psyneuen.2015.06.008.

World Health Organization. (2017). *Constitution of the World Health Organization: Principles*. Retrieved from http://www.who.int/about/mission/en/.

CHAPTER 9

Current Trends and Future Directions in Music Therapy

ALEJANDRA J. FERRER, PHD, MT-BC

A DAY IN THE LIFE: EXPERIENCES OF MUSIC THERAPISTS IN THE UNITED STATES

The daily experiences of music therapists working across the United States could be described as incredibly meaningful, rewarding, and fulfilling, although undoubtedly challenging, encompassing periods of frustration, isolation, and demoralization. Many music therapists would agree that it is not easy to be a clinician. Constantly feeling that others do not understand one's role, scope of practice, knowledge, skill set, and educational training can take a toll on the emotional health of even the most resilient, confident, and levelheaded music therapist (Ferrer, 2012). The purpose of this chapter is to provide readers with a comprehensive understanding of the current status of the field of music therapy by exploring important topics such as workforce characteristics, rewards and challenges faced by music therapists across the country, professional issues that may lead to attrition, the education and clinical training of music therapists, and the research that has contributed to the establishment of music therapy as an academic, evidence-based therapeutic modality. To culminate, possible long-term goals for the profession, including advocacy strategies, growth of the workforce, and curricular modifications will be discussed.

The present chapter will also include a discourse on trends observed within the field. The exploration of trends is imperative for a developing profession such as music therapy, as they provide information concerning periods of growth versus stagnation in relation to issues such as size and specific makeup of the professional body, populations served, and repeated challenges faced by clinicians, as well as the strategies that have been implemented across time to ameliorate these challenges, which could then be applied to current or future events. Careful identification of trends can also promote the establishment of both short-term and long-term goals, which, again, provide the much

needed direction for a relatively young field such as music therapy.

Ferrer (2012) conducted a qualitative study where music therapy faculty and present and past board members of the American Music Therapy Association (AMTA) were interviewed regarding the rewarding and challenging aspects of being a music therapist, their strategies for professional growth and how to decrease the likelihood of burnout and attrition, and strengths and weaknesses related to the music therapy curriculum and research, among other important issues. The findings from the said study, including participant quotes, will be used throughout the present chapter.

Music Therapy Today: A Close Look at the Workforce

According to the Certification Board for Music Therapists (CBMT) (2017), there are currently more than 7000 music therapists worldwide who maintain their board certification credential. Of these music therapists, 1749 held membership with the AMTA in 2016. On an annual basis, the AMTA administers a survey to its members that captures relevant, up-to-date information related to therapists' demographics, employment, salaries, and education. The document produced as a result of this survey is titled the AMTA Member Survey and Workforce Analysis: A Descriptive Statistical Profile of the AMTA Membership and Music Therapy Community. Although this is an important document that reveals useful information about the profession, only a small percentage of music therapy professionals actually completed the survey (769 of approximately 7000, or 11%). Because of the low completion rate, it is difficult to draw conclusions that apply to the field as a whole and results must be interpreted with caution (see Fig. 9.1). Over the next several paragraphs, data derived from this survey will be presented and discussed.

According to the *AMTA member survey* (AMTA, 2016), 3957 individuals held membership with the AMTA in

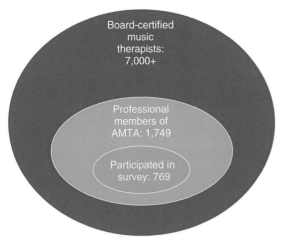

FIG. 9.1 Number of professional members of the American Music Therapy Association (AMTA) who completed the 2016 AMTA member survey relative to the number of board-certified music therapists.

2016. The majority of this membership ($n = 1749$) comprised music therapy professionals (Music Therapist-Board Certified/Advanced Certified Music Therapist/Certified Music Therapist/Registered Music Therapist) followed by students at the undergraduate ($n = 1128$) and graduate ($n = 426$) levels. Approximately 96% of the total members (3810) resided in the United States, followed by members spread across 32 other countries, with the highest international memberships being in Japan (67), Canada (25), and Taiwan (10). Other nations represented in the membership profile included Thailand, South Korea, Hong Kong, Israel, and Australia. The AMTA membership largely comprises individuals holding bachelor's (48%) and master's (40%) degrees, with only 7% holding doctorate degrees. The remaining 5% is assumed to be mostly student members.

Diversity

In terms of gender and ethnic diversity, 89% of the members identified themselves as females and 11% as males. Members identifying as transgender, gender queer, gender nonconforming, or using a different identifier made up less than 1%. Similar to gender, there is little variability in regards to the ethnic makeup of the AMTA membership. Currently, Caucasians/whites comprise the largest ethnic group (89%), followed by Asians/Asian Americans (3%), African Americans/blacks (2%), multiracial (2%), and Hispanics/Latino (2%). American Indian/Alaskan Native, Pacific Islander, and those who identify themselves as "other" compose less than 1%.

The lack of diversity in the field of music therapy results in various challenges (Ferrer, 2017; Groene, 2003). Although this is a large-scale issue, it passively affects each individual music therapist on a daily basis. Per the survey (AMTA, 2016), most practicing music therapists are Caucasian females, between 20 and 40 years of age. Being young automatically results in having fewer years of professional experience. In addition, many clinicians hold only an undergraduate level education (48%) as mentioned previously and therefore may lack an area of advanced competency or expertise. When combined, all of these variables create a difficult and intimidating situation.

In clinical settings, related professionals often have advanced degrees. Sitting within an interdisciplinary treatment team composed of medical doctors (MD or DO), psychologists (PhD or PsyD), mental health/substance abuse counselors, physical and occupational therapists, and speech and language pathologists (all at the master's level or above) could easily result in uncomfortable scenarios for the music therapist related to professional credibility, academic preparation, knowledge and clinical competency, and overall maturity. In addition, there exists the challenge of being a young woman under the age of 40 years with a relatively short professional history in comparison with colleagues. Looking at today's American society, it remains clear that many educational and clinical settings are dominated by middle-aged, Caucasian males, and that inequalities, overt or covert oppression, and discrimination toward minorities, including women, continue to exist (Equal Employment Opportunity Commission, 2016).

A lack of gender and ethnic diversity also poses challenges when trying to find a music therapist who may best fit a job position. For example, it may be that a young Caucasian female is not the most suitable, relatable, or appropriate therapist for a correctional facility setting composed primarily of male clients from diverse ethnic backgrounds. It may be that for this setting, a male music therapist is most preferred (Substance Abuse and Mental Health Services Administration, 2013). It is important that the workforce is representative of the clients served, and that clients and employers have diverse music therapists from whom they can choose to best meet their needs. This means having a workforce that is diverse across the spectrum of age, gender, ethnicity, sexual orientation, religious and spiritual beliefs, and sociocultural backgrounds.

Clinical populations

According to the same report, music therapists serve a diverse group of clinical populations. These

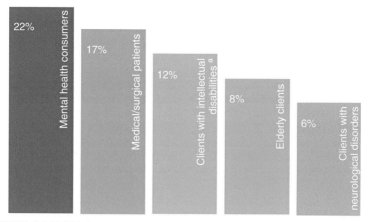

[a] AMTA included individuals who did not have intellectual disabilities in this category. For this reason, a more accurate name for this category that aligns with DSM-5 terminology might be *neurodevelopmental disabilities*.

FIG. 9.2 Most common populations with whom music therapists work, according to the 2016 American Music Therapy Association member survey. (Based on information from American Music Therapy Association. (2016). *The 2016 AMTA member survey and workforce analysis: A descriptive statistical profile of the AMTA membership*. Silver Spring, MD: Author.)

populations have been divided into "umbrellas" or categories, each encompassing multiple diagnoses. The five major umbrellas served by music therapists are (1) mental health (22%), including individuals with behavioral disorders, eating disorders, emotional disturbances, forensic status, mental health diagnoses, posttraumatic stress disorder, and substance abuse problems; (2) medical/surgical (17%), including clients with AIDS, cancer, chronic pain, medical/surgical needs, and terminal illnesses; (3) intellectually disabled (12%), including children and adults with autism spectrum disorders, developmental disabilities, and Rett syndrome; (4) the elderly (8%); and (5) those with neurologic disorders (6%), including clients with Parkinson disease and limited neurologic functioning. The remaining 35% accounts for all other populations served by music therapists that did not fit under the five major population categories. Fig. 9.2 summarizes the five most common population "umbrellas" served by music therapists.

Salary

Data concerning the salary of the AMTA membership are also included within the survey. Salaries varied according to years of experience, population/setting/age group served, geographic location, job title, and type of employment (private practice versus employed by an agency). The average reported full-time salary for 2016 was $50,797. For those music therapists with 10 or fewer years of professional experience, the

average annual salary was $43,872. According to the report, music therapists' salaries tended to be higher if they lived in the Western ($54,333) and Southwestern ($54,286) regions and were employed as a music therapy faculty ($70,457) or categorized themselves as self-employed/consultant ($73,571). Population served also made a difference. Music therapists serving clients with Rett syndrome ($58,727) and medical/surgical patients ($54,329) made approximately $10,000 more than those music therapists serving the dual/diagnosed population ($45,907).

The financial stability of music therapists also comes into play when considering challenges faced by the workforce. Despite working in healthcare settings, being board-certified personnel, and serving vulnerable clinical populations that require a high level of knowledge and skill on behalf of the therapist, music therapists are often grossly underpaid. In 2016, the most commonly reported annual salary (mode) was $40,000 (AMTA, 2016). According to the US Department of Labor Bureau of Labor Statistics (2016), related professionals made higher salaries when compared with music therapists. Per the occupational outlook handbook, physical therapists and occupational therapists had annual salaries of $80,000 and above. For speech-language pathologists, the median annual salary was $74,680. Closer to music therapists' salaries were those of social workers ($46,890), recreational therapists ($46,410), and mental health counselors and marriage and family therapists ($44,170). Although it is true that music therapy professors and administrators make a higher salary, as do some therapists with graduate degrees, the bulk of the music therapists in the United States are not in these positions. Many therapists struggle to make ends meet, pursue higher education, stay in the clinical position that they love, or even continue in the profession because of low salaries and few chances for career advancements (Clements-Cortes, 2013; Ferrer, 2017). In Ferrer's (2012) study, one music therapist reflected on the possibility of moving entry into the profession to the master's level as a possible solution (see Box 9.1).

Job loss and creation

Concerning jobs created and jobs lost, 74 new full-time positions were established in 2015. Of these jobs,

---

BOX 9.1
Quote From Music Therapist on Master's Level Entry

I am hoping that moving to a graduate education entry level will change this [being underpaid] because people with graduate degrees are eligible for higher positions; they get paid more, they have more prestige, more responsibilities in the position. So it is almost like if you create the people who can do more advanced work then the positions will be created for the people to do that work and then people will have a longer career path to follow.

Ferrer (2012, p. 102–103)

---

32 were to "fill a new music therapy position in an existing program" (AMTA, 2016, p. 24). As for jobs lost, five positions were eliminated during 2015. The reasons for eliminating positions included cut back of jobs, closure of music therapy programs, closure of the facility housing the program, and other "undisclosed" reasons. The majority of the new jobs created were located in the Southeastern and Great Lakes regions, whereas the majority of the jobs lost were located also in the Great Lakes region and the New England and Midwestern regions. Compared with years past (see Table 9.1), the number of newly created music therapy positions has been on the rise, and although there were 54 jobs lost in 2012 (AMTA, 2013), only five positions were eliminated in 2015, as compared with 74 newly established positions in the same year (AMTA, 2016).

One possible explanation for the increase in positions could be the greater awareness of music therapy among various professional communities and the general public. This could be the result of strong advocacy efforts led by the AMTA, the CBMT, state task forces, and each individual practitioner (see Box 9.2).

Funding for services

Concerning third-party reimbursement for music therapy services, approximately 30% of the individuals who completed the survey reported receiving some type of third-party reimbursement. The funding sources most frequently reported were private pay (20%), budgeted by facility/hospital (18%), third-party reimbursement (18%), and grants (13%).

TABLE 9.1
Changes in the Music Therapy Profession From 2010 to 2016

	2010[a]	2013[b]	2016[c]
Number of music therapists	Approximately 5000 music therapists	Approximately 6000 music therapists	Approximately 7000 music therapists
Most frequently reported salary	$40,000	$45,000	$40,000
Job created/lost	35 jobs created 19 jobs lost (2009 data)	47 jobs created 54 jobs lost (2012 data)	74 jobs created 5 jobs lost (2015 data)
Received third-party reimbursement	18% of survey respondents	32% of survey respondents	30% of survey respondents
Annual program budgets received from employers	>50% received between $1 and $5000	<50% received between $1 and $5000	>50% received between $1 and $5000

[a]American Music Therapy Association (2010).
[b]American Music Therapy Association (2013).
[c]American Music Therapy Association (2016).

Survey respondents reported obtaining financial assistance from their employers for various professional activities. More than three-quarters of respondents reported receiving assistance such as paid leave for professional events (14%), continuing education (11%),

---

BOX 9.2
Quote From a Music Therapy Professor Who Remains an Active Clinician on the Importance of Increasing Awareness

I would hope that in ten to fifteen years when you tell someone on a plane that you are a music therapist you will not have to go into a long explanation. That is one of my personal goals in life!

Ferrer (2012, p. 112)

---

and attending the AMTA annual conference (10%). Employers also provided monies for music therapy program budgets, with close to half of all respondents reporting having received a purchasing budget of $1 to $5000 from their employer. Similar to jobs created, more music therapists received third-party reimbursement in 2016 as compared with 2010 (See Table 9.1). Per Ferrer's (2012) study, a major goal for the profession is to receive consistent third-party reimbursement for music therapy services to increase the number of clients and facilities that could benefit from the therapeutic modality.

Rewards and Challenges Faced by Music Therapists

The *AMTA member survey* offers important demographic information regarding the music therapy profession. Through the data collected, it is evident that the

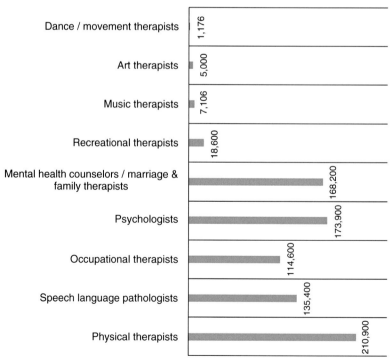

FIG. 9.3 Number of professionals in music therapy and related fields. (Based on data derived from: American Dance Therapy Association. (2017). *Find a dance/movement therapist*. Retrieved from https://adta.org/find-a-dancemovement-therapist/; American Art Therapy Association. (2014). *American art therapy association fact sheet*. Retrieved from http://www.arttherapy.org/upload/aatafactsheet.pdf; Certification Board for Music Therapists. (2017). The certification board for music therapists. Retrieved from http://cbmt.org/; United States Department of Labor Bureau of Labor Statistics. (2016). *Occupational outlook handbook*. Retrieved from https://www.bls.gov/ooh/.)

profession faces multiple obvious challenges. First, the professional body itself is small, with approximately 7000 board-certified music therapists worldwide. Having a relatively small body of board-certified professionals is of significant importance, as music therapists are often easily overshadowed by more robust groups of allied health professionals, including physical therapists, occupational therapists, speech and language pathologists, psychologists, mental health counselors, social workers, and marriage and family therapists. These same fields count with significantly larger workforces. Increased numbers of a particular group of professionals result in increased visibility within a clinical facility and the community at large. Visibility itself leads to more awareness, understanding, and recognition from the general public and various professional communities. It would be difficult to find a person within a medical setting who could not articulate to some degree the duties and responsibilities of a physical therapist or mental health counselor. Most would tend to have a general idea. It is likely that the same would not be true if the same person was asked about a music therapists' work. With greater understanding of a particular field's scope of practice may come increased appreciation and valuing on behalf of related professionals, who could then serve as advocates and champions for the field. This could in turn lead to increased employment opportunities and a more equal role within the interdisciplinary treatment team as others would more fully understand the comprehensive and complex nature of the therapeutic modality. Closer in size to music therapy are fields such as art therapy, dance/movement therapy, and recreational therapy. See Fig. 9.3 for a comparison of workforce sizes for professions related to music therapy.

In addition to easily being overshadowed and outnumbered by more traditional therapies, many healthcare facilities, including large freestanding pediatric hospitals or multisite educational settings, tend to hire only one music therapist, whereas the same facilities will hire several professionals in each field for other related therapies, such as physical therapy. Being the only music therapist in a facility often results in less visibility on patient units or classrooms, reduced attendance at interdisciplinary treatment team meetings, and less time to foster important relationships with colleagues. Music therapists may also feel overworked and spread very thin, as they are responsible for meeting the music therapy demands of an entire facility. On a personal level, music therapists may also experience feelings of isolation if they are the only music therapist working within the facility. Isolation results

> **BOX 9.3**
> **Quote From Music Therapist on Community**
>
> *There's a great quote "in community we divide our pain and we multiply our joy."...What I notice is that music therapists who are plugged into their professional community stick around, and music therapists who are plugged in seem happier, more confident, more accomplished, more successful (2012, p. 68).*

in a lack of like-minded professionals with whom to brainstorm, discuss the daily ups and downs, and share the challenges and rewards ubiquitous to being a music therapy professional. In Ferrer's study, one participant emphasized the importance of surrounding yourself with music therapy peers and developing a strong professional network (see Box 9.3).

Reasons why facilities hire fewer music therapists compared with other professions are not always clear. Is it because music therapists are not viewed equally to other allied health professionals? Is it because most music therapy services are currently not reimbursable by third-party insurance and therefore facilities have the false belief that hiring a music therapist will actually cost them more money than what they receive in return? Could it be that music therapy is perceived as something that is "nice" to have but not as critical as other services? Lack of understanding about what music therapy is, what a music therapist does in practice, and the rigorous educational training music therapy students receive at the bachelor's, master's, and doctoral levels all contribute to this problem. It is no secret that a great level of confusion continues to exist regarding the differences among music therapists, music thanatologists, certified music practitioners, and even the well-intended volunteer musician. Are facilities truly aware of the differences? If they are not, do they care enough or take the time to find out? A music therapy faculty member who is far too familiar with such discrepancies among the general public and professional communities stated "It is such a common thing, the lack of understanding from the public about what music therapy is. That we have to continually educate, and have our elevator speech ready to go at any time" (Ferrer, 2012, p. 76). Another professor with over 45 years in the field expressed similar thoughts by stating:

> *Because of our recent popularity and publicity, everybody thinks they are a music therapist and people really don't understand the exhaustive preparation process and that there is a training program that has as much in therapy and in psychology as it does in music (p. 106).*

BOX 9.4
Characteristics of Burnout

• Emotional exhaustion
• Depersonalization
• Lack of personal accomplishment

Burnout

A discussion about the issues that music therapists face would not be complete if one did not mention the problem of burnout. All professionals are at risk for burnout; however, those in the helping professions are especially susceptible to this phenomenon, as they are often highly committed to their jobs (Fowler, 2006; Larson, 1993 as cited in Clements-Cortes, 2006; Maslach, Schaufeli, & Leiter, 2001; Sprang, Clark, & Whitt-Woosley, 2007). The most frequently recognized explanation of burnout comes from Maslach (1976, 1982, 1998), who describes burnout as consisting of a triad of elements (see Box 9.4). First, there is emotional exhaustion, the most commonly reported and frequently studied dimension of burnout (Maslach et al., 2001). Emotional exhaustion results from heavy workloads, a lack of perceived emotional support, and a heightened and persistent level of job stress and may lead to frequent absences, finding scapegoats for problems, poor productivity, anxiety, irritability, and depression (Bitcon, 1981; Clements-Cortes, 2006; Fowler, 2006; Maslach et al., 2001).

The second component of burnout is depersonalization, an intentional detachment from others, especially those receiving care. In healthcare, depersonalization often begins with good intentions—an attempt at remaining detached from patients to protect oneself from emotional burdens—but can sometimes go too far. In these cases, the healthcare provider has little concern or empathy for patients, leading to negativity, intolerance, and cynicism (Maslach et al., 2001).

It is possible that the aforementioned elements of burnout may lead to the third: lack of personal accomplishment. With this third dimension comes reduced productivity, a lack of professional growth, increased feelings of incompetence, low self-actualization, and inefficacy (Maslach, 1976, Maslach et al., 2001; Wright & Bonett, 1997). Not surprisingly, there is a negative relationship between emotional exhaustion and work performance (Wright & Bonett, 1997). In addition, some of the decline in perceived personal achievement can be attributed to low self-esteem, because even practitioners who are successful in their jobs may not recognize this because of high levels of cynicism and exhaustion. Research has shown that people with high self-esteem have lower levels of depersonalization and exhaustion (Clements-Cortes, 2006).

Little research has been done concerning the burnout music therapists may face; however, what has been done has been congruent with studies in other areas of healthcare. Similar to other fields, the most common stressors for a music therapist are heavy workloads, low pay, conflicting philosophies within the workplace, and few opportunities for advancement (Clements-Cortes, 2013; Ferrer, 2017). Other stressors include inappropriate referrals, overpolicing or neglect by administrators, short staffing, and required overtime (Bitcon, 1981; Clements-Cortes, 2006; Oppenheim, 1987; Vega, 2010). As previously discussed, music therapists often face situations where colleagues or administrators do not truly understand or value the role of music therapy within a patient's treatment. Having to constantly define, defend, and convince others of the importance of one's job can lead to feelings of frustration and inadequacy (Bitcon, 1981; Clements-Cortes, 2006; Vega, 2010). Music therapists have reported receiving comments from colleagues such as "You are so lucky; you get to sing songs all day" (Clements-Cortes, 2006, p. 33). Although such statements are made with the most positive intentions in mind, the music therapist may feel diminished and devalued, as their job has been radically, inaccurately, and inappropriately minimized by peers.

Rates of burnout for music therapists have remained fairly stable over the past few decades. Oppenheim (1987) found that, of 239 music therapists, the majority of the participants scored in the medium range of burnout on the Maslach Burnout Inventory (MBI) (Maslach, Jackson, & Leiter, 1996). Approximately 12% of respondents scored at the high level of burnout. At the time, their most frequently cited criticisms were in regards to poor administrative support, low pay, holding responsibilities outside of their field, and lack of respect from their peers.

Fowler (2006) found that music therapists scored at the midpoint for burnout among other professionals who completed stress profile tests. Results of the study indicated that music therapists have low levels of depersonalization (a higher level of depersonalization would indicate a higher degree of burnout), with no significant difference found between men and women.

Vega (2010) found similar results. In an examination of 137 music therapists from across the nation, she found that 11% of participants had high levels of burnout, as measured by the MBI. Overall, the participants had average scores for emotional exhaustion, and low scores for depersonalization and personal accomplishment. Low scores for personal accomplishment may help give credence to the criticism from many music therapists that there are few opportunities for rewards or professional advancements within the field, one of the major contributing factors to burnout. Indeed, less than 1% of participants had low levels of burnout.

There is evidence that those who have remained in the field the longest have the lowest rates of burnout. Fowler (2006) found that the music therapists who have been in the field the longest have higher rates of cognitive coping strategies and higher feelings of personal achievement, possibly as a result of reporting low feelings of threat and receiving positive feedback over longer periods of time. Fowler also pointed out the methodological limitations of conducting burnout, well-being, and longevity studies, because those music therapists who left the profession as a result of dissatisfaction or other factors are not represented in the samples studied. Overall, however, music therapists are remaining in the field longer now than they once did. In the 1980s, music therapists often practiced for only 3 to 6 years after entering the profession (Braswell, Decuir, & Jacobs, 1989 as cited in Vega, 2010). When surveyed approximately 10 years later, the range had increased from 3 to 6 years to an average of 5 to 10 years (Cohen, Hadsell, & Williams, 1997 as cited in Vega, 2010) to what is now estimated to be 13 to 14 years at the point of survey (AMTA Sourcebook, 2004 as cited in Vega, 2010). It could be hypothesized that the challenges faced by music therapists discussed earlier in this chapter (Bitcon, 1981; Clements-Cortes, 2006, 2013; Ferrer, 2017; Fowler, 2006; Oppenheim, 1987; Vega, 2010) contribute to reduced longevity in the profession. Could it be that music therapists prefer to pursue different career options rather than cope with the common stressors faced on a daily basis by many members of the workforce? A close examination of music therapists who have left the field (including their challenges, reasons, current status, etc.) would be of significant usefulness (Ferrer, 2017).

Rewards

Although the challenges faced by music therapists are many, the rewards are presumably greater for those who have chosen to stay within the profession. Upon seeing a music therapist engage in practice, it is often evident that they approach their work with passion, dedication, and tremendous levels of respects. Ferrer (2012) found that music therapists often considered working with clients, observing their transformations, and seeing their positive responses to music as the most rewarding aspects of their professional experience. Witnessing developments

in the field and achieving professional milestones such as becoming a professor, obtaining a leadership role within the AMTA, or having the opportunity to serve as editor of important documents pertinent to the field of music therapy such as journals and other AMTA governing documents were also mentioned. In the same study, personal and professional rewards also resulted from influencing others to pursue music therapy as a field of study and serving as a mentor to students and interns, knowing they were affected in a positive manner. One study interviewee shared:

Something that has been rewarding is seeing some people that I had previously spoken with or had shadowed me decide to take on music therapy as a career…. That says that I had some sort of an influence on them, deciding what their career path would be.

FERRER (2012, P. 73)

Learning and drawing inspiration from both students and clients, being recognized through awards, publications, unique employment positions, conference invitations, and being in the company of other highly respected music therapy professionals were mentioned as other rewards that music therapists experience. One music therapist interviewed shared the experience of participating in an AMTA committee early on in her career and the excitement she felt while working with other music therapists she had always admired: "I remember sitting there thinking 'who am I to be sitting in a room with these people? Let alone weekends with these people for four years?'… I felt it was such a huge responsibility" (Ferrer, 2012, p. 73). For those music therapists who serve as professors, seeing their students develop skills often results in much satisfaction. One professor stated:

I like working with students who are just starting out and have so much enthusiasm…. I get to see them transform and grow, both personally and professionally as they move through the program. To me that is exciting and probably why I continue to teach.

FERRER (2012, P. 74)

Burnout prevention

It may not be possible to reverse the effects of burnout (West, 2009), so it is imperative that music therapists are trained in coping strategies before entering the field, in addition to engaging in supportive sessions throughout their career. Rowe (1999) found that healthcare providers who received short, but frequent, coping refresher sessions over the span of 2 years showed consistent declines in burnout. Their peers who received one longer, more intense course showed temporary declines in burnout, but burnout levels increased again over time. Both courses taught participants how to create coping strategies and how to address problems in the workplace proactively and positively. See Fig. 9.4 for a list of ways in which music therapists can practice self-care at work.

In-service training that is as specific to one's field as possible may also be beneficial to music therapists. Music therapists who work with geriatric populations may take the same undergraduate coursework as those who work with children; however, there are different emotional and cognitive challenges within both areas. Coping strategies targeted for one area of professional work may help to alleviate emotional exhaustion in music therapists. This is confirmed by Sprang et al. (2007), who found that healthcare professionals in trauma-related fields who received training specific to trauma work had higher levels of compassion satisfaction (the positive end of the compassion fatigue spectrum) than their peers without such training.

Additional coping strategies offered by those who have practiced music therapy for several years include keep in touch with other professionals, maintain a healthy diet, read for fun, exercise, allow unplanned chunks of time in one's schedule, take vacation time, learn to perceive office work as integral to one's job—not just a frivolous task, make music, develop a hobby, continue one's education, conduct research, set personal and professional goals, prioritize time for family and friends, attend professional conferences, and maintain a sense of humor (Bitcon, 1981; Clements-Cortes, 2006; Fowler, 2006; Wilhelm, 2004). Fig. 9.5 summarizes self-care strategies that apply outside of work.

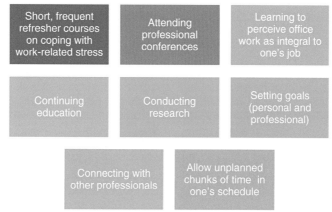

FIG. 9.4 Self-care strategies music therapists can implement at work.

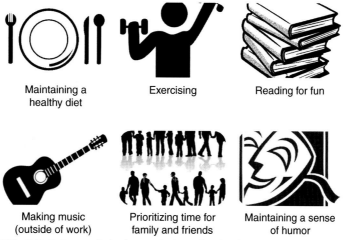

Maintaining a healthy diet

Exercising

Reading for fun

Making music (outside of work)

Prioritizing time for family and friends

Maintaining a sense of humor

FIG. 9.5 Self-care strategies music therapists implement outside of work.

MUSIC THERAPY EDUCATIONAL CURRICULUM

The vast majority of literature concerning the undergraduate music therapy curriculum was published between the late 1970s and mid-1990s. Recent literature focusing on music therapy curriculum is scarce, particularly when compared with the large body of published research regarding clinical applications of music therapy or studies investigating the effectiveness of music therapy intervention. The existing literature primarily focuses on problems within the curriculum, particularly the discrepancy between what is often emphasized and taught, versus what is actually needed as a professional music therapist (Brookins, 1984; Nicholas & Gilbert, 1980).

Madsen (1965) published an early article suggesting changes in the curriculum. He argued that the music therapist "is not a physician, psychologist, psychiatrist, social worker, and, specifically, he is not an applied performer or conductor" (p. 83). Rather, the music therapist combines elements from these different fields in the therapeutic process. Therefore, it must be determined whether the existing music therapy curriculum will provide the student with the necessary tools needed to perform such unique work. Madsen suggested concentrating on essentials and eliminating nonessentials. In 1965, his proposed changes included reducing the music history requirements to one general music history course, which would cover a vast amount of the literature and would be taught by a music therapist. Madsen stated that "the music therapist is not an aesthetician or historian, he is a therapist" (p. 84). Additional suggestions included reducing the years of applied music studies to 1 year: "the primary job of a music therapist is not performer or composer in residence within the clinical institution; he is a therapist" (p. 84) and reducing the years of music theory to only one. Through a series of follow-up studies, it was found music theory is "one of the least essential requirements even for the band, orchestral, or choral teacher" (p. 84).

Alley (1978) discussed the state of the music therapy degree in the late 1970s, pointing out that the curriculum requirements had remained virtually unchanged since being established in 1952. She attributed this lack of change in the curriculum to the music therapy program being housed within schools of music and being subject to National Association of Schools of Music (NASM) requirements, as the primary focus falls on applied music expertise, extensive music theory and history studies, and functional instruction in secondary instruments.

Jensen and McKinney (1990) collected music therapy curricula information from 66 colleges and universities.

They compared their results to the curriculum standards set by the former National Association for Music Therapy. As in earlier studies (Braswell, Decuir, & Maranto, 1980; Braswell, Maranto, & Decuir, 1979; Petrie, 1989), Jensen and McKinney found that certain areas bearing little direct application to the work of a music therapist were highly emphasized, whereas other areas considered *crucial* and *central* to the practice of music therapy were given little emphasis. It is difficult to pinpoint exactly *who* decides what should be emphasized within a particular university's curriculum as multiple stakeholders, including music therapy program directors, university course requirements, deans of the schools of music, NASM requirements, and the field's governing organization(s), play important roles in determining such stipulations and processes. In a more recent study, Groene and Pembrook (2000) found that music therapy faculty continued to desire changes toward more coursework promoting practical music skills "such as hand percussion, functional guitar, functional piano, improvisation, electronic sensory music systems, popular music ensembles, and similar courses" (p. 98). Because these studies were published several decades ago, the situation regarding multiple stakeholders at hand and the challenges this poses to making changes to the curriculum remains virtually unchanged (Ferrer, 2012). There is a need for additional research on music therapy pedagogy and curricular issues. As this book goes to press, there is a great deal of discussion taking place about the undergraduate music therapy curriculum as the AMTA considers moving toward master's level entry, and changes to the music therapy curriculum are likely to occur within the next decade (AMTA, 2017).

RESEARCH IN MUSIC THERAPY: FACING THE FUTURE

The music therapy profession has placed tremendous importance on research activity since its inception as a formal field of study. Two major peer-reviewed journals published by the AMTA, *The Journal of Music Therapy (JMT)* and *Music Therapy Perspectives (MTP)*, share the contributions of researchers in the field of music therapy and related professions. Music therapy research is as diverse as the theoretical approaches to music therapy. There are studies using quantitative, qualitative, and mixed methods designs. The modes of inquiry include philosophical, descriptive, experimental, and historical studies (Wheeler, 1995).

In 2005, the AMTA designated research as a strategic priority and developed an operational plan which "addresses the direction of research in support of evidence-based music therapy practice and improved workforce demand; and recognizes and incorporates, where necessary, federal, state and other entity requirements for evidence-driven research as it relates to practice policy and reimbursement" (AMTA, 2005, para. 2).

More recently, in 2015, members of the AMTA, including clinicians, educators, students, and researchers, convened for an innovative research symposium designed to provide guidelines for future research, promoting dialogue and diversity in thinking, practice, and methodologies and stimulate discussion about generating high-quality research in music therapy (AMTA, 2015). The symposium, titled *Improving Access and Quality: Music Therapy Research 2025* (MTR 2025), resulted in a series of discussions on various themes, including the importance of having input from consumers and practicing music therapy clinicians throughout the research process; the importance of including economic analyses regarding the benefits of protocols and interventions where appropriate; the value of continuing to collaborate with clinicians, educators, and researchers from other disciplines; and "the need to further develop, integrate, describe, and link theory and theoretical models in music therapy research with well-articulated and defined music therapy interventions" (AMTA, 2015, p. 11).

Music therapy educators, clinicians, and researchers alike have discussed the challenges involved with enhancing the music therapy research literature, offering suggestions to increase the caliber of the studies, which could result in greater acceptance from other professional communities. Music therapists have discussed the importance of conducting studies where the music therapy process is clearly described (Ferrer, 2012). This is congruent with the *Journal of Music Therapy* new author submission guidelines, which asks contributors "to provide more detailed description of the music interventions and conditions under investigation" (Robb, 2012, p. 2). Increasing the subject pool size, having different members of the research team provide the treatment and collect and analyze the data, and consulting with experts in research design and implementation (see Fig. 9.6) have also been suggested (Ferrer, 2012).

LONG-TERM GOALS FOR THE MUSIC THERAPY PROFESSION

Advocacy: Recognition and Acceptance Among Various Professional Communities

Many members of the music therapy community wish to be considered by the general public and members of various professional communities at the same level as such related fields as speech and language pathology, physical therapy, and occupational therapy. "I would love to see in all agencies where there is occupational therapy, physical

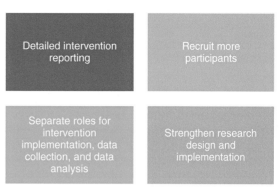

FIG. 9.6 Ways to improve future music therapy research.

therapy, and speech therapy, which are always the standard three, I want to see music therapy as part of that, as the norm" (Ferrer, 2012, p. 111). Music therapists wish for the treatment modality to be readily available to all clients, "so that they can make a choice whether to have music therapy" as part of their medical treatment (p. 111). Another music therapist adds, "My humble wish would be that we will be treated the same as other professionals in the healthcare and educational field" (p. 111).

Many music therapists believe that aside from the AMTA and the CBMT, it is the daily responsibility of all music therapists to advocate and educate others about the field and that when doing this they should clearly articulate the education and clinical training involved in becoming a music therapist. The *Standards of Clinical Practice, Professional Competencies, Code of Ethics,* board certification examination, and research findings should all be incorporated into these conversations. It is important that music therapists do their best to *kindly* educate others and to never take a defensive stand, as it could lead to loss of credibility. As one music therapist in Ferrer's study stated, "You can be a great clinician but it doesn't matter at all if you don't know how to articulate what a great clinician you are" (Ferrer, 2012, p. 133). Some music therapists believe that the lack of understanding surrounding the field of music therapy both from the medical profession and the general public leads to not being viewed as an equal therapy to more commonly known fields such as physical and occupational therapy. This lack of knowledge and acceptance may also contribute to the low reimbursement rates that music therapy services currently receive. One music therapist stated:

> That is kind of a benchmark we are looking for to show that we have been fully accepted as a part of the treatment process. We have done remarkably well not to be getting that reimbursement. There are people who pay for these services.
>
> FERRER (2012, P. 111)

BOX 9.5
Strategies for Improving Music Therapy Advocacy

Continue to expand research and clinical practice with new client populations.

Train and empower music therapists so that they are strong advocates for the profession.

Increase availability of music therapy information to the general public.

Recruit music therapy students from related fields such as music education, music performance, nursing, and psychology.

Ensure that the music therapy major is visible across university and college campuses.

Promote music therapists, rather than just the use of music.

BOX 9.6
Quote From a Music Therapy Educator on Increasing the Number of Music Therapists While Maintaining Quality of Services

I think the demand (for music therapy) is really burgeoning. People say "I'd like to have that service," and the availability of a board certified music therapist is not always adequate to the number of places where people would like to have the service, so they may go with something else, a sound healer, a music practitioner, people that we would consider lesser trained. So it is very important that we keep our standards up and our enrollments as high as we can, even though we have to maintain our quality, so that we can fill the available positions and develop the desirable positions.

Ferrer (2012, p. 103)

In addition to struggles with reimbursement, other financial challenges that may be a product of lack of understanding and value on behalf of employers and consumers include maintaining a successful private practice, dealing with waiver/grant issues, having low salaries, and losing hourly contracts and part-time or full-time positions because of budget cuts. Similar to the arts in educational settings, music therapists have witnessed one too many times their positions being among the first ones to be eliminated. "I have been around long enough to have seen this before, but you get to the point when you say 'when is it that we are not just going to automatically be cut?'" (Ferrer, 2012, pp. 76–77).

As stated before, it is crucial that the music therapy community of practitioners take matters into their own hands and lead in advocacy efforts alongside the AMTA and the CBMT. Box 9.5 highlights suggestions for improving music therapy advocacy. Universities and colleges offering music therapy degrees, clinical facilities that employ music therapists, and related professionals who have witnessed the work of music therapists must also take part in these efforts. One can also never underestimate the power of music therapy consumers and their family members, as they are the first to know and understand the benefits of the therapeutic modality. Music therapy is in great need of champions, allies, and supporters, and these can come both from the outside and from within (Box 9.6).

Growing in Size: Retaining and Increasing the Number of Music Therapists

It is imperative that the profession of music therapy continue to grow in size. An increase in the number of music therapists nationwide would likely lead to an increase in the diversity of the workforce, greater visibility among professional communities and the general public, stronger advocacy and formal/informal outreach efforts, and, most importantly, an increase in the access to quality music therapy services. When asked "Where do you hope to see the field in 10 to 15 years?" and "What needs to happen within the profession for future growth and progress?," music therapists overwhelmingly referred to the need for significant growth in the workforce (Ferrer, 2012). One participant stated, "I would like to see the number of board certified music therapists triple. I'd like to have the problem of too many music therapists" (p. 111). A greater number of music therapists would automatically result in greater exposure for the field, meaning more and more people would become aware of music therapy as a formal academic field of study and viable treatment option. Fig. 9.7 highlights the importance of growing the profession while keeping the standards high.

Growing the music therapy workforce is not an easy feat. Considering past studies on professional issues (Cohen & Behrens, 2002; Ferrer, 2012; Groene, 2003), including the areas of burnout and attrition, there are numerous possible avenues for growing the profession, several of which are summarized in Fig. 9.7.

SUMMARY

The field of music therapy will continue to face numerous challenges over the next few years. Among the most important challenges will be growing the size of the profession by retaining professionals, enhancing the work

Increase professional advocacy efforts	Recruit diverse music therapists	Provide alternative routes to becoming a music therapist
Make changes to the music therapy curriculum to aid in recruitment and retention	Help music therapists practice self-care to prevent burnout	

FIG. 9.7 Strategies for growing the profession of music therapy.

experiences of music therapists by elevating their status so that they are alongside other allied healthcare professionals, considering and possibly making changes to the undergraduate curriculum to increase its relevance to current practice needs, and continuing to improve the research and relationships with related professional communities and the general public. As music therapists face these challenges, they will undoubtedly continue to do what they do best, which is to bring meaningful, enriching, evidence-based music therapy interventions to individuals of all ages and walks of life, seeking to improve their clients' lives, whether cognitively, physically, socioemotionally, or spiritually.

REFERENCES

Alley, J. M. (1978). Competency based evaluation of a music therapy curriculum. *Journal of Music Therapy, 15*, 9–14. http://dx.doi.org/10.1093/jmt/15.1.9.

American Art Therapy Association. (2014). *American art therapy association fact sheet*. Retrieved from http://www.arttherapy.org/upload/aatafactsheet.pdf.

American Dance Therapy Association. (2017). *Find a dance/movement therapist*. Retrieved from https://adta.org/find-a-dancemovement-therapist/.

American Music Therapy Association. (2005). *Strategic priority on research overview*. Retrieved from http://www.musictherapy.org/research/strategic_priority_on_research/overview/.

American Music Therapy Association. (2010). *The 2010 AMTA member survey and workforce analysis: A descriptive statistical profile of the AMTA membership*. Silver Spring, MD: Author.

American Music Therapy Association. (2013). *The 2013 AMTA member survey and workforce analysis: A descriptive statistical profile of the AMTA membership*. Silver Spring, MD: Author.

American Music Therapy Association. (2015). *Improving access and quality: Music therapy research 2025 proceedings*. Retrieved from http://www.musictherapy.org/assets/1/7/MTR2025proceedings.pdf.

American Music Therapy Association. (2016). *The 2016 AMTA member survey and workforce analysis: A descriptive statistical profile of the AMTA membership*. Silver Spring, MD: Author.

American Music Therapy Association. (2017). *Masters level entry considerations*. Retrieved from https://www.musictherapy.org/careers/mle_considerations/.

Bitcon, C. H. (1981). Guest editorial. *Journal of Music Therapy, 18*, 2–6. http://dx.doi.org/10.1093/jmt/18.1.2.

Braswell, C., Decuir, A., & Maranto, C. D. (1980). Ratings of entry skills by music therapy clinicians, educators, and interns. *Journal of Music Therapy, 17*, 133–147. http://dx.doi.org/10.1093/jmt/17.3.133.

Braswell, C., Maranto, C. D., & Decuir, A. (1979). A survey of clinical practice in music therapy, Part II: Clinical practice, education, and clinical training. *Journal of Music Therapy, 16*, 50–69. http://dx.doi.org/10.1093/jmt/16.2.50.

Brookins, L. M. (1984). The music therapy clinical intern: Performance skills, academic knowledge, personal qualities, and interpersonal skills necessary for a student seeking clinical training. *Journal of Music Therapy, 21*, 193–201. http://dx.doi.org/10.1093/jmt/21.4.193.

Certification Board for Music Therapists. (2017). *The certification board for music therapists*. Retrieved from http://cbmt.org/.

Clements-Cortes, A. (2006). Occupational stressors among music therapists working in palliative care. *Canadian Journal of Music Therapy, 12*, 30–60.

Clements-Cortes, A. (2013). Burnout in music therapists: Work, individual, and social factors. *Music Therapy Perspectives, 31*, 166–174. http://dx.doi.org/10.1093/mtp/31.2.166.

Cohen, N. S., & Behrens, G. A. (2002). The relationship between type of degree and clinical status in clinical music therapists. *Journal of Music Therapy, 39*, 188–208. http://dx.doi.org/10.1093/jmt/39.3.188.

Equal Employment Opportunity Commission. (2016). *Charge statistics FY 1997 through FY 2016*. Retrieved from https://www.eeoc.gov/eeoc/statistics/enforcement/charges.cfm.

Ferrer, A. J. (2012). *Music therapy profession: Current status, priorities, and possible future directions*. (Doctoral dissertation). Retrieved from https://etd.ohiolink.edu/.

Ferrer, A. (2017). Music therapy profession: An in-depth analysis of the perceptions of educators and AMTA board members. *Music Therapy Perspectives*. Advance online publication. http://dx.doi.org/10.1093/mtp/miw041.

Fowler, K. L. (2006). The relations between personality characteristics, work environment, and the professional well-being of music therapists. *Journal of Music Therapy, 43,* 174–197. http://dx.doi.org/10.1093/jmt/43.3.174.

Groene, R. W. (2003). Wanted: music therapists: A study of the need for music therapists in the coming decade. *Music Therapy Perspectives, 21,* 4–13. http://dx.doi.org/10.1093/mtp/21.1.4.

Groene, R. W., & Pembrook, R. G. (2000). Curricular issues in music therapy: A survey of collegiate faculty. *Music Therapy Perspectives, 18,* 92–103. http://dx.doi.org/10.1093/mtp/18.2.92.

Jensen, K. L., & McKinney, C. H. (1990). Undergraduate music therapy education and training: Current status and proposals for the future. *Journal of Music Therapy, 27,* 156–178. http://dx.doi.org/10.1093/jmt/27.4.156.

Larson, D. G. (1993). *The helper's journey: Working with people facing grief, loss and life-threatening illness.* Champaign, IL: Research Press.

Madsen, C. K. (1965). A new music therapy curriculum. *Journal of Music Therapy, 2,* 83–85. http://dx.doi.org/10.1093/jmt/2.3.83.

Maslach, C. (1976). Burned out. *Human Behavior, 9*(5), 16–22.

Maslach, C. (1982). *Burnout: The cost of caring.* Englewood Cliffs, NJ: Prentice-Hall.

Maslach, C. (1998). A multidimensional theory of burnout. In C. L. Cooper (Ed.), *Theories of organizational stress* (pp. 68–85). Oxford, UK: Oxford University Press.

Maslach, C., Jackson, S. E., & Leiter, M. P. (1996). *The Maslach burnout inventory* (3rd ed.). Palo Alto, CA: Consulting Psychologists Press.

Maslach, C., Schaufeli, W. B., & Leiter, M. P. (2001). Job burnout. *Annual Review of Psychology, 52,* 397–422. http://dx.doi.org/10.1146/annurev.psych.52.1.397.

Nicholas, M., & Gilbert, J. (1980). Research in music therapy: A survey of music therapists' attitudes and knowledge. *Journal of Music Therapy, 17,* 207–213. http://dx.doi.org/10.1093/jmt/17.4.207.

Oppenheim, L. (1987). Factors related to occupational stress or burnout among music therapists. *Journal of Music Therapy, 24,* 97–106. http://dx.doi.org/10.1093/jmt/24.2.97.

Petrie, G. E. (1989). The identification of a contemporary hierarchy of intended learning outcomes for music therapy students entering internships. *Journal of Music Therapy, 26,* 125–139. http://dx.doi.org/10.1093/jmt/26.3.125.

Robb, S. L. (2012). Gratitude for a complex profession: The importance of theory-based research in music therapy. *Journal of Music Therapy, 49,* 2–6. http://dx.doi.org/10.1093/jmt/49.1.2.

Rowe, M. (1999). Teaching health-care providers coping: Results of a two-year study. *Journal of Behavioral Medicine, 22,* 511–527. http://dx.doi.org/10.1023/A:1018661508593.

Sprang, G., Clark, J. J., & Whitt-Woosley, A. (2007). Compassion fatigue, compassion satisfaction, and burnout: Factors impacting a professional's quality of life. *Journal of Loss and Trauma, 12,* 259–280. http://dx.doi.org/10.1080/15325020701238093.

Substance Abuse and Mental Health Services Administration. (2013). *Addressing the specific behavioral health needs of men. Treatment improvement protocol (TIP) series 56.* HHS Publication No. (SMA) 13-4736. Rockville, MD: Author.

United States Department of Labor Bureau of Labor Statistics. (2016). *Occupational outlook handbook.* Retrieved from https://www.bls.gov/ooh/.

Vega, V. P. (2010). Personality, burnout, and longevity among professional music therapists. *Journal of Music Therapy, 47,* 155–179. http://dx.doi.org/10.1093/jmt/47.2.155.

West, R. (2009). *Music therapists' burnout and job satisfaction levels across work settings* (Master's thesis). Retrieved from ProQuest Dissertations and Theses database. (UMI No. 1471898).

Wheeler, B. L. (Ed.). (1995). *Music therapy research: Qualitative and quantitative perspectives.* Phoenixville, PA: Barcelona Publishers.

Wilhelm, K. (2004). Music therapy and private practice: Recommendations on financial viability and marketing. *Music Therapy Perspectives, 22,* 68–83. http://dx.doi.org/10.1093/mtp/22.2.68.

Wright, T. A., & Bonett, D. G. (1997). The contribution of burnout to work performance. *Journal of Organizational Behavior, 18,* 491–499. http://dx.doi.org/10.1002/(SICI)1099-1379(199709)18:5<491::AID-JOB804>3.0.CO;2-I.

Glossary

A cappella: Singing without instrumental accompaniment.

Active music making: Engaging in singing, playing instruments, or composing music.

Active music therapy: Interventions in which patients actively participate, usually by playing, singing, or composing.

Acute care: Short-term treatment for a severe injury, episode of physical or mental illness, or urgent medical condition.

Acute myocardial infarction (AMI): Also known as a heart attack. Occurs when blood flow to the heart is blocked.

Adjunct therapy: Treatment offered in conjunction with primary treatment.

Adjustment disorder: A disturbance that is short-term, stress related, and nonpsychotic in nature whereby an individual experiences significant distress related to an event or situation.

Advanced Certified Music Therapist (ACMT): A credential for music therapists that was issued by the former American Association for Music Therapy until 1998. This certification will be valid until 2020, after which all music therapists will use the board-certified music therapist (MT-BC) credential.

Afferent: In neurology, afferent refers to the conduction of information toward the central nervous system.

Altshuler, MD, Ira: Psychiatrist at Detroit's Eloise Hospital who, in 1938, initiated one of the first music therapy programs for mental health patients. Considered a pioneer of 20th century music therapy.

American Association for Music Therapy (AAMT, 1971–1997): A professional organization for music therapists in the United States established in 1971 as the Urban Federation of Music Therapists. AAMT was established because a group of music therapists was guided by a philosophy different from that of the existing professional organization for music therapists, the National Association for Music Therapists (NAMT). In 1980, AAMT established the journal *Music Therapy*. In 1998, AAMT and NAMT combined to form AMTA (http://www.musictherapy.org/about/history/).

American Music Therapy Association: A professional organization for music therapists in the United States. The mission of the American Music Therapy Association is to advance public awareness of the benefits of music therapy and increase access to quality music therapy services in a rapidly changing world (http://www.musictherapy.org/).

Amplification: The process of increasing loudness or intensity of sound.

Amygdalae: Two almond-shaped structures located medially within the base of the temporal lobe, one on each cerebral hemisphere, which are involved in experiencing emotions. The amygdalae are part of the limbic system. They help detect and assess emotional salience.

Anorexia nervosa: An eating disorder characterized by excessive weight loss or, in children, failure to gain weight.

Anterior cingulate cortex (ACC): The frontal portion of the cortex that surrounds the corpus callosum, which contains areas concerned with autonomic functions and higher-level functions. As a connector between higher-level cortical functions and lower-level subcortical functions, the ACC helps regulate attention, emotion, reward anticipation, decision making, and autonomic functions.

Anterior frontomedian cortex: The area of the prefrontal cortex implicated in social cognition. Makes evaluative judgments and self-initiates cortical processes.

Anxiety disorders: Conditions in which worry or fear causes distress that interferes with one's ability to lead a normal life, including panic disorder, social anxiety disorder, specific phobias, and generalized anxiety disorder.

Arousal: A state of responsiveness to sensory stimulation.

Assertive community treatment (ACT): A service delivery model in which people with serious and persistent mental illnesses receive the multidisciplinary services typically provided in a psychiatric unit within their own homes.

At-risk children: Youth who have one or more documented risk factors of poor outcomes related to health, mental health, or academic performance.

Atlee, Edwin: Student of Dr. Benjamin Rush and author of the first medical dissertation on the therapeutic value of music, published in 1804.

Attention: The ability to orient and focus on a stimulus or task, sustain that focus, and selectively control and switch the focus. The initial orienting and focusing response involves the parietal and frontal lobes, whereas the ability to control and switch focus of attention involves subcortical and cortical areas, including the anterior cingulate cortex, anterior insula, prefrontal areas in the frontal lobe, and the striatum.

Attention deficit hyperactivity disorder (ADHD): A condition characterized by an ongoing pattern of inattention and/or hyperactivity-impulsivity that impedes functioning or development.

Attenuation: The process of reducing loudness or intensity of sound.

Auditory association area: The part of the posterior section of the superior temporal gyrus that is implicated in processing of sound signals.

Auditory transduction: The process by which mechanical energy, in the form of sound waves, is converted to electrical energy, in the form of electrical signals traveling along the auditory nerves, which can be processed by the brain.

Autism spectrum disorder (ASD): A range of conditions characterized by some degree of difficulty with social skills, communication, and repetitive behaviors.

Autogenic relaxation: A technique in which one learns to relax and control functions such as breathing and heartbeat by responding to verbal suggestions and imagery.

Basal ganglia: A subcortical cluster of nuclei with input and output connections to several cortical and subcortical areas, including the cortical motor response areas and the substantia nigra. Plays a role in regulating the intensity of voluntary motor movements, learning complex movement patterns, and initiating movements. In auditory perception, the basal ganglia is important for relative, or beat-based, timing, which occurs when we perceive the timing of rhythmic intervals based on an existing beat. Also involved in procedural learning and emotions. The basal ganglia include the striatum.

Basilar membrane: The structure in the cochlea of the inner ear that oscillates in response to mechanical sound energy. Contains the organ of Corti and separates the scala tympani from the scala media.

Biofeedback: A process in which electronic monitoring of typically autonomic bodily functions (e.g., respiration, heart rate) helps an individual learn some voluntary control over that function.

Bipolar disorder: A condition characterized by extreme shifts in mood, energy, and activity levels, including emotional highs (mania or hypomania) and lows (depression).

Blackwell's Island, New York: Location of the first recorded music therapy intervention in an institutional setting.

Body percussion: Using the human body to produce sounds similar to those produced by hitting, scraping, rubbing, or shaking percussion instruments. Stomping, patching, clapping, and snapping are four common types of body percussion, although there are numerous others.

Bonny Method of Guided Imagery and Music (BMGIM): An approach to music-centered psychotherapy developed by Helen Lindquist Bonny in which music experiences are used to bring about therapeutic change.

Bordun: A drone accompaniment that uses the first and fifth scale degrees, either played simultaneously (as in the chord bordun and the level bordun) or sequentially (as in the broken bordun and the crossover borduns).

Brainstem: The central trunk of the brain, which connects the spinal cord to the cerebrum. The brainstem includes the medulla oblongata, pons, and midbrain.

Broca's area: A region of the brain involved with expressive communication. Located in the frontal lobe, usually in the left hemisphere (for right-handed individuals). Named after French physician and anatomist Pierre Paul Broca.

Burnout: A type of occupational psychological stress characterized by emotional exhaustion, depersonalization, and lack of personal accomplishment.

Cabasa: A percussion instrument traditionally made from a dried gourd strung with beads, similar to the shekere. The afuche-cabasa adapted by Martin Cohen for Latin Percussion in the 1960s has a wide cylinder, around which loops of steel ball chain are wrapped, attached to a long, narrow handle, and is frequently used by music therapists.

Cerebellum: Latin for "little brain," the cerebellum is a two-hemisphere, subcortical structure that sits at the base of the brain. It is implicated in coordinating and regulating motor movement and motor learning.

Certification Board for Music Therapists (CBMT): Credentialing body for music therapists in the United States. CBMT issues the music therapist-board certified (MT-BC) credential.

Certified music practitioner (CMP): A specially trained musician who provides live acoustic music at bedside, one on one, for therapeutic purposes (see www.mhtp.org). Distinct from music therapy, which is delivered by board-certified music therapists (MT-BC) and has a different scope of practice.

Certified Music Therapist (CMT): A credential for music therapists that was issued by the former American Association for Music Therapy until 1998. This certification will be valid until 2020, after which all music therapists will use the MT-BC credential.

Chronic obstructive pulmonary disease (COPD): A group of progressive lung diseases characterized by increasing breathlessness. Includes emphysema, chronic bronchitis, and refractory asthma.

Cingulate cortex: The medial portion of the cerebral cortex surrounding the corpus callosum. Helps link behavior to motivation and implicated in executive functions.

Closed group format: A type of mental health or counseling group with a fixed number of group members who join the group at the same time and attend the group regularly for a specified duration of time, during which no new members may join.

Cochlea: Latin for *snail*. Fluid-filled, snail-shaped chamber within the inner ear that receives mechanical energy from the middle ear and converts it into electrochemical energy, which is transmitted to the brain.

Cochlear nerve: A part of cranial nerve VIII. Carries electrical signals from the cochlea to various nuclei in the brainstem when stimulated by glutamate in the process of auditory transduction.

Cochlear nucleus (CN): An auditory pathway relay station within the brainstem. Consists of the ventral (ascending) cochlear nucleus and the dorsal (descending) cochlear nucleus. Helps decode intensity, duration, frequency, and the start/end of a sound stimulus.

Columbian Magazine: The journal in which the first recorded reference to music therapy appeared in 1789, in the form of an article called Music Physically Considered (author unknown).

Communication: Involves the meaningful conveyance of information, ideas, or feelings through verbal or nonverbal means.

Community music therapy (CoMT): Providing music therapy to people in a community context and/or using music therapy to effect change in a community.

Composition: A music therapy intervention in which the client engages in creating new, original music.

Conduct disorder: A mental disorder evidenced by a pattern of behavior that violates others' basic rights, social norms, or rules.

Connectivity: In neurology, connectivity refers to communication between neural networks, which are structures and areas in the brain responsible for specific behaviors or tasks. Functional connectivity and effective connectivity are subtypes commonly studied via brain imaging technology.

Contingent music: An intervention in which getting to participate in musical experiences is dependent on the presence or absence of a specific behavior. Contingent music may consist of (1) music listening initiation (e.g., beginning to play music immediately following a desired behavior), (2) music interruption (e.g., stopping music with onset of an undesirable behavior), or (3) music performance (e.g., an opportunity to actively engage in music making following a desirable behavior).

Continuing Music Therapy Education (CMTE): Postcertification education credits for music therapists. Board-certified music therapists must earn 100 CMTE credits every 5 years to maintain certification.

Coronary artery bypass graft (CABG): A surgery often used to treat people with severe coronary heart disease that improves flow of blood to the heart.

Coronary heart disease: A condition resulting from coronary artery disease, in which cholesterol and plaque accumulate inside the coronary arteries (atherosclerosis) to the point that the heart does not receive adequate blood or oxygen.

Corning, James Leonard: Conducted research on the use of music to affect dream states during psychotherapy, the first documented systematic music therapy experiment.

Correctional facility: An institution that confines and rehabilitates prisoners. May refer to a jail, prison, or detention center and may be classified as minimum, medium, or maximum security.

Cortisol: Sometimes referred to as the stress hormone, cortisol regulates and mediates biological responses to real or perceived threats. Cortisol is associated with activation of the hypothalamo-pituitary-adrenal (HPA) axis, the neural network underlying the body's stress response.

Creative arts therapy: Formalized disciplines that apply creative interventions within psychotherapy and counseling. Includes art therapy, music therapy, drama therapy, dance/movement therapy, and poetry therapy. Also called expressive therapies.

Crisis stabilization: A model of care to assist individuals experiencing acute mental health crises, often through short-term hospitalization, therapy, medication changes, and case management.

Declarative memory: Also known as episodic memory. Involves the learning of conscious, verbal, and mental imagery information, including general knowledge of the world (semantic memory) and autobiographic information (episodic memory).

Depression: A state of severe sadness. Sometimes used to refer to major depressive disorder, which is characterized by feelings of sadness and lack of interest in previously enjoyable activities, to the degree that they impede a person's ability to function.

Detection of danger response: Humans' ability to identify potential danger in their surroundings. Detection of danger via auditory signals is possible because neurons from the inferior colliculus and the medial geniculate body, both of which are part of the auditory pathway, project to the amygdala, which is involved in perceiving emotional salience in the environment.

Detoxification: A medically supervised treatment for drug or alcohol addiction in which the patient withdraws from intoxicating or addictive substances as an initial step in overcoming addiction.

Disenfranchised grief: Feelings of deep sorrow related to a loss that is not recognized by society.

Dissociative disorders: Conditions characterized by a disconnection between thoughts, identity, awareness, and memory. Includes dissociative identity disorder, dissociative amnesia, dissociative fugue, and depersonalization disorder.

Dopamine: A neurochemical implicated in reward, motivation, pleasure, working memory, and reinforcement learning.

Dorsolateral prefrontal cortex (PFC): Located on the upper side of the prefrontal cortex. An area of the brain associated with cognitive executive functioning, working memory, motor planning, and social cognition.

Dose-response relationship: The change in effect on a person based on different levels of exposure to a substance or treatment.

Drum circle: Playing percussion instruments in a group format.

Dual diagnosis: Describes a person who has a mental illness and a co-occurring substance use disorder.

Dual Diagnosis Recovery Counseling (DDRC): An approach to treating patients with mental illness and substance use disorders that integrates individual and group addiction counseling and psychiatric treatment.

Ear canal: Also known as the meatus or the external auditory meatus. Part of the outer ear that connects the pinna to the tympanic membrane.

Ear drum: Also known as the tympanic membrane. Connects the ear canal (external auditory meatus) of the outer ear to the ossicles of the middle ear.

Effectiveness research: Attempts to answer the question, "does the treatment still work when used by the average clinician with the average patient?" Typically follows efficacy research and precedes efficiency research.

Effective connectivity: Explores the causal influence of one neural structure over another.

Efferent: In neurology, efferent refers to the conduction of information away from the central nervous system.

Efficacy research: Attempts to answer the question, "is the treatment superior to a placebo or control in randomized controlled trials?" Typically precedes effectiveness and efficiency research.

Efficiency research: Attempts to answer the question, "what level of resources are required to produce benefit?" Typically follows efficacy and effectiveness research.

Elemental music: A term used in the Orff Schulwerk approach to describe music that incorporates multiple elements, including movement, dance, instruments, and/or speech, in addition to music.

Emotion: Brief but intense affective reactions that typically involve subjective feeling, physiological arousal, expression, action tendency, and regulation.

Emotional disturbance: According to the Individuals with Disabilities Education Act (IDEA), an emotional disturbance is a condition characterized by an inability to learn not explained by intellectual, sensory, or health factors, as well as inappropriate behavior or feelings and difficulty maintaining interpersonal relationships. Sometimes called emotional or behavioral disorders (EBD).

Emotional or behavioral disorders (EBD): See emotional disturbance.

Empathy: The capacity to be aware of and understand another person's feelings and emotions.

Entrainment: See rhythmic entrainment.

Episodic memory: A type of declarative memory that is autobiographic in nature. Learning and storage of episodic memory is mediated by the hippocampus and prefrontal cortex.

Evidence-based practice: Basing treatment decisions on the best available research, clinical expertise, and patients' values.

Executive functioning: The management of cognitive processes. Involves the ability to formulate goals, anticipate consequences, initiate behavior, plan and organize behavior, and monitor or adapt behavior to fit a particular task or context. Incorporates skills such as problem solving, decision making, planning, goal setting, behavior regulation, attention regulation, organizing, and reasoning.

Explicit memory: See declarative memory.

External auditory meatus: Also known as the ear canal or meatus. Part of the outer ear that connects the pinna to the tympanic membrane.

Fill-in-the-blank songwriting: A technique in which client-generated words are substituted for selected original song lyrics.

Fellow of the Association for Music and Imagery (FAMI): Specialized training for music therapists who have undergone advanced training in the use of the Bonny Method of Guided Imagery and Music (BMGIM).

Family-based psychoeducation: A model in which mental health professionals work with families of individuals with mental illness to coordinate treatment and provide support.

Forensic psychiatric facility: An institution that houses people with mental illness who have been accused of a crime and are awaiting trial and/or people who have been convicted of a crime and are serving time.

Frequency: The rate at which vibrations occur, measured in cycles per second or Hertz (Hz).

Frontal lobe: A pair of lobes at the front of the brain (one in each hemisphere) that contain areas involved with behavior, learning, personality, speech production, and voluntary motor movements.

Functional connectivity: Explores how spatially separated brain regions work together to accomplish specific functions. Studied by using statistical measures to investigate shared timing of neural activity in separate areas of the brain.

Gaston, E. Thayer: Music educator who started the United States' first graduate program in music therapy at the University of Kansas. Considered by many to be the "father of music therapy."

Glockenspiel: A musical instrument with metal bars of graduated length that are struck by mallets. Smaller and higher in pitch than a metallophone.

Glutamate: As concerns auditory processing, a neurotransmitter that stimulates the cochlear nerve, cranial nerve VIII.

Goal: An expected outcome, purpose, or direction for music therapy, stated in general terms (as opposed to an objective, which is more specific).

GORSKI-CENAPS Model for Recovery and Relapse Prevention: A model for diagnosing and treating substance use disorders and dual diagnosis.

Grapheme: A letter or group of letters that represent a sound (phoneme). The smallest meaningful unit in written language.

Hair cells: Highly sensitive sensory receptors on the organ of Corti that, when deflected against the tectorial membrane, depolarize and release glutamate.

Harp therapy: The use of harp music performed at bedside in healthcare settings. Harp therapy is a type of therapeutic music administered by Certified Music Practitioners (CMP), Certified Clinical Musicians (CCM), Certified Therapeutic Harp Practitioners (CTHP), or Certified Harp Therapists (CHT), but it is distinct from music therapy, which is delivered by board-certified music therapists (MT-BC) and has a different scope of practice.

Health: A state of complete physical, mental, and social well-being and not merely the absence of disease or infirmity.

Heschl's gyrus: Also known as the transverse temporal gyrus. Found in the primary auditory cortex of each hemisphere, Heschl gyrus is the first cortical structure to process afferent auditory information.

Hippocampus: Subcortical structure in the medial temporal lobe of each hemisphere of the brain. Implicated in memory formation and recall, particularly of long-term memory, and emotion.

Hospice: A philosophy of care in which an interdisciplinary group of professionals work together with an individual who is predicted to have 6 months or less to live and their family to alleviate the individual's pain and address physical, psychosocial, and/or spiritual needs.

Hypothalamo-pituitary-adrenal (HPA) axis: An endocrine-related neural network underlying the body's stress response. Includes the hypothalamus, pituitary gland, and adrenal gland.

Hypothalamus: An area of the forebrain underneath the thalamus. Produces hormones that govern homeostasis and coordinate the autonomic nervous system. Controls functions such as body temperature, thirst, and hunger and is involved in sleep and emotional activity.

Illness management and recovery model: Also known as psychosocial rehabilitation, psychoeducation, or psychiatric rehabilitation. This model focuses on psychoeducation, strategies for addressing medication nonadherence, relapse prevention training to reduce symptoms and hospitalizations, and coping skills training to reduce distress and/or symptom severity using cognitive-behavioral techniques.

Ilsen, Isa Maud: Founded the National Association for Music in Hospitals in 1926.

Implicit memory: See procedural memory.

Improvisation: When the client makes up music spontaneously using voice or instruments. Improvisation can be alone, with the therapist, or with other clients. The structure may be free or structured by the therapist.

Incus: Anvil-shaped ossicle (bone) within the middle ear. Works with the malleus and stapes to transmit sound waves from the tympanic membrane to the cochlea.

Individual Music-Centered Assessment Profile for Neurodevelopmental Disorders (IMCAP-ND): A music therapy assessment developed by John Carpente for use with individuals who have neurodevelopmental disorders.

Individualized Education Program (IEP): A legally required individualized student document that guides the delivery of special education supports and services.

Individualized Music Therapy Assessment Profile (IMTAP): An assessment tool created by Holly Tuesday Baxter, Julie Allis Berghofer, Lesa MacEwan, Judy Nelson, Kasi Peters, and Penny Roberts for use by music therapists working with children or adolescents.

Individuals with Disabilities Education Act (IDEA): US law that mandates every child with a disability receive access to a free, appropriate public education in the least restrictive environment.

Inferior colliculus (IC): Bilateral nuclei on the brainstem that is part of the auditory pathway. Connects the nuclei of the lateral lemniscus to the medial geniculate body. Connections between the inferior colliculus and the superior colliculus, part of the visual processing pathway, are responsible for the visual-orienting response in humans. Connections between the inferior colliculus and the amygdala (via the medial geniculate body) are involved in the detection of danger.

Inner ear: The innermost part of the ear, which contains sensory organs for hearing (the cochlea) and balance (the semicircular canals).

Insula: Also known as the insular cortex or insular lobe. Portion of the cerebral cortex deep within the lateral sulcus. Involved in consciousness and emotion, as well as motor and cognitive processing.

Integrated dual-disorder treatment (IDDT): A multidisciplinary model of treatment for individuals with co-occurring mental illness and substance use disorder.

Intellectual disability: A condition diagnosed before age 18 years in which an individual has significant limitations in intellectual functioning and adaptive behavior. This term replaced the term mental retardation in the Diagnostic and Statistical Manual of Mental Disorders, Fifth Edition (DSM-5).

Intensity: In the study of acoustics, intensity is the magnitude of sound wave energy, which is perceived as loudness. Measured in decibels (dB).

Iso principle: A technique in which music stimuli is matched to the client's behavior/mood/physiologic state and slowly adjusted in complexity, volume, and tempo to produce a change in the client.

Journal of Music Therapy (JMT): A peer-reviewed publication of the American Music Therapy Association. JMT's mission is to promote scholarly activity in music therapy and to foster the development and understanding of music therapy and music-based interventions.

Lateral prefrontal cortex (PFC): The area of the anterior portion of the frontal lobe that is involved in executive behavioral control.

Lateralization: A phenomenon in which certain behaviors tend to be more heavily managed by structures in one hemisphere of the brain, either the right hemisphere or the left hemisphere.

Learning: The acquisition of knowledge or skills through experience, through study, or by being taught.

Least restrictive environment: A requirement of the Individuals with Disabilities Education Act that provides students with disabilities—with the use of supplementary aids and services—access to education in the most typical educational environment with students without disabilities, unless the severity of the disability prevents satisfactory education.

Legacy project: In music therapy practice, a legacy project includes audio or video recordings, as well as physical products associated with those recordings, created by clients receiving end-of-life care in collaboration with music therapists and often shared with family members to provide opportunities for creative expression, enjoyment, emotional expression, relationship completion, and life review.

Licensed Creative Arts Therapist (LCAT): A credential administered by the state of New York required for music therapists practicing creative arts therapy in New York state.

Lyric analysis: A type of song discussion that involves a detailed examination of the words of a song as the basis for discussion or interpretation.

Malleus: A hammer-shaped ossicle (bone) in the ear. Works with the incus and stapes to transmit sound waves from the tympanic membrane to the cochlea.

Mathews, Samuel: Student of Dr. Benjamin Rush and author of the second medical dissertation on the therapeutic value of music, published in 1806.

Meatus: Also known as the external auditory meatus, or ear canal. Connects the pinna to the tympanic membrane.

Medial geniculate body (MGB): Also called the medial geniculate nucleus. Part of the thalamus that acts as a relay center for auditory information being transmitted from the inferior colliculus (IC) to the primary auditory cortex.

Medial prefrontal cortex (PFC): An area in the middle part of the frontal lobe. Implicated in empathy and decision making.

Medication management: Service provided by a psychiatrist or another professional qualified to evaluate the need for medication that involves selecting, administering, and monitoring side effects of medications.

Medulloblastoma: A fast-growing, high-grade tumor.

Memory: The capacity by which the mind stores and remembers knowledge or skills.

Metallophone: A musical instrument with metal bars of graduated length that are struck by mallets.

Michigan State University: Location of the first academic training program for music therapists, established in 1944.

Midbrain: (Also known as the mesencephalon.) The central part of the brainstem that consists of the tectum and tegmentum. Involved with eye movement, regulating muscle movement, reward and motivation, and hearing.

Middle ear: The portion of the ear separated from the outer ear by the tympanic membrane and from the inner ear by the oval window. Contains the ossicles and the auditory (Eustachian) tube.

Mood: Affective states that are lower in intensity and longer lasting than emotions.

Motivation enhancement therapy (MET): An approach to counseling that helps individuals with substance use disorders resolve ambivalence about engaging in treatment.

Motor-reticular response: Behavioral response in which our motor system synchronizes to a steady rhythmic pulse without learning or conscious awareness. This response is possible because of auditory neurons that project from the cochlear nucleus to the spinal cord via the reticular formation.

Music and art: An intervention in which music is paired with drawing, painting, or making collages. Making musical instruments may also be included.

Music-assisted imagery: A type of music-assisted relaxation in which visualizations and/or imagery are accompanied by music. Also called music and imagery.

Music-assisted relaxation (MAR): Music paired with relaxation techniques such as verbal suggestion, breathing exercises, and imagery.

Music-based life review: (Also called musical life review.) The use of music, typically with people receiving end-of-life care, to facilitate discussion of present and past events, concerns, and attitudes. Often occurs as part of a legacy project.

Music discussion: A broad term that describes listening to and discussing any type of music, instrumental or with lyrics.

Music medicine: The use of recorded music listening in a healthcare setting, implemented by a healthcare professional who is not a music therapist.

Music thanatology: A musical/clinical modality that utilizes harp and voice at the bedside of people at the end of life. Performed by Certified Music-Thanatologists (CM-Th) (see www.mtai.org). Distinct from music therapy, which is delivered by board-certified music therapists (MT-BC) and has a different scope of practice.

Music therapy: The use of music and the therapeutic relationship with a credentialed music therapist to accomplish nonmusic goals.

Music Therapy **(journal):** A peer-reviewed journal published by the former American Association for Music Therapy (AAMT) from 1981 to 1996.

Music Therapy Perspectives **(MTP):** A peer-reviewed publication of the American Music Therapy Association that focuses on the clinical benefits of music therapy, serving as a resource and forum for music therapists, students, educators, and other professionals.

Music Therapy Special Education Assessment Scale (MT-SEAS): A formal music therapy assessment developed by Colleen Bradfield and colleagues for use in special education settings.

Music therapist-board certified (MT-BC): A credential granted by the Certification Board for Music Therapists (CBMT) to denote music therapists who have shown the knowledge, skills, and abilities needed to practice music therapy.

Musical check-in: A brief process that incorporates instrument playing while having clients identify and share their current emotional and/or cognitive state.

Myelin: A fatty substance that surrounds the axon of certain neurons, providing insulation and increasing the speed and efficiency of neural impulse transmission.

Myelination: A process by which neural connections are strengthened through the production and increase of the myelin sheath.

National Association for Music Therapy (NAMT, 1950–97): A professional organization for music therapists; it created a constitution, bylaws, standards for education and clinical training of music therapists, and a registry for music therapists. Research and clinical training were priorities for NAMT, and they established two scholarly, peer-reviewed journals: *Journal of Music Therapy* and *Music Therapy Perspectives*. When the Certification Board for Music Therapists (CBMT) was established in 1985, NAMT leadership helped establish board-certification requirements. In 1998, NAMT and AAMT merged to become AMTA.

National Association of Schools of Music (NASM): Organization that establishes the national standards for undergraduate and graduate degrees and other credentials for music.

National Standards Board for Therapeutic Musicians (NSBTM): An organization that develops and maintains standards for therapeutic musician training programs. Therapeutic musicians have scopes of practice that are distinct from that of music therapy.

Neurochemical mechanisms: As concerns music-based interventions, the shared chemical and hormonal changes that occur when engaged in music and influence nonmusical behaviors. The production and release of neurochemicals help mediate the connectivity between neural networks.

Neurocognitive disorders (NCD): Conditions characterized by acquired cognitive impairments. Includes NCD caused by Alzheimer's disease, Parkinson's disease, and traumatic brain injury.

Neurodevelopmental disorders: Conditions that manifest in early development, characterized by developmental deficits that produce impairments in personal, social, academic, or occupational functioning.

Neurologic Music Therapy (NMT): An approach to music therapy that includes standardized clinical techniques for sensorimotor, speech and language, and cognitive training or rehabilitation. NMT may also refer to the designation denoting Neurologic Music Therapists who have undergone specialized training in neurologic music therapy.

Neuroplasticity: The ability of the brain to change based on experience. The human brain continues to reorganize itself throughout the lifetime based on environment, behaviors, thoughts, and emotions. Plasticity can occur at the neuronal level and the structural level.

Neuroplasticity model of music therapy: Presented by Elizabeth Stegemöller in 2014, this model purports that music can boost neuroplasticity in one of three ways: by (1) increasing dopamine levels; (2) synchronizing neural firing patterns, creating and strengthening connections between neurons; and (3) providing a clear signal that is easy for the human brain to process, because music is an acoustically organized and structured stimulus.

Neonatal Intensive Care Unit Music Therapist (NICU-MT): A designation denoting music therapists who have undergone specialized training in the music of music therapy to address developmental needs of infants in the neonatal intensive care unit.

Nonnutritive sucking: Sucking not related to or providing nutrition. For premature infants, this often involves a pacifier and can lead to improved bottle feeding.

Nordoff-Robbins music therapy (NRMT): Also known as creative music therapy. An approach to music therapy developed by Paul Nordoff and Clive Robbins in which clinical improvisation is used to develop clients' inner potential.

Nuclei of lateral lemniscus (NLL): A tract of axons in the brainstem that serve as an auditory pathway relay station, connecting the superior olivary complex to the inferior colliculus.

Nucleus accumbens (NAc): An area within the ventral striatum that is implicated in reward and motivation by mediating dopamine release.

Objective: A specific therapeutic aim, stated as a clearly observable outcome.

Open group format: A type of mental health or counseling group in which new members can join at any time.

Optimal complexity theory: Based on the research of D. E. Berlyne. When applied to music preference, the optimal complexity theory suggests that the perceived complexity of music determines the preference or rejection of the music. Enjoyment of music will be diminished if the music is too simple or too complex.

Orbitofrontal cortex: The portion of the medial prefrontal cortex involved with emotion regulation, cognitive processing, sensory integration, and decision making.

Orff media: Speech, movement, singing, and playing instruments.

Orff Schulwerk: A common international approach to music education developed by composer Carl Orff (1895–1982) in the 1920s that is founded in the philosophy of learning by doing. Principles of the Orff Schulwerk approach are often used in music therapy treatment with children in educational settings, and less frequently with adults in other settings.

Organ of Corti: A structure situated on the basilar membrane within the scala media of the cochlea, upon which sits highly sensitive sensory receptors (hair cells).

Ossicles: Three small bones within the middle ear (malleus, incus, and stapes) that transmit vibrations from the tympanic membrane to the cochlea.

Outer ear: The external part of the ear, made up of the pinna and the external auditory meatus.

Oval window: A membrane-covered opening connected to the stapes that separates the middle ear from the scala vestibuli of the cochlea.

Oxytocin: A neurochemical associated with maternal behaviors, regulation of social behavior and trust.

Pacifier Activated Lullaby (PAL) device: A medical device that uses lullabies as a reward for nonnutritive sucking in premature infants, ideally at 34 gestational weeks, to promote nonnutritive sucking.

Palliative care: An approach that improves the quality of life of patients (adults and children) and their families who are facing problems associated with life-threatening illness. It prevents and relieves suffering through the early identification, correct assessment, and treatment of pain and other problems, whether physical, psychosocial, or spiritual.

Parahippocampal gyrus: The area of the brain surrounding the hippocampus. A part of the limbic system. Involved in memory encoding and retrieval, particularly episodic memory, as well as visuospatial processing and processing contextual associations.

Parietal lobe: A pair of lobes at the top of the brain (one in each hemisphere) that include areas implicated in reception, perception, and integration of sensory information.

Parkinson's disease: A neurodegenerative disorder characterized by motor symptoms, as well as gradual changes in cognition, speech, mood, and autonomic functions.

Passive music therapy: Interventions in which patients listen to music, live or recorded, that is selected and/or implemented by a music therapist. Although music therapy interventions involve interaction with a music therapist, some studies inaccurately refer to music medicine interventions, which do not involve interaction with a music therapist, as passive music therapy.

Personality disorders: Conditions characterized by rigid and unhealthy patterns of thinking, functioning, and behaving that cause significant problems in relationships, social activities, work, and school. Includes paranoid, schizoid, schizotypal, antisocial, borderline, histrionic, narcissistic, avoidant, dependent, and obsessive-compulsive personality disorders.

Phoneme: A sound or group of sounds that function together to give words meaning. Changing a phoneme alters the meaning of a word (e.g., changing the /b/ phoneme in the word *bat* to a /p/ phoneme changes the meaning).

Piggyback songwriting: See song parody.

Pinna: The external part of the ear that captures and funnels sound waves into the ear canal.

Pitch: Perceived frequency of sound.

Posttraumatic stress disorder (PTSD): A condition that may develop after a person has experienced a frightening, shocking, or dangerous event. Includes reexperiencing symptoms (e.g., flashbacks), avoidance symptoms (e.g., avoiding thoughts related to the event), arousal and reactivity symptoms (e.g., being easily startled), and cognition and mood symptoms (e.g., distorted feelings such as guilt or blame).

Posterior lobe of the cerebellum: (Also known as the neocerebellum.) The portion of the cerebellum behind the primary fissure. Receives input from the cerebral cortex and the brainstem, and is involved in motor coordination.

Prefrontal lobe (cortex): The anterior part of the frontal lobe. Carries out functions related to executive functioning, planning complex cognitive behaviors, personal expression, decision making, and mediating social behavior.

Premotor cortex: Located in the frontal lobe, the premotor cortex is implicated in planning of precise motor tasks and initiation of voluntary motor movements.

Primary auditory cortex: The area of the superior temporal gyrus in the temporal lobe that processes auditory information, which arrives via the medial geniculate body (MGB) of the thalamus. Implicated in detecting and processing characteristics of the auditory signal. Involved with analyzing acoustic features of frequency, intensity, and timbre; storing auditory sensory memory; discriminating and organizing sounds and sound patterns (known as stream segregation); and transforming the acoustic features (e.g., frequency) into perceptual ones (e.g., pitch).

Primary motor cortex: A part of the frontal lobe that generates voluntary motor movement instructions.

Procedural memory: Also known as implicit memory. Involves the learning of an automatic or subconscious cognitive or motor skill, or of a conditioned response.

Process, Orff Schulwerk: The series of steps through which the teacher/therapist guides the student to reach the short- or long-term goal.

Production music therapy techniques: Music therapy interventions that focus on emotional expression and musical improvisation.

Psychoeducation: The process of providing education and information to mental health consumers and their families.

Psychotic disorders: Severe mental illnesses that cause abnormal thinking and perceptions and a lack of connection with reality. Two common symptoms of psychosis include delusions and hallucinations. Include schizophrenia and schizoaffective disorder.

Receptive music therapy techniques: Music therapy interventions that involve listening to live or recorded music to increase awareness or promote relaxation. (Also called reception techniques.)

Recorder: A woodwind instrument that is played vertically (as opposed to the flute, which is held transverse). The soprano recorder is often used in music education and in music therapy in educational settings.

Recovery-oriented systems of care (ROSC): Networks of organizations, agencies, and community members that coordinate a wide spectrum of services to prevent, intervene in, and treat substance use problems and disorders.

Recreational music making: Enjoyable, accessible, and fulfilling group music-based activities.

Registered music therapist (RMT): A credential for music therapists that was issued by the former National Association for Music Therapy until 1998. This certification will be valid until 2020, after which all music therapists will use the MT-BC credential.

Reproduction music therapy techniques: Music therapy interventions that focus on playing or singing precomposed music.

Reissner's membrane: (Also known as the vestibular membrane.) Membrane inside the cochlear of the inner ear. Separates the scala vestibuli from the scala media.

Resource-oriented music therapy: An approach to music therapy that focuses on strengths while also addressing problems and striving to empower individuals through collaboration.

Reticular formation: A group of interconnected nuclei located throughout the brainstem. Involved in generating reflexive motor responses, awareness, and consciousness.

Rhythmic auditory system (RAS): A neurologic technique in which auditory rhythmic entrainment is used to rehabilitate biologically rhythmic movements, particularly gait.

Rhythmic entrainment: Phenomenon of auditory-motor coupling in which the motor system synchronizes to a steady rhythmic pulse.

Rolandic fissure: Also known as the fissure of Rolando or the central sulcus. Separates the frontal and parietal lobes of the brain.

Rolandic operculum: Also known as the frontal operculum. Area of the frontal lobe that partially covers the insula that holds representations of motor movements of the lips, tongue, and pharynx muscles.

Round window: A membrane-covered opening that separates the middle ear from the scala tympani of the cochlea.

Rush, MD, Benjamin: Physician and psychiatrist who supported the use of music in medical treatment in the early 1800s.

Scala media: A central fluid-filled compartment within the cochlea, separated from the scala vestibuli and the scala tympani by the Reissner membrane and the basilar membrane, respectively. Contains the basilar and tectorial membranes.

Scala vestibuli: The upper bony fluid-filled compartment within the cochlea, separated from the scala media by Reissner membrane.

Scala tympani: The lower bony fluid-filled compartment within the cochlea, separated from the scala media by the basilar membrane.

SCERTS model: An educational model developed by Barry Prizant, Amy Wetherby, Emily Rubin, and Amy Laurant for use with children who have ASD. Often used by music therapists. The acronym SCERTS stands for Social Communication, Emotional Regulation, and Transactional Support.

Schizophrenia: A chronic and severe mental disorder that affects the way a person thinks, feels, and behaves. May include positive symptoms (e.g., hallucinations, delusions), negative symptoms (e.g., reduced speaking), and/or cognitive symptoms (e.g., poor executive functioning).

Secondary auditory cortex: The area of the temporal lobe involved with sound localization, analysis of complex sounds, and auditory memory.

Self-esteem: The extent to which people value, approve of, or like themselves.

Semantic memory: A type of declarative memory that describes general knowledge of the world.

Semi-closed group format: Similar to a closed group, except that new members may join when there is an opening in the group.

Severe and enduring mental illnesses (SEMI): Long-term mental illnesses that produce severe and debilitating symptoms and require extensive services over time. Often includes schizophrenia and other psychotic disorders, as well as bipolar disorder.

Seymour, Harriet Ayer: Founded the National Foundation of Music Therapy in 1941.

Shekere: A West African instrument made by taking a dried, hollow gourd and covering it with a netting of beads. May be shaken like a rattle or pounded (on the bottom) like a drum, or the netting can be smoothed over the gourd like a cabasa.

Sing-along: Live singing of patient-preferred music.

Social cognition: The mental processes underlying social interactions. Our capacity to predict other people's intentions, motivations, and actions, and how this ability influences social practices.

Social Stories: A social learning tool developed by Carol Gray to improve the social skills of individuals with autism spectrum disorders.

Song discussion: An intervention in which a client and therapist listen to a preselected song and discuss elements of the lyrics and the musical elements to explore the meaning of the song to the client.

Song parody: A songwriting technique in which client-generated lyrics are substituted for original lyrics.

Songwriting: The process of creating, notating, and/or recording lyrics and music by the client or clients and therapist within a therapeutic relationship to address psychosocial, emotional, cognitive, and communication needs of the client.

Sound wave: A longitudinal pressure wave consisting of cycles of compression and rarefaction that travels through an elastic medium, such as air.

Special Education Music Therapy Assessment Process (SEMTAP): A formal assessment tool created by Kathleen Coleman and Betsey King for use by music therapists working in special education settings.

Stapes: Stirrup-shaped ossicle (bone) in the ear. Receives mechanical sound wave energy from the tympanic membrane (via the malleus and the incus) and transmits it to the cochlea.

Stream segregation: The perpetual discrimination and grouping of sounds and sound patterns that occurs when processing a complex auditory signal.

Stress: Physical, mental, or emotional strain or tension.

Striatum: The subcortical area of the forebrain involved in the reward system. Part of the basal ganglia.

Stroke: Also called cerebrovascular accident (CVA). Occurs when there is a disruption in blood supply to the brain, either because a blood vessel is blocked or because a blood vessel ruptures.

Substance use disorders (SUD): Conditions in which the recurrent use of drugs and/or alcohol causes significant impairment or distress. The most commonly used substances that result in SUDs in the United States include alcohol, tobacco, cannabis, stimulants, hallucinogens, and opioids.

Substantia nigra: The area in the brainstem, considered part of the basal ganglia, that produces dopamine. Plays an important role in motor planning, as well as in reward and motivation.

Superior colliculus: Bilateral nuclei in the brainstem involved in, among other behaviors, gaze control. Connections between the inferior colliculus, which is part of the auditory pathway, and the superior colliculus are responsible for the visual-orienting response in humans.

Superior olivary complex (SOC): The auditory pathway relay station within the brainstem. Consists of the medial superior olive, which helps measure the difference in timing of arrival of sounds between the ears, and the lateral superior olive, which helps measure the difference in intensity of sound between the ears.

Superior temporal gyrus: The top ridge of the temporal lobe that contains the primary auditory cortex.

Superior temporal sulcus: The first groove below the lateral fissure, separating the superior temporal gyrus from the middle temporal gyrus. Activated during music improvisation and social cognition.

Supplementary motor area (SMA): Located in the frontal lobe, the SMA is implicated in planning and initiation of voluntary motor movements. Activated during beat-based timing, as well as during beat perception.

Supportive employment: Services provided to individuals with disabilities and mental illnesses to assist with obtaining and maintaining employment. Models of supportive employment include job crews, enclaves, and working with employment specialists.

Synapse: A small gap between two neurons through which a chemical or an electrical signal is sent from one neuron to another.

Synaptic connections: (see also synapse) Interactions and neurochemical communications that occur between neurons.

Synaptic pruning: The process by which the brain sheds synaptic connections that are old or weak because of lack of use.

Tectorial membrane: The structure against which hair cells on the organ of Corti (within the scala media of the cochlea) shear during the process of auditory transduction. The deflection of hair scales against the tectorial membrane causes the hair cells to depolarize (or hyperpolarize) and release glutamate, which stimulates the cochlear nerve, cranial nerve VIII.

Tempo: (plural: tempi) The speed or pace of a piece or section of music. Typically measured in beats per minute.

Temporal lobe: A pair of lobes in the brain situated beneath the temples in each cerebral hemisphere. Includes the superior temporal gyrus, which contains the primary auditory cortex. Involved in cortical processing of sound and speech.

Temporal pole: The anterior end of the temporal lobe. Integrates complex perceptual information (auditory, olfactory, and visual) with emotions. Activated during music listening and implicated in social cognition.

Thalamus: The area of the brain that serves as a relay center for sensory and motor signals traveling between subcortical areas and the cerebral cortex.

Timbre: The character or quality of a sound as distinct from its pitch and intensity. Sometimes called tone quality, tone color, or resonance. A sound's timbre is determined by the acoustic characteristics of spectrum and envelope.

Transdiagnostic theory: Psychiatric group music therapy treatment philosophy that emphasizes commonalities between individuals with various mental disorders within groups regardless of diagnosis.

Transdisciplinary: Model of treatment in which the disciplinary lines become blurred or eliminated because of members' strong understanding of and collaboration with each discipline and an emphasis is placed on the student, client, or patient rather than professional identities.

Transition songs: Songs that are designed and used in a systematic way to aid students during transitions. Transition songs provide structure and cues to indicate what is coming next, are predictable because of the inherent qualities of the music, and can be paired with visual cues.

Traumatic brain injury (TBI): When an external force, such as a blow to the head or an object penetrating the skull, causes brain dysfunction.

Tubano drums: Tube-shaped drums with feet that can be comfortably played while seated; made by Remo.

Twelve-step (12-step) treatment: A frequently used model for addiction recovery grounded in spirituality and peer support. Originated with Alcoholics Anonymous (AA) but is also used in Narcotics Anonymous (NA), Heroin Anonymous (HA), and Gamblers Anonymous (GA).

Tympanic membrane: Also known as the ear drum. The membrane that connects the ear canal (external auditory meatus) of the outer ear to the ossicles of the middle ear. Vibration of this membrane moves the ossicles.

Unpitched percussion: Instruments that make sounds of indeterminate pitch when struck, scraped, rubbed, or shaken.

Urban Federation of Music Therapists: Original name of the American Association for Music Therapy (AAMT); founded in 1971.

van de Wall, Willem: Author of the first instructional text for music therapists, entitled *Music in Institutions*, published in 1936. van de Wall advanced the practice of music therapy in state-funded facilities.

Ventral striatum: The part of the basal ganglia that mediates reward, reinforcement, and motivation. Includes the nucleus accumbens.

Ventral tegmental area: The part of the reticular formation implicated in reward and motivation by producing dopamine.

Ventral thalamus: A narrow area between the dorsal thalamus and the hypothalamus. Sometimes called the subthalamus, and sometimes considered part of the basal ganglia. Involved in motor control.

Ventromedial prefrontal cortex (PFC): The area in the middle, underside of the frontal lobe involved with emotion regulation, empathy, and social decision making.

Verbal processing in music therapy: Conversation that facilitates therapeutic progress during, and in response to, music making or music listening.

Vescelius, Eva Augusta: Founded the National Society of Musical Therapeutics in 1903.

Visual-orienting response: Behavioral response in which humans automatically turn to look for the source upon hearing a sudden loud sound. This reflex occurs because of connections between the inferior colliculus and superior colliculus.

Well-being: The presence of physical, psychosocial, and spiritual health.

Wellness: An active process through which people become aware of, and make choices toward, a more successful existence.

Xylophone: A musical instrument with wooden bars of graduated length that are struck by mallets.

Index

Note: 'Page numbers followed by "f" indicate figures, "t" indicate tables and "b" indicate boxes.'

Printed in the United States
By Bookmasters